Social Policy for Nurses

This book is dedicated to my late husband Derek and to Gareth, Gayle, Brendan and Sarah. With love also to my wonderful grandchildren – Maisie, Grace, Harry and George

Social Policy for Nurses

ANITA FATCHETT

polity

First published in 2012 by Polity Press

Polity Press
65 Bridge Street
Cambridge CB2 1UR, UK

Polity Press
350 Main Street
Malden, MA 02148, USA

ISBN-13: 978-0-7456-4919-1
ISBN-13: 978-0-7456-4920-7 (pb)

A catalogue record for this book is available from the British
Library.

Typeset in 9.5 on 12pt Utopia
by Servis Filmsetting Ltd, Stockport, Cheshire
Printed and bound in Great Britain by
MPG Books Ltd, Bodmin, Cornwall

The publisher has used its best endeavours to ensure that
the URLs for external websites referred to in this book are
correct and active at the time of going to press. However,
the publisher has no responsibility for the websites and can
make no guarantee that a site will remain live or that the
content is or will remain appropriate.

Every effort has been made to trace all copyright holders,
but if any have been inadvertently overlooked the
publishers will be pleased to include any necessary credits
in any subsequent reprint or edition.

For further information on Polity, visit our website:
www.polity.co.uk

Contents

Preface

> 'The National Health Service ranks as one of the most successful innovations in social policy of the 20th century. It represents a brave assertion of the equal value of human life, by ensuring that patients get the treatment they need, rather than the treatment they can afford.'
>
> (Cook, 1994)

Thanks to the National Health Service (NHS), the population of the UK has largely been entitled to healthcare, free at the point of need, for more than 60 years. It is something of which we can be justifiably proud in this country, reflecting as it does a society expressing a practical concern for the health and well-being of all its citizens.

It has of course accumulated its own fair share of faults, two of which in particular are worthy of mention at this stage. First, a lower priority in practice has been given to the prevention of ill health, with the greatest attention and status given to the treatment of illness and hospital care. Second, the glamour and prestige of surgery, high technology and the creation of ever more splendid hospitals have swallowed up a disproportionate amount of healthcare resources. This has sidelined, effectively for decades, attention away from the broader, more socially useful primary healthcare setting, in which the majority of the population experience their healthcare at primary, secondary or tertiary levels.

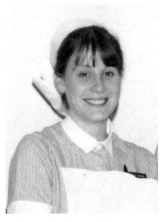

Anita, student nurse. St Bartholomew's Hospital, London. November 1965.

Now well into the second decade of the twenty-first century, with another new government at the helm, there are many issues to be addressed within the NHS, not least the direction which the new policy imperatives will take and shape the service and those of us who work within it. That said, while political aspirations and promises may strike a positive chord, the challenge for nurses is to influence moves beyond the slogan, and to ensure both the continued contribution of a professional nursing workforce and an effective national health service.

Acknowledgements

I would like to thank Margaret Faull, Ulrike and Charles Maltman, Jane Pinder, John Puntis, Catherine Samiei and Julia Weldon.

Thanks to Mid Yorkshire Hospitals NHS Trust and also to Leeds Metropolitan University for use of the images on the cover and page 270.

The author and publisher would also like to acknowledge the following permission to reproduce copyright material:

Page 2, 4 (right), 6, 25, 37, 44, 79, 127, 186, 210, 248 © Wikimedia Commons; 4 (left) © World Economic Forum; 20, © David Joyner/ istockphoto.com; 46, © Nils Jorgensen/Rex Features; 66, © Cathal McNaughton/ Reuters/ Corbis; 97, © Dean Mitchell/istockphoto. com; 103, © Alina Solovyova-Vincent/ istockphoto.com; 126 (left), © Adivin/istockphoto.com; 126 (right) © Mutlu Kurtbas/istockphoto. com; 153, © Chris Schmidt/istockphoto.com; 162, © Diana Hirsch; 178, © Bettmann/CORBIS; 212, © Lars Christensen/istockphoto.com; 218, © Burger/ Phanie/ Rex Features; 229, © Mark Papas/ istockphoto.com; 235, © Alex Macnaughton/Rex Features.

List of Tables, Figures and Boxes

Tables

Figures

Boxes

1 Introduction

Aims

- to introduce students to the National Health Service in the UK
- to show why this knowledge is relevant for nurses

'From the cradle to the grave, the NHS is there for all of us. It supports people at those moments in life when they find themselves at their most vulnerable, providing a service to everyone that is free at the point of need. It is not just an organisation, but a cherished and ingrained part of life in our country.'

(Andy Burnham, cited in Darzi 2009a)

'It has been described as still "far and away the most popular of public services – a jewel in the crown of welfarism, and very much the envy of billions of people around the world whose health services are less developed, less accessible, more expensive, and more exclusive".'

(Lister, 2008)

The NHS has changed, grown and developed both in size and complexity over six decades, witnessing major advances in clinical care and applied technology; it has remained as it began in 1948, the subject of often furious arguments over its policies, resources and future. Importantly, it is an institution much loved by the population. As such, each successive government in recent decades, whether Conservative, Labour or Conservative–Liberal Democrat Coalition, has stated its continued support for the development of a thriving NHS (DOH, 1997; DOH, 2010c). Important for us to note are the differing diagnoses of its problems by successive governments, and of the many solutions nurses are tasked to deliver to improve its health and that of the population.

The Labour government's health policy in 1997

The change of government from Conservative to Labour on 6 May 1997, after a period of 18 years in opposition, offered the opportunity for the new administration, apparently with a different ideological perspective and mission, both to halt and to redirect the process of fundamental change and reform within the NHS. This was aimed at changing both the context and the content of healthcare delivery within the NHS from that which had developed from 1979 under the Conservative prime ministers, Margaret Thatcher (1979–90) and then John Major (1990–7).

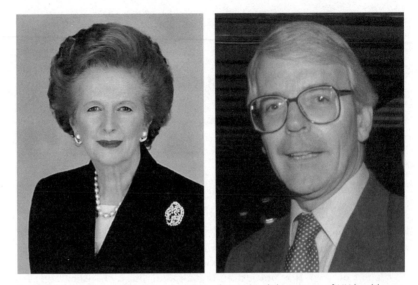

1.1 Successive Conservative governments determined the course of UK healthcare policy for 18 years, first under Margaret Thatcher (1979–90) and then under John Major (1990–7).

The then newly appointed Prime Minister, Tony Blair, speaking on behalf of the new Labour government on 6 May 1997, referred supportively to the NHS in his opening address to the nation on the steps of 10 Downing Street. He said: "A new Labour government . . . remembers that it was a previous Labour government that formed and fashioned the welfare state and the National Health Service. It was our proudest creation. It shall be our job and our duty to modernize it for the modern world." This statement of intent both reflected the Labour Party's general election manifesto commitment for a new and changed health service agenda and pointed towards immediate policy activity to be announced in the Queen's Speech at the State Opening of Parliament 12 days later. As the Queen pronounced: "My Government is committed to the development of the National Health Service, as a service providing care on the basis of need to the whole population. They will bring forwards new arrangements for decentralisation and co-operation within the service, and for ending the internal market" (14 May 1997, House of Lords).

Under the previous four successive Conservative governments (1979–97), all professionals, including nurses, midwives and health visitors, and non-professionals alike had felt the impact of major political and managerial change within the NHS, whether in acute or in primary healthcare settings. Increasingly, they had all found themselves working within a more commercialized and fragmented organization, feeling the impact of a much sharper financial environment right across the NHS.

Whether right or wrong (depending on your political persuasion, belief or understanding), this period had been neither comfortable nor easy, particularly for those in face-to-face contact with the patients and users of NHS services. The specific promise of more power and choice for all had not been matched by the means to meet this idealistic aim, not least against a backcloth of encouragement for raised consumer expectations and demands. In one sense, nurses and other health service workers had found themselves in an invidious situation – being asked to deliver the potentially impossible, often with very little in the way of the requisite resources and backup.

As a result, professional morale and self-belief had been frequently challenged during the 18-year period of Conservative health changes. Mixed messages had done little to help. On the one hand, the NHS Management Executive had set out ambitious and positive-sounding strategies for nurses throughout the reform programme, reminding them and others that 'improving health and making care services better was heavily dependent upon their contributions' (NHSME, 1993). On the other hand, the credibility of all healthcare professionals, including nurses, had frequently been challenged. Like many of the disappointed 'consumers', many nurses had often felt let down and discouraged as a result of the Conservative governments' reforms.

The subsequent election of a Labour government in May 1997, with a landslide majority, 'carried with it the hopes and expectations of millions of health workers, patients, carers and campaigners for the NHS' (Lister, 2008). While it may have been tempting for this new government to tear up all old health policy roots and start again, this was not in reality to be the case. In spite of the many acknowledged difficulties and ideological differences for Labour opposition members surrounding the Conservative health service reforms of the 1980s and 1990s, certain aspects of a clearly positive nature were to be maintained – from both an organizational and a professional perspective.

Much progress had clearly been achieved on both counts, and it was only pragmatic and sensible, indeed inevitable, for this new Labour administration to hold on to that which was constructive and positive, and to seek to reverse only those aspects it considered antipathetic to high-quality professional practice and to the provision of high-quality care for all within the NHS. Surely, only a professional or political dinosaur would have wished at that stage to return to the previous status quo of the late 1970s, or indeed to 1948 – even if such options had been possible to achieve.

Picking up the pieces and moving on – new directions or more of the same?

The proposed Labour health policy programme of 1997, on the face of it, looked more sympathetic in scope, and gentler in its ideological interpretation of solutions to the many problems facing the NHS. It promised to replace the competitive internal healthcare market of

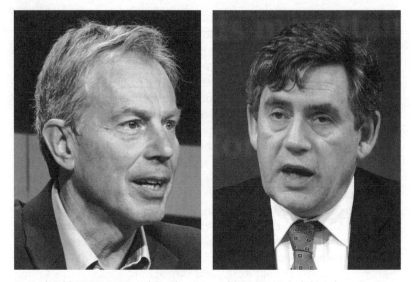

Tony Blair (L) 1997–2007 and Gordon Brown (R) 2007–10, led the Labour Party's government programmes for health.

previous times, with its often perverse outcomes, with a collaborative structure. It also appeared to offer an opportunity for nurses and nursing to regain and develop some new professional high ground. It referred very supportively to nurses and doctors 'taking up the reins' of service development 'together', and of the government really 'listening' to their views as promised during the run-up to the general election of 6 May 1997 (DOH, 1997).

However, in government, Labour's programmes for health have been described as 'cautious' and a far cry from the party's former pre-election promises both to move away from the market approach and to cut back the massive bureaucracy that had built up in the NHS (Lister, 2008). The promise of competition being replaced by cooperation was in many respects broken. As pointed out by *The Economist* (1997), the government opted to live with the market in the NHS rather than abolish it. Rather than its being scrapped, the market was modified, in some ways for the better, in others for the worse.

On one hand, important national standards for care delivery, targets to be achieved and the national inspection of activities give a flavour of this whole period and emphasize the importance given to the attempted delivery of equitable standards of good quality and safe healthcare across the UK. On the other hand, we see the increased development of a healthcare market with a diversity of new organizations, including NHS Trusts, third-sector bodies and the encouragement of the private sector.

After publication of *The NHS Plan* (DOH, 2000b), there was a rapid succession of reorganizations, structural reforms, increasing levels of privatization and the use of private sector providers. Secretary of State Alan Milburn (2000) argued that the 1948 NHS model was 'simply inadequate' for a modern NHS. The government believed that 'it was time to move away from the 1940s, top-down centralized NHS towards a devolved health service, offering wider choice and greater diversity bound together by common standards, tough inspection and NHS values' (DOH, 2002a).

Healthcare provision and services were increasingly rationed, with the open exclusion of a growing number of elective treatments from the NHS. The clear implication was that services not provided by the NHS would have to be bought from the private sector by those patients who could afford them: presumably others would have to do without and suffer the consequences – a potential reversal of the concept of comprehensive healthcare for all, free at the point of need.

At the same time, the initial years of the Labour government also had many positive aspects both for the NHS and for nurses. Its reforms were underpinned by significant investment, a focus on building appropriate infrastructure, the recruitment of more doctors, nurses and allied health professionals and a review of pay and conditions. It also set about meeting the concerns of patients and the public: improving access to healthcare and reducing waiting times. It moved on to update and review systems and processes that were more appropriate to a modern consumer society which was increasingly knowledgeable about how care should be provided.

Importantly for the nursing profession, nurse-led developments and opportunities were made available and grasped by many throughout the whole period of Labour governments. This included new roles in the acute, primary and community care sectors, a shift to university education, the introduction of healthcare support workers and assistants, role substitution, the ability of nurses to prescribe certain medicines, increased numbers of nurse specialists, practitioner and consultant roles, increased interdisciplinary teamwork and multiprofessional care across all sectors – statutory, private and third sectors.

Many of these varied developments in England, whether organizational or professional, were applied (or not) during Labour's tenures in office (1997–2010), depending on the distinct social, cultural and logistical issues within the health services of Scotland, Wales and Northern Ireland. The devolution of powers to the elected Scottish Parliament and the National Assembly of Wales from 1998, and the devolution of powers to the Northern Ireland Assembly in May 2007, opened up the possibility for, and delivery of, increasingly distinctive health policy development and delivery in each of the other three countries in the UK.

The election of the Coalition government in May 2010

Andrew Lansley, appointed in 2010 by Prime Minister David Cameron as Secretary of State for Health, just like all earlier health ministers, described the NHS as a great national institution. He referred to the continued importance of its founding principles: free at the point of use and available to everyone based on need, not the ability to pay (DOH,

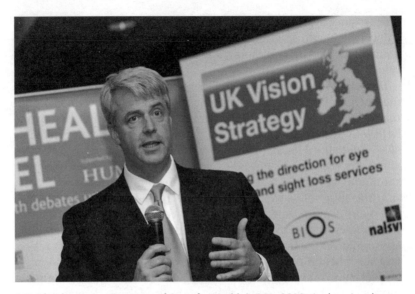

1.2 After becoming Secretary of State for Health in May 2010, Andrew Lansley
introduced several major reforms to the NHS.

2010b). However, the new Conservative–Liberal Democrat Coalition
government believed 'it could be made so much better – for both
patients and professionals alike. He had an ambition for excellence
. . . buoyed by the knowledge that, the NHS had medics, nurses and
scientists as good as anywhere in the world' (DOH, 2010c).

David Cameron and Nick Clegg (Deputy Prime Minister) emphasized the strength of a combined package of Conservative and Liberal
Democrat health policy reforms, underpinned by Conservative thinking on markets, choice and competition and mixed with Liberal
Democrat belief in advancing democracy at a much more local level.
This 'win–win' united approach aimed truly to radicalize the NHS and
move on from the Blair and Brown governments' approach from 1997
to 2010.

The Coalition's policy intentions, as set out in the initial health White
Paper, *Equity and Excellence: Liberating the NHS* (DOH, 2010c), were
presented as 'a bold vision for the NHS – rooted in the Coalition's core
beliefs of freedom, fairness and responsibility'. The policy developments and changes proposed were set against a difficult backcloth of
financial deficit and a growing debt within the public services. This was
not going to slow down their reforms – rather the opposite. It gave them
the necessary impetus for a gear change in the pace of reform. As they
made clear:

> We arrive at this programme for government, as a strong, progressive
> coalition inspired by values of freedom, fairness and responsibility.
> This programme is for five years of partnership government driven by
> those values. We believe that it can deliver radical reforming govern-
> ment, a stronger society, a smaller state, and power and responsibility
> in the hands of every citizen. Great change and real progress lie ahead.
> (HM Government, 2010)

What did it mean for nurses?

Healthcare delivery and professional nurse practice, then as now, need to move with the times and to respond to the changing environment of health needs and economic realities. It was, and is, increasingly evident that we will only gain the right to develop professionally under this government, or indeed any government, if we take on the responsibility of coordinating appropriate and ever more modern responses to the complex health needs of the twenty-first-century UK. The need for constant policy change and development is a given – however challenging.

To be able to manage this often uncomfortable reality, all nurses need to have a broad understanding of the combination of forces that have led to the situation in which they now find themselves. Indeed, a failure to understand and to learn lessons from recent history could well result in a failure to survive as a profession or, indeed, to be able to provide nursing care to the professional standards to which nurses currently aspire for their patients and the public.

Admittedly, this particular challenge is not an easy one to achieve. While the health agenda of a new and differently focused coalition administration has offered us a new programme of activity, it does not give the promise of an easy ride for anyone – public or professional alike (DOH, 2010C). The reform programme was designed to touch every part of the NHS and to have an impact on every organization that delivers NHS care. The striving for financial efficiency and the search for proof of the effectiveness and value of care delivery in every area of the health service will continue, as will the requirement for all professionals, of whatever discipline, to prove that there are values and benefits that result from the high cost of their expert contributions.

The right to claim such status, and all that this implies, will in the foreseeable future only be granted to those who are prepared to change. They will have to take up responsibility for the continued development of both their knowledge and skills to postgraduate level, and certainly well beyond that of initial qualification and appointment to practice. Resting on well-worn professional laurels, however good in practice terms, is a recipe for professional and personal failure in the developing NHS world, and no individual, group or discipline is immune.

There is clearly a need to break out of the now increasingly outdated NHS straitjacket of traditional nurse disciplines and titles, and to look towards the creation of more relevant professional 'role bundles'. New and different combinations of skills and knowledge will be required, combined with the ability to offer flexibility and creativity in care, appropriate to and focused upon assessed local needs and circumstances. This will require an ever greater individual responsibility for lifelong learning, and an ability to reflect on practice and to develop new ways of working, not least within the new and growing NHS family of care sectors. Those who are now making little effort to redefine and to develop their current roles may well lose out to others, and with this the opportunity for work enrichment and satisfaction as professional nurse players in the developing twenty-first-century NHS.

It will involve nurses in carrying out and using research and information technology; increasing their understanding of, and influence upon, health policy-making; and adopting the ability to manage change both for themselves and for/with others. Importantly, adapting to new ways of working as a professional nurse in all the currently developing settings of health and social care delivery will rely upon the ability to work effectively and in close collaboration with many other professional and non-professional carers, employed by any sector.

This book will consider many of the issues raised so far in greater detail. In Chapters 2 to 12 the discussions will try to help nurses clarify what has been going on around them in recent years. Consideration will be given to the historical background and political reasoning behind the changes, the major themes for the NHS, and the issues that are now in the ascendancy and are of concern to both nurses and patients alike. These issues will all be examined from the point of view of nurses.

The book will encourage the development of strategies that will enable nurses to direct the future for themselves and to avoid being pushed into a shape created by others, who may neither support the continuation of a national health service nor indeed understand the role and importance of the continued maintenance of professional nursing care. We all need to take part in, and to influence, the political debates around healthcare and to help shape our own professional futures. There is a need to demonstrate that the nursing profession intends to learn from past experiences and to use both its political and its professional muscle to good effect in the future under the current Coalition government.

What's in the book ?

We will now note briefly the focus of the chapters to follow. While ideally it might be helpful to read each chapter sequentially, they can also be read as free-standing discussions. Ideas raised, however, may well build on earlier discussions and definitions. So you will have to refer back to earlier in the book for clarification of points which need further explanation.

Chapter 2: Policy and Nursing

This chapter will explore the concepts of policy and policy-making and the potential role of the nurse in influencing and implementing policy in practice. It will be proposed that the nursing profession has the potential to ensure a relevant and constructive balance in the how, what and who of healthcare delivery, development and change. Nurses can both influence and implement policy; as such, not only can they protect health services for the public, but they can also influence the future shape and remit of professional nursing in the UK.

To achieve these aims, nurses need to take the initiative, help each other to become involved and push together for policy changes that benefit both the public and the profession. It is to be hoped that understanding how to be involved will equip the reader with an ability to adapt and respond appropriately to the broad spectrum of changing patient needs and policy imperatives, and to ensure that health services are led and managed in ways which support compassionate, safe and effective care within the twenty-first-century UK NHS.

Chapter 3: Reforming the National Health Service: 1948–2010

This chapter will begin to set the scene for the discussions to follow. It will highlight important periods of NHS reform from its beginnings in 1948 to the early 1980s and the impact of the managerial and more commercialized changes under four consecutive Conservative governments. It will then look at the run of three Labour governments from 1997 to 2010, which saw the continuation of similar (if differently named) themes allied to the development of an even more diverse, fragmented market-like approach to NHS healthcare delivery and services, involving the statutory, private and third sectors. This chapter will conclude by drawing together the strands of the main challenges and issues which were handed over to the incoming Conservative–Liberal Democrat Coalition government led by David Cameron and Nick Clegg on 6 May 2010.

Chapter 4: The Coalition Agenda, May 2010: Themes Arising

This chapter will set out and review the implications of the Conservative–Liberal Democrat Coalition's initial health policy changes. These merit serious consideration by nurses who are looking for professional development and enrichment in their future nursing lives. We will look at the changes that were proposed, the challenges created and the potential implications for patients, the public, the nursing profession and for the NHS as a whole.

Chapter 5: Working in Partnership and the Policy Agenda

This chapter will explore the concept of partnership working and its application in practice. It will be argued that all professions within the NHS need to work together, not just to implement and to create effective health and social care policy responses, but also to harness the help and support of users and carers, for the survival of both a good national health service and the professional nursing care which the public want and enjoy.

This will involve a good understanding of the broad diversity of policy agendas requiring implementation in all health and social care fields. As the financial situation tightens, it will be ever more important that health workers and social carers operate together to make the best use of scarce resources, developing, for example, an increasingly joint approach to supporting service users and patients with multiple and complex long-term needs.

In parallel, pressures for further integration are also emerging from initiatives such as the continuation of the transformation of community services, vertical relationships between the acute trusts, primary and community care providers, and the push for cross-sector provider organizations. Successful integration will require mechanisms for facilitating this process, not least to overcome the obstacles of competition between providers and other allied vested interests.

Chapter 6 – Policy and Technology: A Developing Relationship in the NHS

This chapter will discuss the importance of technology, both for information and communication and also as an enabler in healthcare delivery within the NHS. The developing use of technologies to inform and to provide supportive evidence for change, and also for speeding up care delivery within the NHS, is now commonplace. It can improve communication between professionals, patients and others in different locations, facilitate the sharing of information and expertise and, very importantly, help to pull together the complex web of issues and people involved in influencing and changing policy directions in healthcare delivery and organization.

We will consider the practicalities, responsibilities and difficulties of nurse professionals working within an increasingly high-technology NHS environment. Nurses who want both to be part of the new policy challenges and to ensure a strong professional future need to be fully involved in the current technological developments and to understand the implications for practice, both for now and for the future.

Chapter 7: Empowering Patients and the Public

A patient-led agenda within current healthcare delivery remains a central theme of the Coalition government's health programme. It is envisaged that this will better inform service development and change, improve the health of the population, reduce health inequalities and ensure the provision of cost-effective and efficient professional care. This wide-ranging package of expected outcomes is predicated on the idea that patients and the public, as 'consumers' of healthcare, can and do behave like consumers purchasing clothes or cars. This notion will be discussed against the backcloth of policy efforts over time by previous governments to make the users of NHS services central to professional care, service development and change. Some exploration of this challenge will be considered in the light of the currently reforming NHS as set out in the Coalition government's White Paper, *Equity and Excellence* (DOH, 2010C).

Chapter 8: Health Policy: Building a Healthier Nation and Reducing Health Inequalities

Improving public health and reducing health inequalities remain major policy challenges. The Coalition's decision to transfer public health teams to the local authorities, with a 'health premium' designed to promote action to improve population-wide health and reduce health inequalities, will be explored, not least in the light of the other primary and acute care developments (DOH, 2010d).

Current changes in healthcare delivery may not improve the situation. Community nurses as valued and known health promoters could be functionally split away from the new local authority public health hubs, not least as new employers (for example, acute foundation trusts) may require their own pressing health agendas to be addressed in the first instance. In addition, concerns have been expressed at the increasing government interest in care services being provided by other non-statutory sectors in order to save money and professional nursing care being passed to the unqualified.

An effective health promotion agenda, not least with the aim of reducing health inequalities within the diverse UK population, needs to be well managed and resourced, and not subject to the vagaries of a mixed economy of providers, who may or may not see these issues as an important or prime responsibility. Having a diversity of providers working in a fragmenting NHS environment may prove to be counterproductive, both for patients and the public and for the nursing profession as a whole. A managed, well-resourced, organized and overarching public health agenda is surely the way forward, with the NHS as the appropriate vehicle.

Chapter 9: Working with Diversity and the Policy Agenda

This chapter will discuss the concept of diversity and its application in practice for patients, the public and colleagues alike. Consideration will be given to the implications of the changing NHS for the future delivery of a diversity-sensitive service. While the government's initial Health White Paper lacked any specific mention of the diversity agenda, other than in an oblique sense, the NHS itself currently has much work to do in addressing the issue in any serious way. Attempts to reduce health inequalities, to promote good health and to work in effective partnerships with patients, colleagues and local communities are all predicated on understanding and applying the requirement of law, professional code and policy to treat others fairly, in the role of both nurse and citizen within the diverse population of the United Kingdom.

Chapter 10: Supporting People with Long-Term Conditions: A Policy Perspective

Caring for the health of people with long-term conditions (LTCs) is one of the three major challenges facing the UK health service today. The other two relate to the health needs of the ageing population and the lifestyles people adopt across all ages. In combination, success in meeting any or all of these challenges rests upon the ability to deliver the policy imperatives as set out in the previous chapters – working in partnership, promoting health and reducing health inequalities, listening to and being responsive to patients, being diversity-sensitive and harnessing the benefits of new technologies to expedite and improve care, improve communication and develop trust in and a desire for modern professional nursing.

The Coalition's health programme is very demanding in its remit, both for the NHS as an organization and for those who work within it. These changes are taking place against an exceptionally tight financial backdrop. The delivery of an effective response to the increasingly growing, and very costly, LTC issue is a must if the financial challenge is to be met within the NHS. At the same time, the complex health responses needed to manage the issue require professional nurses who have the high level of skills, knowledge and abilities required to achieve success. While no doubt less costly, non-professional carers can provide functional and much-needed support, the more expensive professional nurse, with a broader vision and understanding, can provide much more. In this situation, it is vital that nurses influence the direction and implementation of currently proposed policy, not least by demonstrating and articulating the benefit and added value of their special professional contribution. This notion is developed further in the next chapter.

Chapter 11: Policy and Nurse Professionalism Today: A Threat or a Promise?

We will now consider the concept of professionalism and its application to the nursing profession. An understanding of its many interpretations and attributes will aim to inspire nurses to defend and to promote the professional status of nursing and also to support the continuation of a professional nurse workforce within the NHS. The nursing profession is challenged to become involved in the making and shaping of health policy – an important theme in both protecting and developing professional nurse practice and also in improving and maintaining high standards of care for the population as a whole within an effective and efficient national health service.

Chapter 12: Learning from the Past, Looking to the Future

In essence, then, as with many previous books concerned with nursing policy and politics, nurses continue to be confronted by the often uncomfortable realities of their changing working lives. They are being invited to think about these challenges in relation to the survival of a nursing profession as they would like it to be – an often difficult task, set as it is against an ever-changing policy backcloth. Inevitably, the vision for today will be replaced by a new perspective tomorrow. Having acknowledged this, the concluding chapter will discuss some potential future strategies, and encourage, like others before, a collective response from nurses.

Using the Book

Although many terms, such as 'consumer', 'service user' and 'client', have been used interchangeably in recent years, reflecting the changing status and expectations of people accessing the health service, the term 'patient' retains its dominance in everyday use and features prominently in all recent literature concerned with nursing. So the term will continue to be used in this work.

In addition, the generic term 'nurse' will be used throughout as a means to cover every field of nursing – mental health, child health, learning disability and adult nursing, as applied in both hospital and community settings. It would be too difficult to name all the many important sub-specialities. So, if this offends you, please accept my apologies. In essence, as professional nurses, we all work in some way or another with people 'from the cradle to the grave' – an apt notion for a book on the National Health Service, professional nurse care and the impact of policy change and development.

While much of the legislation and many of the key policies discussed in the book are primarily set in England, the themes discussed are still relevant across all the countries of the UK, and the specific application of these details and developments can be sourced at www.dh.gov.uk, with relevant Acts of Parliament available on www.opsi.gov.uk/. The structures and issues of importance for each country have, at times, both converged and diverged. This is no surprise, as this reflects the specific and often-changing complexity of issues facing each country. The devolution of government to Scotland, Wales and Northern Ireland has offered the opportunity for each country to apply its own cultural flavour and choice to health policy (see Williamson et al., 2010: 37).

All the chapters that follow are very broadly themed and the ideas are of relevance to every professional nurse, irrespective of time, place or person. Directed learning activities, usually comprising questions for reflection or discussion with fellow students or colleagues, will be given in each chapter. These need to be considered in the context of your own specific professional practice and related to the developments in your particular country in the UK. It is hoped that this will help you to reflect and to clarify the policy developments that are affecting you, your patient group and your community. In turn, you may be better able to decide on what is working effectively, what needs to be improved and changed, and how you might be able to do things differently and better in the future, both for your patients and for yourself as a professional nurse.

2 Policy and Nursing

Aims

- to define policy – the who, what and how of policy-making;
- to discuss how to be involved in the policy-making process at many different levels;
- to explain why all nurses should be involved in making and implementing policy.

'Health care is unquestionably one of the major fields of public and social policy and is often at the heart of political debate. There are obvious reasons for this, not least the fact that access to healthcare services is vital for our general well-being. Indeed it is central to our basic human rights – including the right to life – and Article 25 of the Universal Declaration of Human Rights (UN Assembly, 1948) states that both access to medical care and, more generally, a standard of living adequate for health and well-being are fundamental rights.'

(Hudson et al., 2008)

'For some nurses, their commitment to caring goes beyond the bedside into trying to make things better for everyone . . . We can all make a difference. Just stand up and make your choice.'

(Whyte, 2010a)

Nursing does not take place in a political or economic vacuum; it is shaped by the prevailing political, cultural and socio-economic circumstances (Fatchett, 1998; Fatchett et al., 2002). Ackers and Abbott (1998) concur with this view and acknowledge that, while people become nurses because of a desire to care for others, their ability to do so is crucially determined by social policies. The ways in which services are actually organized and provided are determined not by the immediate providers of the services, but by government policies.

Changes in policy invariably impinge on the service providers as well as on the recipients of care in both positive and negative ways. While, for example, laudable aims are constantly expressed in successive government policies for health and healthcare, a deeper understanding of the reality of policy-making activity is of relevance and importance. In the real world of policy-making, the 'could' and 'should' may never become 'can', 'will' or 'is' until the proposed activity and focus are perceived as relevant, achievable and, most importantly, affordable by those who make and implement policies for the nation's health.

Aims, however good and right, have to be translated from inspiring international declarations, government legislation, acute or primary-care policy, professional code – or even wishful thinking – into reality in practice for the patient, user or carer who needs to access health and social care services. The bridging of the gap between policy statement, guidance or directive and their effective implementation at street-level care requires understanding, motivation, involvement, enthusiasm and energy from all interested parties – the public, professionals and policy-makers alike.

That said, as nurses we have a dual responsibility and interest, not only to work towards the provision of high-quality care, wherever and whenever it is needed, but also to develop and strengthen the nursing profession and its future. In turn, we need to be very aware that we will only gain the right to develop under this or any future government if we take on responsibility for influencing, creating and coordinating appropriate and modern professional nurse responses to the demands of the many complex health issues facing our communities today.

As Anne Milton, Conservative health minister and former nurse, made clear, delivery of the Coalition government's health programme (DOH, 2010c) relies on there being an active role for nurses, not just in their continuing provision of the excellent clinical care that is the hallmark of the profession, but also in their increased involvement in commissioning, education and leadership in the NHS (Milton, 2010d).

So, what is policy?

Like so many terms we come across in nursing, the concept of policy is open to a wide variety of interpretations and nuances. As such, the potential for an uncritical acceptance of any definition is likely to be, and probably is, unhelpful. Unless its attributes, characteristics and uses in practice are examined carefully, then any serious wish for effective involvement in the policy-making process is unlikely to be achieved. Hill (1990) explained that achieving policy change is never an easy process – to make a contribution towards this end requires not only a knowledge of alternatives and a commitment to putting them into practice, but also an understanding of what policy is and how it is made and implemented.

📋 Activity

- What do you think policy is? See how many definitions you come up with in discussion with your colleagues or fellow students.
- What sort of areas did you think about?

You have probably found that the concept of policy is interpreted in many different ways. Colebatch (2002) would agree with your findings. He described policy as being encountered in a wide range of contexts – in different fields of action, different times and circumstances – and that it is impossible to discuss all types. In fact it is a term widely used and applied in many areas of life, for example in industry, the environment, housing, immigration, defence, childcare, criminal justice, political parties, sport, religion, the voluntary sector, education and, of course, in healthcare.

Policy is created and implemented on both the international and the national stages, as well as on a smaller scale at local level, ranging, for example, from the World Health Organisation (WHO) through national, regional and local government, the media, professional bodies and trade unions, the business sector and voluntary organizations to the village cricket team, hockey club, Brownie pack and playgroup. All of these will both create and implement policies to organize and to achieve their stated goals and targets.

As such, Colebatch (2002) says policy is concerned with ordering an activity, implying a systematic and consistent approach. This is usually legitimized by the authority of individuals, offices or organizations. It also implies the presence of expertise or special ability. According to Baggott (2007), a policy is a position taken on an issue by an organization or individual in a position of authority. It can refer to a statement, decision, document, guideline, protocol or programme of action. It may not always be a positive action: it could be a form of inaction or a deliberate attempt to block a decision. In these ways, all of us are likely to have been involved in making policy or, indeed, in carrying it through in some way or another. As nurses working in healthcare delivery, we are involved both in implementing and creating policy every day of our working lives.

It can often be a difficult balancing act, as different policy mechanisms will advantage or disadvantage different groups of people, and reconciling different and competing interests is far from easy. Providing information on health matters and services online, for example, may be fine for many in the population, but not for those who have no access to a computer or, indeed, who are unable or do not want to use a computerized service. We will explore this issue further in Chapter 6.

Levin (1997) set out a variety of usages of the concept of policy, which he grouped under four helpful headings:

1 Policy as a stated intention.
2 Policy as a current or past action.
3 Policy as an organizational practice.
4 Policy as an indicator of the formal or claimed status of a past, present or proposed course of action.

Let us explore these descriptions of policy in more detail below.

Policy as a stated intention

This relates to the taking of a particular action, or to the influencing or bringing about of a situation or change in activity. We can examine the stated health-policy intentions of the political parties in their general election manifestos. The incoming Labour government of 1997 looked towards a more integrated and less competitive environment than had been encouraged by the previous four Conservative administrations. It subsequently encouraged nurses to take up the reins of policy-creation alongside the medical profession and to head up new initiatives in healthcare delivery. 'Local doctors and nurses who are in the best position to know what patients need will be in the driving seat in shaping services' (DOH, 1997).

The current Coalition government in their initial White Paper (DOH, 2010c) referred to empowering professionals, giving them freedom to use their professional judgement in doing what was right for patients. Healthcare was to be run from the bottom up, with ownership and decision-making in the hands of professionals and patients. We will explore what has happened to these stated policy intentions in the chapters that follow.

Policy as a current or past action

This concerns continuing policy activity, or some aspects of policy which have been developed in the past and, indeed, may still be effecting change. As an example, we could look back across the past half-century or so to national government efforts to reduce health inequalities within and between population groups. Efforts to achieve this policy aim continue to be addressed by the current Coalition government (DOH, 2010d: 9) as inequalities have continued to widen (Marmot, 2010).

Policy as an organizational practice

This concerns the implementation of policy by the use of some established practices for an organization, the rules and regulations, the ways things are done, and attitudes customarily taken by those carrying out the given policy imperatives. The NHS Constitution for the UK, enacted on 1 April 2009, set out a broad agenda of behaviours and expectations for the delivery of healthcare and policy implementation (DOH, 2008b). On coming into office, Secretary of State for Health Andrew Lansley confirmed the Coalition government's continuing support: 'We will uphold the NHS Constitution, the development of which enjoyed cross party support' (DOH, 2010b).

The broad intentions include an emphasis on the requirement for user centredness and involvement in all healthcare planning and delivery, not least in the pursuit of care which is cost-effective, research-based and flexible. In turn, there is an understanding that, while the users of the service have *rights* to high standards of professional care, they also have *a responsibility* to behave in appropriate ways – whether *towards* and *with* their carers or in their own personal health-promoting behaviours. They have a right to be '*helped to health*', but also a responsibility to '*help themselves to health*' by taking advice and playing their part (DOH, 2010b).

Policy as an indicator of the formal or claimed status of a past, present or proposed course of action

In this case, the term denotes a claim to status by being a product of deliberation and announcement – for example, by central government involving Cabinet deliberations and ministerial announcements. An example of this includes the 'must do' annual verification and proof of achievement of standards, targets and evidence of good outcomes across a wide range of healthcare activities. The NHS Commissioning Board, for example, is held to account for the delivery of improvements against the agreed outcome indicators, the delivery of choice and patient involvement and in the maintenance of financial control as set by the Treasury (DOH, 2010c: 33). As Peter Levin (1997: 18) explained: '[I]f a policy can successfully be labelled "government policy" . . . that policy will have a valid claim to priority over others not so labelled in the allocation of money or other scarce resources. This can be seen in the process of deciding public expenditure.' Further, Levin explains that commitment and status often go together – 'decisions and announcements create commitment too'. The publication of the National Service Frameworks (NSFs; DOH, 2000), which covered certain, but not all, areas of healthcare activity, have helped ensure financial and other organizational support for developments – often at the expense of others not selected for NSF attention.

Ham and Hill (1993) similarly describe policy as a web of decisions and actions that allocate values and as a set of interrelated decisions concerning the selection of goals and the means of achieving them within a specified situation. A policy is then formulated to achieve certain aims and goals in response to some problem or issue. It is hoped that this will reflect both the contributions of those with specific expertise and knowledge of the issues and the end product of an exercise in skilled problem-solving. It involves the creation of an ordered response, drawing a range of varied activities and personnel into a common framework for action. Endorsement confers both status and authority upon it, although not always the required resources of finance, people and time to ensure its effective implementation.

The process of policy-making

So far, then, the creation or making of policy seems to imply the deliberate and focused imposition of order for activity within and between organizations and personnel. It appears to emerge as a response to particular interests as expressed by any number of individuals, whether at political, institutional, professional or public levels. Policy is described as a product of debate or of a rationale; as a selective response to interests; as the outcome of a process; and as a reflection of power structures.

As such, it is not surprising that the process of making policy is often perceived as synonymous with politics, political ideology and activity – concepts which have often been perceived as nothing to do with nursing (Toofany, 2005). The words are often used interchangeably and, unfortunately, incorrectly. Price (2010) refers to those who might imagine that policies are made elsewhere, sometimes far removed from practice. There is considerable scope, however, for all nurses to influence and develop relevant agendas for their communities, their patients and themselves (O'Connor and Purves, 2009; Whyte, 2010a). Because of this, we need to be very clear about definitions if we are to become involved in the process and to be successful.

Let's define politics

Politics is variously described as the study of institutions, rules, structures, norms, activities and procedures that are concerned with the allocation of resources. Colebatch (2002) refers to politics as being about the 'struggle' for a particular policy end. In turn, then, political activity (politics) is about *who* gets *what, when, where,* and *how.* For example, over the past century and, markedly in this country, the political struggle has taken place within the overall framework of a constitutional monarchy between the competing political formulae of liberalism, conservatism and socialism – all of which have different perspectives on resource allocation for the benefit of the population. For example, we can relate this to healthcare delivery in the UK. Note the different ways in which the NHS has been led, funded and supported by different governments since its inception in 1948.

Despite all the ideological differences, principles and nuances that have underpinned the focus of the policy directions taken over time, the national government of the day is seen as the final arbiter and decision maker. It settles the complex political disputes of the day and allocates resources within a framework for action. We can see this happen by watching the political debates on healthcare delivery in the House of Commons and then reading any subsequent documents, reports or government White Papers which set out what is required or what needs to happen for delivering healthcare to the population. The policy-making process is the means used to achieve this end.

The Chief Nursing Officer at the Department of Health is a good source of information on such matters and provides a useful, continuing interpretation for nurses across the UK of the current government's intentions for care delivery right across the fields of health and social delivery (www.dh.gov.uk/cnobulletin).

Policy-making by government

The government promotes legislation in Parliament, introducing Bills and taking them through the prescribed formal stages, doing its best to secure the necessary majorities when voted on in the various divisions, to the bestowing of Royal Assent – at which point the Bill in its final form gets on to the 'Statute book': it becomes an Act of Parliament, a legislative measure (Naidoo and Wills, 2005). Take a look at the flow diagram shown in Figure 2.1, which sets out the process that takes place in the Houses of Parliament.

The political ideology or beliefs which underpin the government of the day with the majority political voice in the House of Commons are usually able to override and vote against the political views and ideologies of the elected opposition politicians. For this reason, policy developments and changes in healthcare delivery and organization over time are a manifestation of what takes place when a political party takes over in government following a general election and pursues new, and sometimes very different, political views and aspirations from those of its predecessor.

While all political parties (and aspiring governments) may well currently support a national health service, the ways in which, or indeed the degree to which, they wish to do this in the future might easily vary considerably. Chapters 3 and 4 reflect further on this theme. Look at what has happened to the NHS since 1948 and note how it has been made to change in both structure and organization by government after government right up to the present day.

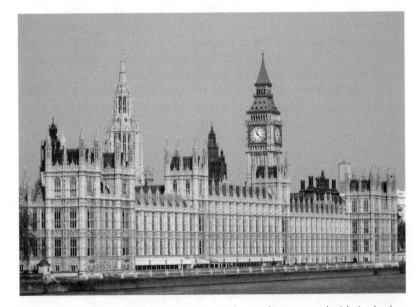

2.1 The Houses of Parliament in Westminster house the supreme legislative body of the United Kingdom.

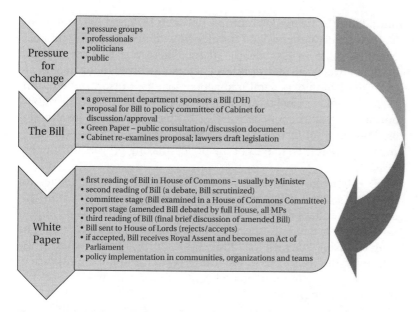

Figure 2.1 Policy creation and legislation in the Houses of Parliament

In broad and simplistic terms, while politics, political ideologies and political activity are labels used to describe the steering of organizations in particular ways, policy and policy-making are described as providing *order* and *organizational focus*. This is a notion that is often questioned by those who may at times feel overwhelmed by the ever-developing policy requirement to do things differently or to achieve new targets or goals – it's like trying to stand still on ever-shifting sands (Glenn, 2010; Upton and Brooks, 2000).

Wildavsky's (1979) definition of policy-making, for example, certainly captures the slippery and complex nature of the concept and its real-life application in healthcare practice. He describes its aim as being 'to ameliorate problems through a process of *creativity, imagination* and *craftsmanship*'. Schaffer (1977) too, describes public policy-making in similarly lyrical and positive terms: 'The public policy process is then a multi-person drama going on in several arenas, some of them likely to be complex large-scale organizational situations. Decisions are the outcome of a drama, not a voluntary, willed, individual, interstitial action. The drama is continuous.'

As such, policy-making by government in the field of health and all other areas too involves a continuing and developing pattern of events; a 'drama' with participants from both within and outside the sphere of central government playing their part. The process begins long before the announcement of any formal policy statement from the government, and its implementation, development and re-evaluation continue long after its initial announcement and legislation.

Think back over the long period of the Conservative governments' internal healthcare market reforms. Between 1979 and 1997, for example, their objectives grew and developed with new and different goals becoming more or less clearly stated. There was also overlap and conflict between the many parties ('actors') involved in the healthcare arena: for example, general managers, doctors, nurses, trade unionists, professional associations, support workers, politicians, the public, community health councils (CHCs), hospital trusts and local councils. This 'cast' of just some of the many protagonists demonstrates how many people were part of the policy-making process during that period.

The Labour governments since 1997 similarly made policies for healthcare services which reflected the same approach. It is within this context that nurses clearly have had, and continue to have, an important role to play and an informed contribution to make. As noted by many (Crinson, 2009; Green, 2007; Price, 2010), nurses make up the majority of the workforce in the health service and the importance of the nursing voice in influencing healthcare services and delivery has been widely recognized.

Milton similarly emphasized this view following the publication of the White Paper, *Equity and Excellence: Liberating the NHS* (DOH, 2010c). She looked to nurses to take on the new opportunities within the proposed Coalition programme for the NHS, and placed great reliance on their considerable expertise and proven experience of making the most of all opportunities to improve care for patients under each and every government to date. She looked to proactive engagement by nurses in taking up the challenge, in delivering the government's policy objectives, offering 'fantastic opportunities for those who were prepared to take them up and run with them' (Milton, 2010b).

The development of the hospice and palliative care movement under the charismatic leadership of Cecily Saunders in previous decades is a good example of such an approach. Indeed, the subsequent greater attention given both then and now to cancer and palliative care demonstrates the need for the continued push by many players, including nurses, to place and maintain cancer and palliative care at the centre of NHS policy-making. This development has, of course, spanned several governments, albeit of different political persuasions, since Saunders's interventions in the 1960s and beyond. It also reflects the persistent nature of the many different and interested players at all levels who have wished to influence and to maintain health policy in favour of the cancer and palliative care agendas.

Implementing policy and influencing change – becoming involved

Ham and Hill (1993) highlighted the overwhelming importance of negotiation and bargaining which have to occur throughout the policy-making process, the struggle between interests and the need

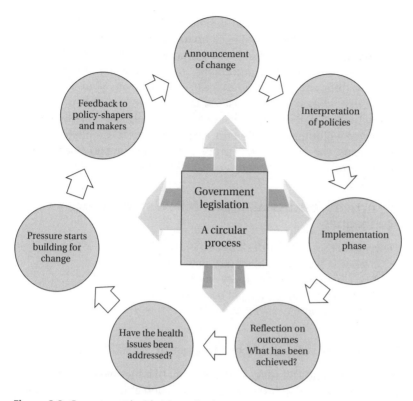

Figure 2.2 Government legislation: a circular process

to negotiate and compromise, which all add up to the reality of the process of making and implementing policy. Unfortunately, this has often been said to have been a stumbling block for many nurses, who frequently wish to avoid the perceived rough and tumble of politics (Toofany, 2005). As Alison Dunn reminded us (in Maslin-Prothero and Masterson, 1985), it is, however, the means by which power and influence are gained and held, in order to pursue particular goals, to shape health policy and to influence the redistribution of resources in ways which reflect the assessed health needs of the users of our care services.

The Nursing and Midwifery Council Code (NMC, 2008), 'our badge of professional integrity', however, surely supports our being clearly involved and proactive at all points in the process. Look at Figure 2.2 and consider where you might be able to contribute, either in a *proactive* or in a *reactive way*. There are no fixed points for involvement. As such, you need to seek out the appropriate opportunities, both to influence the implementation of policy in practice and to push for emphasis to be placed on your particular issues of interest in relation to your professional work, focus and circumstance.

Figure 2.2 is a representation of how legislation is passed down from the government through the NHS structure to be implemented at local levels within our teams. Evaluation and reflections on this will in turn inform discussion and debates on its success and relevance, which will and can be passed back up to government for amendments and change. New ideas can also be proposed at local level and pushed upwards for consideration and change. It is possible to influence policy at many different levels and stages, whether from your local team in practice, with your patients, via professional association or trade union, by discussions with local or national political representatives, interested voluntary groups and many others. As Colebatch (2002) reminds us, the public policy process is a multi-person drama going on in several areas – it is continuous, large-scale and cyclical in nature.

Activity: discuss with your fellow students or colleagues

- With your specific area of care in mind, consider where you might be involved in the process as set out in the diagram above.
- Who else might be involved with you?
- What are the different ways of being involved?
- With whom do you need to work?

How to be involved and be successful

In 1993 Ham and Hill suggested a number of issues which were important to understand in order to be involved and able to influence policy successfully – whether in its implementation in practice or in influencing its change and development. If you want to become involved, it is important to understand the context within which you wish to make changes and the other potential policy-making players. You must have a good understanding of the foci of the different levels of your organization and which might be the most appropriate one(s) to approach. You need to know about the decision-making structures and how, by whom and where decisions are made. This will help you to understand the power relationships within and between groups, and with whom to align and whom to challenge. This also includes knowledge of the connection between internal organizational power and structures and those of external contexts – which external players might or might not be supportive.

Colebatch (2002) and Levin (1997) refer to many groups, all of whom may be involved in developing, implementing and evaluating policy imperatives and activities and whom you may wish to approach for help and support. These exist both inside the NHS and outside within the wider network of policy-makers interested in healthcare delivery. These include the authorized decision-makers; the government, health authority or trust board, other statutory, private or voluntary sectors, and other agencies; the drug industry and other commercial sectors, other levels of government, and national and international participants; and the European Community, World Health Organization and

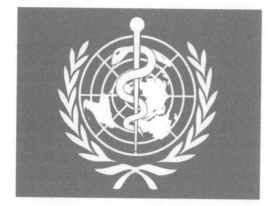

2.2 International bodies such as the World Health Organization form a crucial part of the broader context for healthcare policy.

United Nations. Other important networks of support include political parties, pressure groups, trade unions and professional associations, the media, newspapers, professional and other journals, television, radio, the internet, social networks and contacts. You may also wish to use the machinery for monitoring, coordination and communication in the NHS.

This list reminds us that it is important to remember that policy-making is clearly not just the remit or province or concern of those who are most often formally identified as making and implementing policy, for example the MPs or perhaps NHS managers. As has been described, there is an array of people (including nurses) with varying levels of interest – and expertise – in different health-policy issues, and with quite distinctive perspectives on offer. In addition, while the formal authority of the government and its members in the two Houses of Parliament may be the authorized makers of health and social policy, the expertise of those with knowledge both of and in practice (nurses) is an equally important basis for participation in the policy-making process. As Levin (1997: 20) explained:

> It is not ministers and officials who look after sick people, educate children, run homes for the elderly, and dispense social security benefits. Those tasks are organized and carried out by other people in other organizations: in health authorities and trusts, hospitals, surgeries and clinics, local authority education, housing and social services departments, schools, colleges and universities; not-for-profit and commercial organizations; and executive agencies (like the Benefits Agency and the Child Support Agency).

When any health or social policy is adopted by government, its subsequent effectiveness and success will rely on the active support and involvement of those who are required to implement it from the centre, down to street-level practice and the general public (Lipsky, 1980). Indeed, without a continuing close relationship between all the interested participants, any proposed policy activity, however good in intent, may flounder or even fail. Nurses need to maintain their vigilance and be active in seeking the required resources (whether persons or finances) to implement or indeed to influence the creation of policies that actually meet the needs of their patients. Without such efforts, other current and equally pressing healthcare agendas may well take precedence.

It is worth reiterating that entry into and continued successful participation in the policy-making process require knowledge, motivation, continued enthusiasm and energy. While it is unsurprising that many nurses feel they have too much to achieve in practice to become involved in the broader and more contentious contextual issues, they do nevertheless have much to offer.

All professional nurses have the potential – and, indeed, the responsibility – to provide those of their nursing colleagues who are desirous or more able to take up the more prominent roles on the policy stage with all the evidence and support they need to influence health policy in the desired directions. As Miatta Gbanya strongly reminds us all (in Whyte 2010a: 17): 'Nursing is more than just a profession. It touches the lives of patients and communities. It is about sacrificing to help others and understanding the difficulty that patients have in accessing healthcare. It involves critical thinking when there seems no way out, and it brings satisfaction when you can help people who have no hope' – a telling statement from a nurse who worked in a Liberian hospital at the height of the civil war there. As Saunders (1999) pointed out: 'everyone should do something to advance the care agenda, however small' – it all counts.

📋 Activity: discuss with your fellow students or colleagues

Have a look at the debates in the House of Commons, on television or website on days when health is being discussed, and read the reports about them in the newspapers. Some of the broadsheets have special health days for reporting on health and social care issues. These will keep you updated about new policies being introduced or how earlier policies are being implemented currently. They can also inform or remind you of the issues which you might, could or should be introducing into your practice. We can then begin to consider how we might respond and make a difference.

It becomes very obvious from watching the debates in the House of Commons, listening to the news and reading the papers that, despite the widespread support for the NHS, there are regular arguments and discussions about its shortcomings, shortfalls and ways of organizing and providing health services. It is clear that, in spite of all the technological developments and possibilities, means of diagnosis, medications, treatments and surgery, rationing is inevitable. It is not possible to provide everything that might be needed and consequently hard choices have to be made, with, by definition, some people losing out.

The financial parameters and the organizational structures for care are set out by the government of the day. It is up to the government to decide on what can be provided, how it will be delivered and when. Many questions remain today. Will the major health concerns of the day, not least the widening gap in health inequalities and the growth in the numbers of people with long-term conditions, be effectively managed by the current government as a result of its wide-ranging health reforms? What sort of health service will we have in the future? Are we seeing the beginnings of the slow privatization of national health services with the emergence of a safety net of provision for the weakest and most vulnerable in society?

Within the United Kingdom, the state is currently the near monopoly provider of healthcare. It owns the majority of facilities, employs most health professionals and funds the service through taxes, national insurance and some charges. Everyone (currently) is entitled to use the services, which are free at the point of use and given on the basis of need. At the moment, public sector healthcare is a major responsibility of the government, and public provision of care tends to crowd out private and third-sector providers (see Table 2.1). However, current government health policy looks to be changing this balance with its very overt support for an influx of 'willing providers' from the other sectors (DOH, 2010c). The issues arising from all the changes and developments will have an impact on the services provided, for the patients and for nurses. We will discuss these in the chapters to follow, but for now let us consider how we might be involved and make a difference.

What do we need to influence policy?

Butterworth and Bishop (1995) looked at what they consider to be prerequisites for the delivery of optimum practice. These include the following, all of which are clearly necessary in order to implement new policies or, indeed, to influence the development of different and perhaps more relevant policy and responses to the assessed health needs of the patients and users of our care services:

- a supportive environment;
- supportive management;
- active team education;
- active patient education;
- standards set around quality;
- political awareness;
- an awareness of and active involvement in research activities.

Table 2.1 Key participants in healthcare provision in the UK

Participant	Function
Public sector (BusinessDictionary.com)	Part of the national economy providing basic goods or services that are either not, or cannot be provided by the private sector. It comprises national and local governments, public organizations and quasi-autonomous non-governmental organizations (QUANGOs).
Private sector (BusinessDictionary.com)	Part of the national economy made up of, and resources owned by, private enterprise. It includes the personal sector (households) and corporate sector (firms), and is responsible for allocating most of the resources in the economy.
Third sector (www.cabinetoffice.gov.uk/ third_sector/about_us/index. asp)	Those organizations that are neither private nor public. Defined as non-governmental organizations which are value driven and which principally reinvest their surpluses to further social, environmental or cultural objectives. Includes voluntary and community organizations, charities, social enterprises, cooperatives and mutuals.

Gough et al. (1994) believed that studying politics and policy-making was similarly important. By these means, they believed that nurses could gain a greater understanding of the processes by which decisions are made and implemented at the macro (government) policy level and the consequences of that decision-making on individual practitioners and patients. Through such study, nurses individually and collectively should become more able to influence the decision-making process itself and not merely react to an agenda that is controlled and set by others – an accusation frequently made about nurses (Gough et al 1994; Maslin-Prothero and Masterson, 1998; Rafferty, 1992; Robinson et al., 1992).

While some, however, still question the ability or desire of nurses to take part in the policy-making process, Broome (1998) and others (Fatchett, 2002; Wright, 1998) argue strongly for such involvement. They relate broadly to a number of reasons. Nurses have an in-depth knowledge of care in practice and are familiar with the healthcare system in all its many manifestations. The professional role of nursing is acknowledged as one of influence, as demonstrated by government support for nurses both to make and to implement policy for the benefit of patients. The bottom line, however, is that nurses have a professional responsibility to take part in, if not to lead, the policy process. If you are passionate about improving health, you have to look at a broader perspective – uphold the principles and integrity of the profession by taking action and helping to ensure that high standards of care are maintained. By definition you are involved and a policy-maker.

As Broome (1998) further explains, organizations must depend on the people in their systems to develop a culture of innovation and change. While structures and organizations are reworked and legislation introduced – combined, it is to be hoped, with the requisite financial support – changing care practice is reliant on people within organizations. As Broome says, 'it is the people who will push for change not systems or technology' (1998:1). It is people who are needed to carry through the proposed policy agendas or, indeed, to challenge bad policies and propose other more relevant and achievable means of delivering good-quality healthcare.

McCarthy and Holt (2007) refer to nurses as catalysts for change in the evolving health sector. So how can *you* make your contribution to the health policy-making machine count? How can you bridge the gap between the worthy policy statements of the ideal and the reality in practice for your patients, users and carers?

Some words of encouragement

Becoming involved and trying to influence the direction of policy travel within healthcare, in whatever discipline, is not likely to be an easy ride. After all, there will always be others with competing and similarly pressing arguments for their own particular agendas. As such, you will have to harness the interest and as much support as possible from others around you towards the same policy goal. In turn, this will need to fit in with the general aims of current policy developments within your own organization. It is much more likely to be accepted if it fits as part of the continuing current agendas.

Going out on a limb, however good and right the intention may be, is a much harder pursuit. That is not to say that bold and more unusual ideas should be shelved because they are not a local imperative in terms of delivery. They may have to be pursued in other ways, perhaps by taking smaller steps or indeed marshalling other external support and planning for when the time is right to push them back onto the agenda. Involvement in the process may well involve taking different routes from your immediate care environment or team, as noted earlier. This could involve working with other professionals, trade unions and professional associations, politicians and the wider

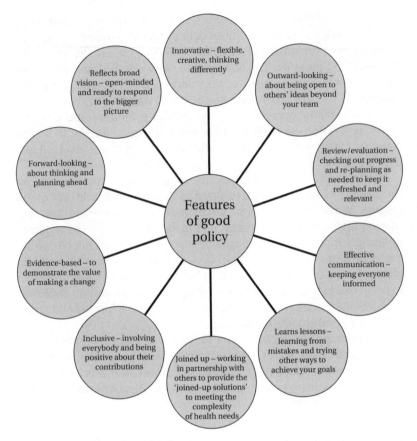

Figure 2.3 Features of good policy

interested public organizations, groups or individuals with similar interests.

Generally then, for whatever policy change you wish to pursue, it is a good idea to look for the appropriate timing to ensure that the policy change you wish to deliver is applicable to your audience, relevant to the current circumstances, reflects assessed needs, is evidence-based and acceptable to potential users – whether clients or colleagues. Importantly, you need to work in partnership with others to ensure that what you wish to achieve can demonstrate Wildavsky's (1979) notions of creativity, imagination and craftsmanship. In terms of policy-making and healthcare delivery, it cannot be a one-man show.

Good policy-making, according to the Civil Service (1999, 2002, 2008), has a number of features which we need to remember as we consider how best to work through the process and to achieve our policy goals (see Figure 2.3). With all this in mind, we can now begin to work through how we might implement a new policy or, indeed, influence a change in policy. Either way, careful preparation is the key to success.

🗒 Activity: discuss with your fellow students or colleagues

- Select a policy which you have found out about in your reading and would like to implement. If you need an idea, you could think about the drive to make patients central to decision-making in clinical practice.
- Relate it to your practice area and to your patients.
- What changes might be needed to implement the policy?
- What issues will you need to address to implement it?
- Where might you start?

'It ought to be remembered that there is nothing more difficult to take in hand, more perilous to conduct, or more uncertain in its success, than to take the lead in the introduction of a new order of things' (Machiavelli, 1532). With this famous quotation in mind, let us just reflect on how others might respond to your wish to implement some new policy, or, indeed, to marshal support for making a change to the status quo, whether in your local team or at a national level. Either way, it might be difficult, as individuals may resist your best-laid plans. Why might this be?

They may view the proposed changes in policy direction as a criticism of the currently accepted focus and implementation of practice and/or administration. As Wright (1998) explains, 'it is an attempt to alter or replace existing knowledge, skills, norms and styles of individuals and groups'. It may affect their current status and they may suspect a hidden agenda on your part, with an alteration in organizational plans, values or activities. As a result of poor or misunderstood communication, there may be a lack of trust in what you will achieve, or wish to achieve, and in your implied intentions. Broadly then, they may feel unable to function in the proposed new environment or to carry through something different, reflecting a fear of the untried or unknown.

In the light of all of this, the first requirement is to have explored thoroughly and to have a very clear understanding of the details of the change you wish to make. In addition, you need to understand and know your team and the likely responses from each individual. You may well be faced with a variety of potentially negative responses – a lack of interest, scepticism, anger, noncommittal, withdrawal, shock, disbelief, unhappiness, anxiety, worry, boredom, querying of everything, subversion, sabotage, destructive or disruptive behaviour, or even outright refusal to listen or discuss.

Although very disquieting, it is useful to have some understanding of why you may be faced with such responses, because again you need to think ahead and to plan how you might respond and get everyone on board. So, how to move forwards?

You need to create a sense of ownership, by discussion and encouragement of active participation. Try to remove any sense of threat and explain the positives and benefits clearly. You also need to have a good grasp of the disadvantages likely to be perceived and already to have thought through your reasons and responses to the many questions that may be asked. You need to sound convincing and be clearly organized.

Identify your supporters and those who may help. Also, identify resisters and find out the reason for this resistance. Consider ways of creating a more positive response by responding to their expressed concerns and explaining the benefits. It is important to communicate your ideas very clearly and check that you are being heard and understood correctly, and make sure everyone is kept informed. It is very important to identify any required learning and other information needs.

Making progress

It is a good idea to have a time span in mind for achieving and/or checking on progress being made in moving the agenda forwards. This will of course depend upon the size of your goal. Implementing or creating a small policy change is clearly different from carrying through a much larger project. It is worth remembering that any involvement in helping to shape some aspects of policy differently can be a task of days, weeks or even a lifetime. So, in moving forward with others, a number of broad themes apply. It is important to work with others and together create a timed strategy to implement or to create the new policy or initiative. Consider all options, share out the work and identify who will do what and when and how (Andrews, 2009).

Maintaining momentum

Your continuing enthusiasm and motivation is essential, so meet regularly. The evaluation of progress should be a regular occurrence, with honest and specific feedback given. Listen and respond to your colleagues, involving people in decisions, encouraging ideas and the sharing of information. Keep up to date with your knowledge and understanding of other allied or similar policy developments and revisit, change and update as necessary any aspect of your policy goal. Listen and respond to the recipients of your changes and ideas and work hard with them to help achieve success. Most importantly, celebrate your successes, share them with others and thank people personally for their hard work and support.

A way forward

The important contribution of all nurses to the achievement of modern and effective health services has been made very clear by successive governments. In addition, opportunities for professional advancement for those who have the skills and the willingness to rise to the challenges are clearly available (Milton, 2010d). All nurses, of whatever discipline, need to ensure their continued participation in any or all of such developments, both on behalf of their patients and for themselves. As proposed, the understanding of the what, why and how of making policy is an essential start. By acquiring and developing this knowledge, nurses should not only be more able to strengthen their influence on health policy development and practice, but they could simultaneously take up the reins more strongly in relation to the profession's future.

There is of course, however, another side to this interesting equation. While there is little doubt of the importance of all nursing contributions to policy-making – both great and small – the nursing profession cannot influence and achieve policy change alone. At the same time, governments and society at large also have a duty to provide nurses with the recognition they deserve – and patients with the care they need. If the goal for the future is to develop high-quality and more equitably provided healthcare services for all in the UK, this does not just rest within itself, but in a reciprocal relationship with the whole community.

Learning outcomes

- an understanding of the who, what and how of policy-making;
- an understanding of the potential for nurse involvement at many different levels in the policy-making process;
- an understanding of why all nurses should be involved in making and implementing policy and how this might be achieved.

Further reading

Alcock, C., Payne, S. and Sullivan, M. (2000) *Introducing Social Policy.* Prentice-Hall.

Baggott, R. (2007) *Understanding Health Policy.* Policy Press.

Greener, I. (2009) *Healthcare in the UK: Understanding Continuity and Change.* Policy Press.

Hudson, J., Kuhner, S. and Lowe, S. (2008) *The Short Guide to Social Policy.* Policy Press.

Rafferty, A. M. (1996) *The Politics of Nursing Knowledge.* London: Routledge.

3 Reforming the National Health Service: 1948–2010

Aims

- to explore the historical development of the NHS;
- to consider the policy drivers, changes and developments;
- to reflect on the impacts of these for the patients, the service and for nurses;
- to note good progress made and mistakes to be avoided in the future.

In this chapter we will explore what has happened in the NHS from its beginnings in 1948 until 6 May 2010, when the Coalition government took office under the leadership of David Cameron and Nick Clegg. In Chapter 4 we will look at the Coalition's proposed health service changes to date, not least with the benefit of the knowledge gained from our earlier exploration of NHS policy activity under previous governments.

The National Health Service (NHS) has experienced continuing change and reform over the decades. These have included the introduction of general management, a managerial and more financially aware approach, an internal healthcare market and the current development of a diverse, multi-organizational approach to healthcare delivery, embracing statutory, private and voluntary sector organizations (Barnett, 2008; Heaney, 2010). These changes have coincided with, and provided the backcloth for, a number of well-promoted and important policy themes for all nurses to deliver in their practice, whatever the discipline or setting within the UK.

Significant issues include a developing need for effective multidisciplinary and multi-sector teamwork within the mixed economy of healthcare providers. Users and carers are to be empowered with the provision of healthcare that respects and responds to the diversity of need in the population and to the reduction in health inequalities. Modern technology is to enhance and accelerate healthcare delivery, with the setting of quality standards, audits of clinical delivery and effectiveness, the achievement of targets and evidence of good outcomes to provide a focus for public expenditure and activity. Appropriate and affordable healthcare responses to emerging health trends are to be underpinned by national health promotion strategies and an emphasis on individual self-help within local communities. This has been described as encouraging engaged, active citizenship by everyone as part of delivering David Cameron's concept of a 'Big Society' (see Chapter 5).

Interestingly, these themes have developed and grown alongside a change in the power base and focus of healthcare organization and delivery from that of the traditional hospital-led service of 1948, to one which is now general-practice-led, multi-centre-based and fragmented. The *right* to healthcare for each individual within the NHS is now balanced by the need for individual *responsibility* for health – whether functionally or even by paying extra for certain aspects of healthcare not now fully provided for everyone within the NHS. A healthcare marketplace with a mixed economy of care providers is slowly repositioning itself across the UK, and a much sharper commercial edge to care delivery within the NHS, free at the point of use, is continuing to develop at a fast pace (DOH, 2010c), as in all other areas of public sector provision.

As ever, the current political and public debates around the NHS and its likely future provide a diverse menu of interesting stories for the whole of the mass media, providing us with important information on a daily basis. The impact of past and current health policies needs to be understood by us all, as these will continue to shape and influence the context of our care and what we can or cannot do in practice for some time to come.

📋 Activity

- For one week, listen to the news on the radio or television, read the newspapers or go online.
- What made headlines in the news?
- What health issues raised relate to your practice area and to the people you meet and work with in your local community?

The answers to the questions in the Activity, from your own professional and personal perspective, may begin to help you to assess the benefits or challenges of any new policy development proposed by politicians and health service managers. That said, we do need to remember that any new changes or promises of change may not or cannot be introduced overnight. A period of transition is probably inevitable in moving and reshaping such a large undertaking as the NHS. It has been likened to an oil tanker, which cannot be turned around at speed. As such, any major change is likely to be incremental and slow in nature, building upon structures and systems created over time.

So before exploring the present day and the potential future of our practice within the NHS, it is worth reminding ourselves of past developments, both positive and negative, and then using this knowledge to reflect and to judge the success or otherwise of any proposed policy developments that we face today. In a sense, we need to know something of the history of the NHS and to learn from its mistakes and successes to date – not least if (as proposed elsewhere) we as nurses are going to be influential in the policy-making process and to contribute to the debates around professional healthcare delivery and its future.

Where did it all begin?

The start of a UK-wide national health service in 1948 after the end of the Second World War represented a rejection of the mixed bag of healthcare services – both public and private – which had developed over many decades. As with education, housing, employment and finance, it was acknowledged that many in the population were not able to protect themselves from the seemingly uncontrollable external factors which impinged upon their health and well-being – wars, economic recessions, unemployment, low incomes, environmental pollution, dangerous workplaces and poor housing, to mention just a few.

The Victorian notions of 'self-care' and 'standing on your own two feet' were seen to have been impossible aspirations for many in the previous decades. A belief had slowly developed amongst politicians, professionals and the public alike that the government should intervene to provide a mechanism that would support the whole population – indeed to *help people to health* in the very broadest sense, not least after fighting a second world war and giving so much to protect the country and its democracy.

The result of this push for change saw the wartime coalition government led by Sir Winston Churchill encourage the development of a major institutional social support system – the welfare state. William Beveridge, an economist, who spearheaded the creation of this new body, aimed to fight the so-called 'five giant evils' in society: Want, Ignorance, Disease, Idleness and Squalor (WIDIS; see Table 3.1). The type of organization he proposed, the welfare state, would provide a response to all of these needs (Beveridge, 1942).

Importantly, it was argued that this development was not about providing something for nothing. It was based on the insurance principle that all should contribute towards its cost, which in turn would give everyone the right to take advantage of its provisions when and if needed. Its aim was to provide a better balance of opportunity than hitherto for all citizens, rich and poor alike, to be able to meet their health and social care needs (see Figure 3.1). At the same time, it represented an acknowledgement that the promotion of good health embraces a wide spectrum of issues and not just healthcare delivery. It was very much the agenda of public health policy (Ramesh, 2010) as we know it today and which we will discuss later in Chapter 8.

The values underpinning the new NHS of 1948 and the other arms of the welfare state reflected an acceptance of, and general responsibility for, each member of society collectively insuring against the personal,

Table 3.1   The welfare state: problems and solutions

Problem	Solution
Want	A system of financial benefits – social security, redistributive taxation and state pensions
Ignorance	State schooling
Disease	A national health service – the NHS
Idleness	Labour exchanges and employment opportunities
Squalor	Adequate housing provision

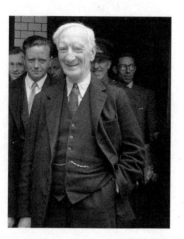

3.1 Pioneered by William Beveridge, the development of the welfare state represented a major shift in attitudes towards issues such as health and social care.

financial and social costs of unexpected ill-health and other misfortunes. Healthcare and good health were not to be seen as a consumer product to be bought and sold in the marketplace, or to be dependent upon any one individual's spending power. Also, unlike buying something like biscuits or clothes, no lay person was assumed to know enough about health to choose between this or that form of healthcare. Similarly, unlike returning and complaining about some faulty shop goods, it was clearly perceived as not easy, or indeed in some cases possible, to trade in or to question defective healthcare, malpractice or some irreversible life-threatening treatment.

The free market mixed economy of healthcare provision in the previous decades had been a failure for a large part of the population. This new collectivist solution to meeting health and social care needs for everyone, and not just for some, was exemplified by the creation of the welfare state system, including the specific introduction of a national health service. It was acknowledged at last that the entire population, to a greater or lesser degree, needed help with their healthcare and

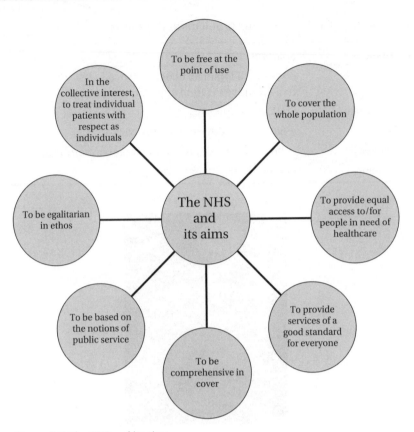

Figure 3.1 The NHS and its aims

good health, and the introduction of the NHS, together with the other supporting mechanisms of the welfare state, would be the vehicle for this. This was 'modernization' 1940s-style, as it was an historic and fundamental break with the past. Lister (2008) aptly reminds us not to underestimate the courage of those who took those first crucial steps along a previously uncharted route.

The NHS was introduced by the Labour government in July 1948, despite much opposition from both Conservative politicians and many in the medical profession. However, the majority in support were jubilant. A nurse called Mary Whitting, writing in the *Nursing Times* on 3 July 1948, said: '

> The great principle has been accepted. Never again need any of us suffer disease through lack of money. Let us be proud that a country still poor after war has taken this courageous step. It [the NHS] will be responsible for its sick without question, because on the health of each member depends the health of the community. We [nurses] are part of the service. This is a great time to be alive!

Some 60 years on, it is very easy (and understandable too) to realize that we may all find it difficult to feel the same excitement about having a national health service. We are probably used to reflecting on and dealing with the downsides of our services, and sadly too easily forget how fortunate we are as a country and a population to have such amazing and all-embracing care provision – irrespective of money, employment, status and culture.

Of course, this ideal description can be challenged, and we will explore the downsides later, not least in relation to health inequalities and diversity in both provision and outcomes (Hills, 2010; Marmot, 2010). A service as large as the NHS, with its seemingly ever-changing policy directions, inevitably has many faults and faultlines but, compared with other more exclusive systems across the world, its attempt to provide for everyone free at the point of need (whatever its shortcomings) is surely worth keeping and nurturing.

📋 Activity

- Reflect on the excitement expressed by both Mary Whitting (1948) and also the people who lived through the Second World War and knew the difficulties of accessing or affording healthcare before the NHS existed.
- Reflect on all the positives of the NHS, which we, as people who have grown up with the service, now expect as a matter of course.
- What do you think is the most important part of the NHS for your patients and why?

The rise and fall of support for a national health service: 1948 onwards

The post-war welfare state, including the NHS, became a welcome and accepted reality by the general population, with earlier opposition from both Conservative politicians and the medical profession declining rapidly. Consequently, the 1950s and 1960s saw a general political consensus in support of the welfare state. This situation was referred to as 'Butskellism' (a term inspired by an article in *The Economist* in 1954, compounding the names of Rab Butler and Hugh Gaitskell), in which all the structures of state health and welfare provision featured as key items in the programmes of the main political parties in the UK.

This consensus or agreement across the political spectrum lasted until the late 1960s, when the apparent underperformance of the economy was seen by the political right as resulting in high public spending and direct taxation. Interest turned back to the use of the market for delivering health and social care services. The importance of individual freedom and responsibility for oneself and one's family, as in previous times, came rapidly back into fashion. This new right-wing thinking continued to gain ground and public support throughout the 1970s, culminating in 1979 in the landslide election victory of Margaret Thatcher as Prime Minister and a strong Conservative government determined to shatter the political consensus of previous years around health and welfare provision.

The main target was wasteful public spending and activity within central and local public sector bureaucracies. They were perceived as being held back by restrictive practices and powerful professional groups, offering no real consumer choice, demonstrating indifference to quality issues, providing a lack of incentives for innovation or efficiency, and displaying a profound reliance on government spending and the consequent high level of tax bills for every individual in work.

Specifically, the NHS was represented as being a vast and growing consumer of public funds. Its activities suffered a sustained attack of criticism. A wide variety of problems and challenges would, if not addressed, consume more and more of the general public sector budget, to the detriment of other important government programmes.

Demographic and other trends of importance causing concerns in the late 1970s

In tandem with this hardening of attitudes towards the ever-rising costs of public expenditure on healthcare were a number of other factors which exacerbated these concerns about the NHS and which are reverberating once again today (see Table 3.2).

The Conservative government of the late 1970s was clearly aware of these issues and indeed concerned about the long-term impact on public expenditure if the ever-increasing spending approach of the previous years was maintained. So, while giving reassurances as to the safety of the NHS in their hands, the government started on the policy changes that would be necessary for the creation of a new business-like, value-for-money health service, one which they felt would be better equipped to deal with the health issues and agendas of the twenty-first century.

The Conservative governments: 1979–1997

The long period of Conservative NHS governance and policy development encapsulated three distinct phases (see Figure 3.2).

Phase 1: A push for change in public sector values and culture

The initial changes involved an attempt to revisit and rework public attitudes in relation to state-provided welfare. It looked to make 'a new contract between public health services and their customers, making a break with the provider-driven, paternalistic welfare approach which had been the dominant modus operandi in health and social care since the second world war' (Hunter, 1993).

Table 3.2 Pressures on the NHS

An ageing population	Demographic trends were then showing an increasing number of people living into old age and a decline in the ratio of working to non-working population (Central Statistics Office, 1993). The consequent proportional decrease in national insurance and tax contributions would mean that the NHS would increasingly be limited in its ability to meet the expected healthcare needs of the growing elderly population. This is a concern which clearly continues to be felt today by the present Coalition government and the Treasury (DOH, 2010c; Gould, 2010).
New developments and more demands for treatment	Advances in medical knowledge and technology, including new innovations in surgery, drug therapies, screening facilities and diagnostic ability, had in turn created new demands and raised the costs to the NHS in paying for these new facilities. As a result the expectations of the public had risen over time as new possibilities in care had been introduced.
More demanding and knowledgeable users	People also had generally become better educated and more informed on health and healthcare matters, so their understanding and expressed needs as healthcare consumers had developed. Specifically, the growing demands of the middle classes, who were both more articulate and knowledgeable than the less able and poorer members of the population, had become disproportionately stronger and had created even greater health inequalities within the population (Black, 1980).

Across all welfare institutions, including health, the government began to push back the boundaries of state provision, tightening up, slowing down and reversing the growth in public spending. Some public services were partly or wholly privatized following the introduction of competitive tendering in 1983 (Gaze, 1992; Laurent, 1990). Increasing use was made of information technology to monitor, distribute and control expenditure on national healthcare services (Luker and Orr, 1992).

According to commentators, during the Conservative administration of the 1970s and 1980s, all aspects of NHS spending were under scrutiny, and efficiency savings were being sought at every opportunity. None of this was of course surprising, as the then Prime Minister,

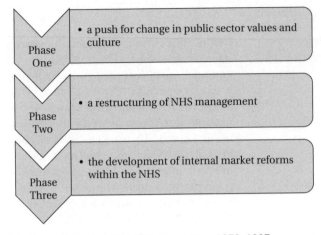

Figure 3.2 Phase of Conservative NHS governance, 1979–1997

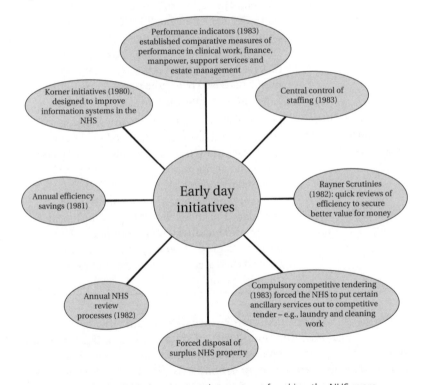

Figure 3.3 Early day initiatives to start the process of making the NHS more business-like

Margaret Thatcher, was openly averse to state-run services (Holliday, 1995). A number of new initiatives clearly reflected the government's intention to change the culture of the NHS to make it more business-like, and were also important precursors to the general management changes which would follow (see Figure 3.3).

📋 Activity: discuss with your fellow students or colleagues

- Reflect on how many of the initiatives described in figure 3.3 have moved on since that time and are now part and parcel of everyday business activity within the NHS.
- Reflect on the advantages and disadvantages for patients.

Phase 2: A restructuring of NHS management

The deliberate restructuring of NHS management at this stage, with the introduction of general managers, was a necessary second part of NHS change, a prerequisite for the internal market reforms to be introduced later following the NHS Review of 1988. The NHS management inquiry team, chaired by Roy Griffiths (Managing Director of the food chain Sainsbury's), was set up to advise the Secretary of State for Health (Norman Fowler) on what action was needed.

The report was published on 25 October 1983, noting 'a lack of clearly defined general management function in the NHS, with responsibility too rarely placed on one person' (Fowler, 1984). As the report put it: 'If Florence Nightingale were carrying her lamp through the corridors of the NHS today, she would almost certainly be searching for the people in charge.'

Changes proposed

The team proposed a series of changes aimed at making the existing organization work better, which included the identification of general managers, regardless of discipline, at regional, district and unit levels of the organization. The general manager would be the final decision-maker for issues normally delegated in the past to the consensus-management team of health professionals and others. It was believed that this approach, which had existed since the inception of the NHS, had led to 'lowest common denominator decisions, and long delays in the management process'. The Health Secretary was in total agreement with this analysis and said that a change to general management leadership would be one of the best contributions to improving patient care.

Reactions to the Griffiths Report

Bodies representing major staff groups in the NHS appeared to accept the inquiry team's critique of management, but criticized the introduction of the general manager concept (Social Services Committee, 1984). Representative bodies for nurses, midwives and health visitors saw the report as both a threat and a snub to the profession. Nurses were mentioned only twice in the report: in the remark about Florence Nightingale and in a passing comment about staffing levels. No real recognition was given to the major role of nursing in the NHS, and

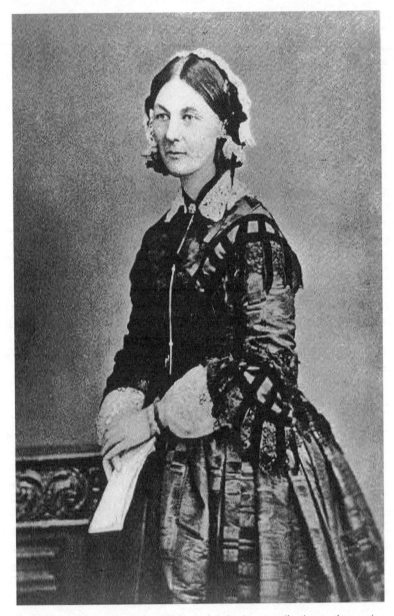

3.2 Florence Nightingale (1820–1910) made a lasting contribution to the nursing profession.

nowhere in the report was there any recommendation that a nurse should be part of the new general manager cadre – a similarly interesting omission in the 2010 White Paper (Snow, 2010b).

Nurses were outraged by the notion of being managed by non-health professionals who, they felt, would be unable to make decisions on what was needed to provide effective patient care, as they believed that nurses and nursing could be led and managed only by someone from within their own profession. This anger was further compounded by the realization that the medical profession had been described as 'natural managers at unit level' in spite of previously expressed doubts as to their management abilities as non-professionally qualified managers.

Can a health service be run like a business?
Overt criticism was made of the appropriateness of the inquiry team and its commercial approach to management. Unlike a commercial organization with profit-making as a clear objective, it was believed the NHS could never have a goal any more closely defined than, for example, the best use of resources or better health for the whole population.

It was argued by nurse and medical representative bodies alike that decision-making in the NHS needed to be a consensus activity, one in which professional and other specialist interests concerned reached agreement on priorities and policy. Failure in a few areas was not a reason to jettison the entire system. Of course, these arguments fell on stony ground. The new system was introduced. Nursing did gain some representation in the general management hierarchy, but in general had to concede the principle of self-government.

📋 Activity: discuss with your fellow students or colleagues

- It is commonplace in the NHS today to have general managers fully involved in healthcare organization and delivery. Indeed many nurses do take on the role. Consider your experiences, both positive and negative, of working with general management.
- Can they understand your needs and those of your patients?

Reactions within the NHS
By the end of the 1980s many NHS employees had had their battles with both the new-style general managers and also with the Secretary of State for Health. There was much employee discontent and periods of industrial action, which also involved many nurses (Fatchett, 1994). The important recurring theme was that of the government's attempts to retrench within the public sector in general, and the related perception of the underfunding of health services (Hoffenberg et al., 1987; Butler, 1992).

It became increasingly obvious that the government needed to draw together all of these issues to provide a political solution that would show leadership and vision, and to prove that the NHS was still safe in its hands. Margaret Thatcher did this by announcing a review of the NHS during a BBC television programme. According to Turner (1998), 'within weeks it was evident this gamble was paying off . . . claims of cumulative underfunding and a complete ministerial muddle were eclipsed by a coherent plan'.

By announcing and commencing a review of the health services, the

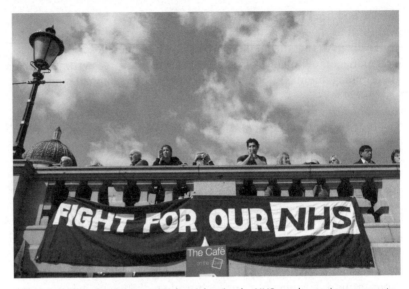

3.3 The 1980s saw widespread industrial action by NHS employees in response to public sector cuts.

government demonstrated that it had taken back control of the health policy debate from professionals and indeed from the trade unions and professional bodies. That said, this did not prevent the tsunami wave of policy-making interests from having their say and trying to influence the direction of travel, not least in making decisions on the way forward for the NHS (Fatchett, 1994). As was proposed in the previous chapter, it is possible for everyone to play a part, however small, in the policy-making process (Fatchett, 2002).

📋 Activity: discuss with your fellow students or colleagues

- Politicians need to appear to be in control of policy issues at national level, and to be able to present well-informed plans for new policy directions, whether for healthcare or indeed for any other sector.
- Have a look at current news and media bulletins around health issues and reflect on the plans being defended or proposed – not least the ones relating to your area of care.
- Are these plans appropriate and workable?
- Are the financial resources available?
- Is the government in control?

Phase 3: The development of internal market reforms within the NHS

Having introduced general managers at all levels of the NHS, the government now turned its focus onto the structure and organization of NHS healthcare delivery. The presentation of the government's strategy for the NHS was made to the House of Commons only one year after the announcement of the review in 1988. The content of the White Paper *Working for Patients* (DOH, 1989c), coupled with those of the NHS Management Inquiry (Griffiths, 1983), provided a template for the greatest changes in the NHS since its inception in 1948.

The new management information systems had revealed clear variations in provision and performance across the country; there were wide differences in costs, drug-prescribing habits, waiting times for operations and referrals for hospital care by GPs. While there were pockets of excellence, the government stated its intention of raising all hospital and general practice standards to that of the best. They said they wished to:

• give patients, wherever they lived in the UK, better healthcare and a greater choice of services;
• give greater satisfaction and rewards to those working in the NHS who successfully responded to local needs and preferences. (DOH, 1989c)

Neither then, nor now, could nurses and other professional colleagues disagree with these objectives, or, indeed, with many of the other positive statements which characterized the then government's new White Paper. That said, it is worth sifting through other more current White Papers relating to your area of healthcare and to remind yourself of other similar-sounding worthy objectives, which abound in all government documents. What we always need to do – then and now – is to blow away the froth and examine the contents.

We need to note the problems highlighted, the solutions on offer and the likelihood of the proposed changes making a difference that is relevant and positive for both our patients and for ourselves as professionals. The general election period of 2010, for example, provided an introductory flavour to the potential health policies of all the political parties. But we can now push away the rhetoric of those election hustings and really examine (with some experience) what the Coalition government's health policies mean for us and for our patients in practice.

Activity: discuss with your fellow students or colleagues

• Examine the outcome of a recent and relevant policy proposal by the government, for example, including lay people in decision-making around the development and delivery of services.
• What sort of difference is it making to your patients' experience of healthcare?

Working for patients: 1989-style concerns – today's also?

The issues seen as needing attention in 1989 are very much issues for today's NHS and for the users of our varied services: long waits for treatment, lack of choice, impersonal and inflexible care services. Much of the content of the White Paper is related to the acute hospital sector, but the issues raised could be broadly applied to all healthcare settings. Generally, the 1989 proposals were looking to provide a more user-friendly, high-quality service – one that is very similar in approach to today's NHS (DOH, 2010c).

The 1989 solutions proposed included the following:

- reliable appointment systems;
- quiet and pleasant public waiting areas, with proper facilities for parents with children and for counselling worried parents and relatives;
- clear information leaflets about facilities, services and procedures, and what people needed to know when they came into hospital;
- clearer, easier and more sensitive procedures for making suggestions for improvements and, if necessary, complaints;
- once someone was being treated, they should receive clear and sensitive explanations of what is happening – on practical matters such as where to go and who to see on clinical matters, such as the nature of the illness and proposed treatments;
- rapid notification of the results of diagnostic tests;
- a wider range of optional extras and amenities for those who wanted to pay for them, such as single rooms, personal telephones, television sets and a wider choice of meals.

Activity: discuss with your fellow students or colleagues

- How are the 1989 proposed solutions currently being handled in today's NHS?
- Have we achieved everything or are there still failings?

It was argued that the problems noted in 1989 could have been solved without major NHS reform. However, the White Paper was not just about dealing with the minutiae of ineffective healthcare services, however important. It was in effect proposing major and far-reaching solutions to the problems of funding, controlling and managing a public institution that was perceived as being grossly out of control. The seven key organizational changes required (see Box 3.1) were more fully set out in a series of follow-up working papers (DOH, 1989b). Interestingly, two decades on, very similar policy imperatives litter the current healthcare agenda (DOH, 2010c).

While freeing up the structures and activities of the NHS, the government also gave explicit support for a new and developing partnership

Box 3.1 The seven key organizational changes in 1989

1 The delegation of power and responsibility to local levels – to include greater flexibility in pay and conditions of staff.
2 The creation of self-governing status for hospitals.
3 The removal of administrative and financial barriers to enable patients to travel to NHS hospitals and centres of their choice.
4 The reduction of waiting-list times, both for outpatient and inpatient care.
5 The ability of general practices to hold budgets and to compete for patients by offering a wider range and better services than other practices.
6 The continued improvement of NHS management effectiveness by streamlining management bodies at all levels.
7 The application of rigorous auditing to help ensure high-quality standards, good health outcomes and the delivery of a value-for-money service.

between the public, private and voluntary care sectors. This was done in the belief that each had much to learn and indeed to gain from the others, not least in providing both mutual support and new-style services. Any work taken from the NHS would, it was believed, not only relieve pressures on the NHS, but also offer greater diversity in provision and choice for all.

Let us now briefly explore some of the main developments which shaped the NHS in the 1990s, further controlled and shaped professional activity and pushed responsibility for health and well-being back onto every individual. Unsurprisingly at that time, many believed that all these ideas offered very clear clues as to the future direction and development of the NHS. As you read through the developments to follow, reflect on the similarities to the changes currently taking place in the NHS.

The internal healthcare market

The development of the internal market in the 1990s provided a new way of managing and delivering healthcare, in which purchasers and providers were separated, with payments determined locally through a system of financial contracts. These formal financial arrangements made at local level removed automatic payment from the centre and provided the means for purchasers to shape, cost and control service delivery. Further to this, all providers had to compete with each other for business. This idea was based on the belief that the competitive environment engendered between purchasers and providers would stimulate greater efficiency, raise standards of care and service, and place the patient centre stage as the 'all powerful consumer' (Dr Alain Enthoven, cited in Robinson, 1989).

Joining the marketplace – purchasers and providers

Two major features of the internal healthcare market included the creation of a new kind of provider, called an NHS hospital trust, and of a new type of purchaser, called a general practice fundholder.

The hospital trusts – the new providers

One of the important aspects of the creation of the internal healthcare market in the early 1990s was the proposal that as many major hospitals as wished should run their own affairs, competing for business on the national stage, while remaining part of the NHS (Clarke, 1989). They were to be called hospital trusts.

The perceived advantages of trust status included the ability to create a stronger sense of local ownership and pride, with an opportunity to build on the enormous fund of goodwill that exists in local communities for the health service. It was also about the stimulation of commitment and the harnessing of the skills of those who provide the services, the development of a more competitive spirit and the encouragement of local initiatives – all themes that clearly resonate today in the current concept of Foundation Trusts (DOH, 2007d).

The budget holding practices – the new purchasers

A second major change involved the option of general practices becoming budget-holders and thereby taking responsibility for purchasing healthcare services from either the NHS or the private sector. The advantages of such a development included the ability to secure the best value-for-money care, a shortening of waiting times for hospital appointments and admissions for care, with improvements in standards of care because of the competition between providers to win the contracts. The ability to advertise for, and to develop, available practice expertise and services also opened up the possibility of greater consumer choice. All these aspects are similarly expected within the currently developing GP consortia services (DOH, 2010c).

Becoming business-like and controlling professional activity

The introduction into the NHS of contracting for healthcare services further extended the cultural shift towards an even more business-like approach. It was clearly seen as a way of providing some much-needed discipline for professionals, who were perceived by the government as profligate users and spenders of health service monies – unlike general managers. If nurses and doctors wanted their discipline or service to survive in the competitive NHS, they had to ensure that their contributions were relevant, research-based, high quality, cost-effective, efficient and consumer friendly. It was up to them to win contracts and to ensure they remained, in effect, in business – an approach that, again, is being mirrored today.

The developing primary-care setting

Simultaneously, and central to the many changes in the NHS during this period, appeared to be the developing government enthusiasm for the primary healthcare setting. While at the inception of the NHS, and certainly during the 1950s and 1960s, the role and status of the hospital sector were paramount, during the 1970s and 1980s the future powerful role of primary care was slowly becoming more evident. There was a belief that the gate-keeper role of general practice could, if it were tightened up and developed along managerial lines, play an important part in holding down the ever-rising costs of healthcare delivery. General practitioners and their teams were to play a key role in deciding who should get what, where and how within the reforming service.

Some of the roots of this shift in policy can be traced back to the publication of the White Paper *Promoting Better Health* (DOH, 1987). This set out the government's intention of improving primary healthcare delivery based on the development of general practice as the new focus for NHS care. The onus was placed on the then family practitioner committees (subsequently primary care groups and then primary care trusts) to ensure that primary-care delivery would develop in a number of important ways.

Efforts were to be made to ensure that services were more responsive to assessed needs and provided a widening range of care services and choices for the users. Clear priorities for care were to be set, with an emphasis on improvements in quality. Special attention was to be given to both health promotion and illness prevention.

It was believed that primary-care teams had the ability and the potential to meet these responsibilities within realistic financial and professional frameworks. In turn, this was seen as likely to generate better-quality services, producing efficient and effective value-for-money care and treatment for individuals, families and communities.

Activity: discuss with your fellow students or colleagues

- List the services now available both in general practice and more generally in the broader community.
- Is the current policy of expanding the service and care remit of general practice as commissioners and members of consortia a good idea?
- Have you been able to develop, even diversify, your professional contribution to the local community?
- With what sectors outside the NHS are you now working?

Impacts of the Conservative policies for reform, 1979–1997

This whole period of upheaval and change saw the development and, indeed, the consolidation of a more commercialized and financially aware NHS. Efforts were made to use all the new structures to deliver the kind of health service it was argued that the public wanted, to move away from arguments about managerial approaches and to focus directly on questions about the provision of quality services and care. After the general election of 1992, and with another Conservative government in power, the reforms developed apace.

The increasingly commercializing focus for health service delivery saw trust status applied not just to hospitals, but also to community and ambulance services. There was a programme of rationalization throughout the whole of the NHS, with closures and mergers and sales of unwanted buildings focused on saving money and removing wastage. Skills in pricing, purchasing, contracting, quality-standard setting and the auditing of all care interventions were developed, aided by the use of new information systems. Desktop communication, processing, publishing, prescribing and pathology systems were all combined to build up, expedite and facilitate both hospital and general practice information, care and services. All activity, whether clinical or not, needed to be of proven value to the service.

Primary care was developed much further, with budget-holding practices creating new and ever more complex and diverse models for care delivery (Dinsdale, 1998). However, 50 per cent of general practices chose not to become budget-holders at that time. It was subsequently found that this led to inequalities in both services and access to hospital care for many patients, with patients from non-budget-holding practices faring worse than those from of budget-holding practices.

There was a massive growth in services offered by general practices, including a range of minor operations and the employment of hospital consultants to provide a convenient service in the practice building – previously only available in an outpatient department and timed to fit with hospital and professional needs, rather than those of the patients. Practice nurses, together with other community nurses and health visitors, began to make an important and growing contribution to the development of service provision by general practice.

In very general terms, this new enthusiasm for the empowerment of primary care began to influence the ways in which the hospital sector behaved. The placement or non-placement of contracts by GPs was a powerful tool, not least in relation to the strongest and the weakest of the hospitals, all competing for business in the new internal market. Consultant-led teams (both medical and surgical, adult and paediatric) began to woo the interests of the purchasers, metaphorically 'outside their hospital walls'.

New and interesting vertical outreach team working began to be developed in many areas – in paediatrics, the care of those with long-term conditions; and for older adults, to provide continuity of care for patients and to develop liaison effectiveness between hospital and community. There was also a need to secure good relationships with a wide variety of purchasers, to gain a competitive edge and to lead the market over other nearby provider bodies with similar care interests and packages on offer.

As purchasers, the new GP budget-holders were enabled and encouraged to select from a broad menu of care services to meet the varied and wide health needs of their practice clientele. This included courses of exercise sessions at local sport centres and surgical or medical treatments in the most appropriate or cost-effective venue. In a sense, the traditional gatekeeper role of general practice was beginning to be visibly enhanced and expanded in nature.

In addition, a more positive health-focused agenda was being promoted, with responsibility for maintaining good health pushed back onto individuals. While the public had a right to healthcare, they had a reciprocal responsibility to help themselves to remain healthy. Policy imperatives, set out in a number of government White Papers, called for a stronger focus on health, health promotion, illness prevention, health-education initiatives, and the use of alternative therapies, rather than an immediate reliance on drugs and referral to the hospital sector (DOH, 1992).

As Holliday (1995) described it, the medical definition of disease, centred on glamorous NHS services provided by hospital consultants, was coming under scrutiny and challenge, as a transfer of emphasis from secondary to primary care began to take place at that time. By May 1997, and with a new Labour government in office, the direction of NHS policy reforms was firmly pointing towards the continued strengthening of general practice and the primary care sector – an environment that was to be developed still further throughout Labour's period in office (1997–2010).

The New Labour government, May 1997: all change or more of the same?

After 18 years in opposition, the newly elected Labour government under the leadership of Tony Blair and his health team faced a very difficult agenda. They had the demanding task of both reviewing and changing a very well-established political approach and ideology, which by then clearly underpinned the management and delivery of healthcare in the NHS.

It was acknowledged at the outset that not everything about the previous system was bad. The separation between the purchasing and providing of care, for example, was to be maintained, but not the competitive element of the internal healthcare market. While it had been introduced as a means to improve care delivery, it was believed to have created many more problems than solutions.

In general, it was argued that the competitive and financially led market mechanisms and processes of the previous years had resulted in a sidetracking of resources and focus away from healthcare delivery and patients, and towards excessive administration. The NHS of

Box 3.2 Inherited problems

- fragmentation of services;
- unfairness and inequalities in service availability across the country;
- distortions in provision, inefficiencies and instability;
- a heavy bureaucracy;
- secrecy between NHS organizations and a lack of sharing of knowledge;
- long waiting times for hospital and other kinds of care;
- highly variable access to care in terms of the range of drugs and treatments on offer in different parts of the country.

(DOH, 1997)

the future was to be run in what was termed 'a third way' (Giddens, 1998; Powell, 2000) – a system based on partnership and driven by performance.

The stated prime effort from that point on was to refocus health-care onto the patients and not on competitive activity between either organizations or professional individuals vying for business. New developments were to be pragmatic and evidence-based, and were expected to be firmly back in the hands of those who knew the patients best – the health professionals (Jay, 1997; Timmins, 2002). Support for an NHS delivering high-quality professionally led nursing care was reinforced by successive Labour health secretaries (Frank Dobson, Alan Milburn, John Reid, Patricia Hewitt, Alan Johnson and Andy Burnham).

The headline themes underpinning the health policy changes that were required from then on were: modernization, investment and development. These were to remain the central foci for the 13 years of Labour government led by Blair and then Brown, and influenced by 26 green and white papers, 14 Acts of Parliament and countless initiatives, crackdowns and targets under six successive health secretaries (King's Fund, 2010a).

The new modern dependable NHS (1997)

The first Labour health White Paper (DOH, 1997) began the reorganization of service delivery and management. This started the dismantling of the previous competitive internal healthcare market, replacing it with a collaborative model, in which NHS organizations worked together, with local authorities and with the private and voluntary sectors.

An initial act was to abolish budget-holding by general practices (Greener, 2009). It was seen as inefficient and inequitable, because of the advantages it had given to patients of budget-holding practices. It had also created an unnecessary and expensive massive bureaucracy. Primary care groups were introduced as the main purchasers and providers of NHS care, subsequently to become primary care trusts, responsible for purchasing integrated community-based care.

The NHS Plan (DOH, 2000b)

The NHS Plan (2000) was hugely significant, as it set out a 10-year plan of activity and investment aimed 'to give people a health service fit for the twenty-first century: a health service designed around the patient' (Milburn, 2000). It looked to sustained increases in funding, far-reaching changes to NHS practices, a patient/public-led service, raised standards of care and major improvements in the general health of the population. Efforts were now focused on replacing old and outdated systems, addressing perceived failings and replacing these with more relevant and modernized approaches fit for a twenty-first-century NHS (see Figure 3.4).

According to Milburn (2000), the basic principles of the NHS were sound, but its practices needed to change. There would be major investment to help this to happen, but it had to be accompanied by service and personnel developments of a very wide-ranging nature, described as the most fundamental and far-reaching reforms the NHS has seen since 1948 (DOH, 2000b).

Developments set out in The NHS Plan

1 A massive growth in professional personnel, support staff, services and infrastructure both in hospitals and general practice.
2 Devolved power to local health services to modernize service delivery and allied activities.
3 National standards set by the Department of Health to be delivered at local level, matched by regular inspection of these by an independent inspectorate, the Commission for Health Improvement.
4 The National Institute of Clinical Excellence (NICE) – to standardize treatment and to get all health services working to the highest standards of evidence-based practice.
5 The Modernisation Agency set up to oversee and spread best practice.
6 High-performing local organizations which performed well for their patients to be given freedom to run their own affairs and to become Foundation Trusts.
7 Central government to intervene rapidly in those areas which underperformed.
8 The development of joint activity and pooled resources between social services and the NHS, to commission health and social care services by a single organization.
9 New contracts for hospital doctors and general practitioners, with an emphasis on quality, increased productivity and evidence of good health outcomes.
10 Nurses and other staff to extend their roles – including specialist and consultant roles, non-medical prescribing, modern matrons and new developments in leadership opportunities.

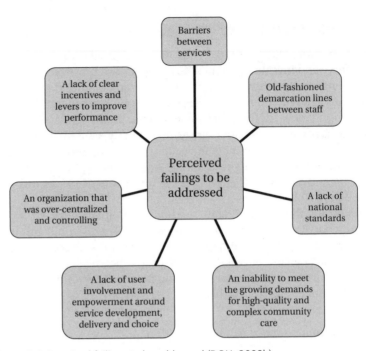

Figure 3.4 Perceived failings to be addressed (DOH, 2000b)

11 A new relationship with the private sector to provide healthcare services on behalf of and alongside the NHS – described as a 'mixed economy of care'.

12 A strong emphasis on giving patients new powers and influence over the way the NHS worked and developed.

Following on from the policy imperatives set out in *The NHS Plan*, we can trace the beginnings of many important changes. There was organizational restructuring and a greater focus on the quality of care, improved information availability and an increasing use of new technologies. There was a growing interest in employee empowerment and rights, combined with responsibilities at both the personal and the professional level. Importantly, very strong emphasis was placed on listening and responding to the users of the service. Later policy reinforcement (DOH, 2004e) set out specifically ambitious pathways and targets for inpatient care, predicated on the need for proven evidence of improved quality, efficiency, productivity, cost-effectiveness and patient safety.

The parallel push to care outside hospital

In tandem with this focus on hospital and acute-care services, we also see the ever-continuing interest in shifting the balance of NHS effort to primary and community care settings (DOH, 2006d; DOH, 2008a; DOH, 2009b). The well-promoted themes were continued evidence of the policy shift away from a predominantly illness and hospital-focused model, to one of individual responsibility, increased self-care, health improvement and greater independence. Transforming community services, together with a change in the population's behaviour, would be the means to deliver an affordable and effective new-style NHS.

Changes to patient care

1 More services to be developed and provided closer to home, with increased patient choice and more innovative service provision.
2 The introduction of professionally managed personalized care packages and better management of long-term conditions (LTCs).
3 Improved coordination of care activity with local authorities and greater integration between health and social care services.
4 Supportive development of the 'third sector' and more work with private organizations to increase care options.
5 Better-quality health information, with improved data on health outcomes and greater financial incentives related to improved patient outcomes.
6 The prevention of ill health – with specific focus on obesity, alcohol consumption, drug abuse, smoking and efforts to improve mental and sexual health.
7 The creation of a 'constitution' for the NHS – to safeguard its core principles and values for the next generation, while setting a clear direction for the future.

Box 3.3 The third sector

- a diverse, active and passionate sector;
- organizations share common characteristics of non-governmental organizations;
- driven by their values;
- reinvest any financial surpluses to further social, environmental or cultural objectives;
- encompass voluntary and community organizations, charities, social enterprises, cooperatives and mutual societies, both large and small.

(www.cabinetoffice.gov.uk/third-sector/about-us)

Box 3.4 The NHS Constitution

- reaffirmation of the right to NHS services, free of charge and with equal access for all;
- enshrined patient rights to choice of services and to NICE-approved drugs recommended by clinicians;
- new and decisive action to be taken against failing services, whether in hospital or the community.

(DOH, 2008b)

Help for NHS nurses and doctors to deliver the new approaches

Lord Darzi (a prominent surgeon, and Parliamentary Undersecretary of State for Health) was commissioned to look to all clinical leadership at grassroots level to support the required organizational changes, promising greater freedoms for frontline staff aspiring to excellence in practice, with investment in training and educational opportunities (DOH, 2008a). Importantly, he noted that the reforms would bring even more opportunities for all nurses to improve care, influence how services would be run and enhance their career paths – a theme which was to be developed in the following year with the publication of *High Impact Changes*, aimed at motivating frontline staff to initiate better ways of working, to meet targets and to reduce expenditure (DOH, 2009a).

Box 3.5 *High Impact Changes*

- no avoidable pressure ulcers in NHS-provided care;
- demonstrate a year-on-year reduction in the number of falls sustained by older people in NHS-provided care;
- stop inappropriate weight loss and dehydration in NHS-provided care;
- promote normal birth;
- avoid inappropriate admissions to hospital and increase the numbers of people who are able to die in a place of their choice;
- reduce sickness absence in the nursing and midwifery workforce to no more than 3 per cent;
- increase the number of patients in NHS-provided care who have their discharge managed and led by a nurse or midwife where appropriate;
- demonstrate a dramatic reduction in the rate of urinary tract infections (UTIs) for patients in NHS-provided care.

(www.institute.nhs.uk/hia)

The ultimate aim was to reduce hospital admissions, encourage a health-promoting culture and thus control costs – a major responsibility for the whole of the NHS workforce and not least for those working outside the hospital sector (DOH, 2008a). The transformation of the NHS in the community, its workforce and its activities were now clearly centre stage and ready for the next moves.

Transforming Community Services (DOH, 2009)

The aim of these changes was to meet the aspirations of the Darzi (2008) vision and also to put in place the new World Class Commissioning agenda (DOH, 2009). The clear vision which spanned three areas

– patient safety, patient experience and the effectiveness of care – required transformational change. This was to be delivered by clinicians, by all other frontline staff, by the organizations providing community services and by the commissioning arms.

The planning and commissioning arms of the primary care trusts were to be separated from those of the now-diverse provider bodies. The aim was to achieve innovative community services that had direct benefits for patients, were responsive to local need, and promoted seamless care through increased integration of health, social care services and other networks. The commissioning primary care trusts were charged with agreeing the new organizational structures and services with the providers with whom they had previously worked by 31 March 2010 (Brindle 2010).

> Where once much effort was put on building capacity and getting people through the door, all thoughts now are on getting more for the public out of what we have got – this means building on our reforms of the last ten years but refocusing them for the new times we are in. It means more choice, more empowerment, more autonomy for the frontline, better focused on the new challenges of a more preventive, more personalised and higher quality NHS. (Burnham, 2009c)

All members of the NHS workforce were being challenged to drive up the quality of care, to obtain value for money and to increase productivity. But it was not to be just about meeting targets and reducing delays in care delivery. As from then, it was about changing the ways health services were provided and managed, with innovation and creativity very much to the fore (DOH, 2006d). Frontline staff were described as key to a successful NHS and the clear drivers for innovation (DOH, 2009a).

🗒 Activity: discuss with your fellow students or colleagues

- Can you be creative and innovative in your practice? – If so, what have you done?
- Are you able to be responsive to ideas from your patients for improving services?

Looking back: 1997–2010

A review of the promised NHS policy developments offers us a judgement on the successes delivered by the Labour health administrations of 1997–2010, and whether 'top-to-toe modernization' had really happened (King's Fund, 2010a). The themes explored focused on England, but are of relevance to all nurses and their patients, whatever their discipline base and circumstances within the United Kingdom. The review provides us with a means of pulling together the many disparate policy developments of the previous 13 years and covered a number of important areas, all of which now rely on continuing investment and effort by the Coalition government.

The issues arising in 2010 and needing continuing attention were as follows:

- accessibility
- consistency of care services
- safety
- health promotion
- management of chronic illness
- clinical effectiveness
- delivery of positive patient experiences
- equitable care
- efficiency
- accountability

Accessibility

Under the Labour administration there had been sustained reductions in waiting times for hospital treatments, combined with the achievement of targets covering a wide variety of issues around care delivery, quality and safety. There remained much room for improvement, but this would prove difficult to achieve if funds continued to be tightened.

Services in primary care had grown in number and in variety. GP appointments and access had been expedited and developed, with many more services provided within practices. Care activities, once the remit of the acute sector, were now provided in a variety of ways closer to home for patients. However, progress was relatively slow in shifting even more healthcare back into the community, because of a lack of the requisite infrastructure. A start had been made in 'transforming' the services and reorganizing community nurse activity, but the future remained uncertain on both counts, in the light of public expenditure cuts and efficiencies required by the new government.

Consistency of care services

The creation of the National Institute for Health and Clinical Excellence (NICE) had helped to ensure the delivery of evidence-based and consistent guidance on the drugs and treatments that were clinically and cost-effective. This had improved consistency of service across the NHS, but variations in prescribing and access had not disappeared.

Safety

Patient safety had been prioritized as a major policy issue. There had been a successful campaign to reduce healthcare-acquired infections and accidents. The National Patient Safety Agency (NPSA) had been established and systems created for collecting and analysing information on adverse events. Efforts had been made to learn from these incidents and to share the information gained with the whole workforce. There was still some way to go, however, in creating a fully open culture of reporting within NHS organizations.

Health promotion

Significant progress had been made in reducing smoking, with smoking cessation programmes and a ban on smoking in public places (DOH, 2007c). Less success had been achieved in reducing alcohol consumption or indeed in slowing down the growing rates of obesity in both adults and children. There had been some improvement in the rates of exercise uptake and healthier eating. The predictions of significant increases in obesity and related ill health meant that the government would need to sustain initiatives in this area, both within the NHS and in all other relevant agencies, if any progress was to be sustained.

Management of chronic illness

There had been a range of initiatives to support those with chronic long-term conditions, backed up by National Service Frameworks (NSFs). GPs had been given incentives to manage long-term care, and achievements had been high against performance indicators. Intensive care and support had been delivered by nurses and other primary care professionals, with modern community matrons appointed to lead developments. Training had been given to patients in self-care and to help others in similar situations (DOH, 2004b). The many developments delivered outside hospital had involved multi-sectoral working and would need sustained investment, development and continued support if they were to continue to be successful.

Clinical effectiveness

The three major health conditions which account for the most NHS spending are: cancer, cardiovascular disease (CHD) and suicides.

Cancer and CHD death rates had come down substantially since 1997. However, in spite of improvements in cancer care both in mortality and survival rates, the UK still lagged behind other European countries. In turn, while there were improvements in the success of cardiac surgery and recommended standards for the treatment of stroke victims, variations persisted in England and in comparison with other comparable countries. On both counts more work needed to be done and financial support continued.

The level of suicides had reduced, with access to specialist early intervention and crisis resolution seen as the best in Europe. The quality and scope of clinical guidelines on all kinds of mental health problems had improved dramatically, with reductions in acute admissions. The long-term reduction in symptoms and improvements in the quality of life of service users would continue to need more help and work. In turn, the rise in numbers of cases of dementia would place high demands on health and social care services, particularly if finances are reduced or withdrawn.

Delivery of positive patient experiences

Overall, public satisfaction with the way the NHS was run had been increasing steadily over the previous years. The total NHS patient experience surveys had provided a great deal of helpful information on which to gauge improvements in activity. Most patients reported that they were treated with dignity and respect, but more work was needed around choice, involvement in care and some aspects of the hospital environment – for example, single-sex accommodation, help with feeding and the maintenance of good nutrition while in hospital.

However, systematic differences in treatment were found according to age, self-rated health status, ethnic group and region. The worst results came from the users of inpatient mental health services. Effort and investment would be needed to get all organizations to build on the progress to date and to create a complete and true picture of the patient experience in what appeared to be growing into a very diverse organization.

Equitable care

From 1997 onwards there had been a clear shift in government policy towards reducing health inequalities. Infant mortality had decreased and life expectancy improved for all social groups. Progress had, however, been much slower in the more socially deprived groups. This had occurred despite efforts to concentrate health initiatives on the most deprived areas of England. Questions still remained as to the sufficiency of funding given to reduce health inequalities and the degree of serious commitment from the NHS in making a difference. More work clearly remained to be done to address this issue, whether by research or by trying different approaches. On either count, more funding and effort would be needed, as inequalities had progressively widened.

Efficiency

Historically there had been weak incentives to improve productivity within the NHS. Since 1997, however, there had been some developments in productivity measures, but further refinements were still needed. Substantial savings had been made in the costs of medicines and of other goods and services. There remained scope, however, for further savings through the more efficient delivery of hospital and other services, greater reductions in lengths of stay in hospitals, an increase in the rate of day-case surgery, the use of lower-cost drugs and the employment of cheaper and fewer staff. It was suggested that this might be achieved by nurses carrying out work currently done by doctors or support workers doing the work of nurses – an issue considered later in chapter 11.

Accountability

The accountability of the NHS to the government had been strengthened. The use of targets had brought benefits, such as shorter waiting times for treatment. NHS trusts had also become accountable to local commissioners. There had been significant developments in creating more locally accountable services through the creation of foundation trusts with their members and elected governors. These developments had improved trusts' relationships with, and awareness of, the priorities of their local populations.

More generally, strong direct performance management, together with independent regulators to inspect and assure the quality of services, had helped to strengthen accountability to the users of the services. The three agencies – the Healthcare Commission, the Mental Health Act Commission and the Commission for Social Care Inspection – were combined into the Care Quality Commission (CQC) from 1 April 2010.

In tandem with these service developments, professional regulation had been overhauled with the aim of making the professions more responsive to public rather than professional interests. Finally, efforts had been made to make the system more accountable to patients, notably through the NHS Constitution (DOH, 2008b). This set out the principles and values of the NHS and brought together in one place the rights and responsibilities of patients and staff.

Thoughts on the review

The analysis above (King's Fund, 2010a) reminds us all of the work that still needs to be done. A major effort is needed to encourage everyone in the population to live healthily and to take responsibility for promoting their own good health and well-being and that of their families. This is set against the potential of both the transformed community services and the acute sector to deliver more innovative, creative and cost-effective care services in partnership with the ever-growing private and third sector organizations. The clear policy challenge for all of us working within the NHS is to do more with less, as the financial environment hardens and difficult choices have to be made on what services can be afforded, who can have them and for how much longer. This debate will no doubt resonate for the foreseeable future. As Ham (2010: 1) aptly reminded us:

The NHS must now transform itself from a service that not only diagnoses and treats sickness but also predicts and prevents it. If the same energy and innovation that went into reducing waiting times and hospital infections could be put into prevention and chronic care, the NHS could become truly world class. This will not be easy and it is vital that politicians engage in an honest dialogue with the public about the changes needed.

📋 Activity: discuss with your fellow students or colleagues

- Imagine you are a politician and reflect on the difficulties for the NHS in providing everything that is invented or found to cure illnesses.
- What do you think should continue to be provided within the NHS today and why?
- What services would you discontinue to save money and why?

2010 and the general election

The 2010 general election saw the early months of that year filled with claims, counterclaims, promises and accusations about the NHS. As ever, all the political parties set out their future vision for healthcare delivery, all set against a backcloth of inevitable public expenditure cuts. The nursing press provided wide coverage of these discussions, in particular from potential MPs with a nursing background (Dean, 2009b).

While many judged the promises and plans for the future, others reflected back on what had happened and, by definition, reminded us of what had worked and indeed where politicians, professionals and the public alike needed to use their energies in the future (King's Fund, 2010a). To coin an old phrase: health was in everybody's interest (DHSS, 1976) – and was clearly set to remain so for the foreseeable future. All the problems and challenges were to be passed on into the hands of the Coalition government.

Learning outcomes

- the historical development of the NHS from 1948 to 2010;
- the policy drivers, changes and developments;
- the impacts of these for the patients, the service and for nurses;
- progress made, mistakes to be avoided and work still to do.

Further reading

Greener, I. (2009) *Healthcare in the UK: Understanding Continuity and Change.* Policy Press.
Hunter, D. J. (2008) *The Health Debate.* Policy Press.

Lister, J. (2008) *The NHS After 60: For Patients or Profits?* Middlesex University Press.

North, N. and Bradshaw, Y. (eds) (1997) *Perspectives in Health Care.* Macmillan.

Ranade, W. (1997) *A Future for the NHS? Health Care for the Millennium,* 2nd edn. Longman Ltd.

Williamson, G. R., Jenkinson, T. and Proctor-Childs, T. (2010) *Contexts of Contemporary Nursing,* 2nd edn. Learning Matters Ltd.

4 The Coalition Agenda, May 2010: Themes Arising

Aims

- to explore the programme of the Conservative-Liberal Democrat Coalition for the NHS as set out in 2010;
- to reflect on the potential impacts of this for the patients, the service and for nurses.

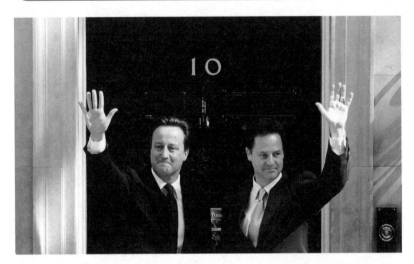

4.1 In May 2010 the problems and challenges facing the UK healthcare system were passed into the hands of a new Coalition government, under David Cameron and Nick Clegg.

Policy developments

Against the backcloth of a huge economic challenge, the King's Fund diagnosis and prescription for the NHS (Ham, 2010) passed into the hands of the new Coalition government on 6 May 2010, under Prime Minister David Cameron (Conservative) and his deputy Nick Clegg (Liberal Democrat). The delivery of this difficult portfolio was given to the new Secretary of State for Health, Andrew Lansley (Conservative), who, with his newly appointed ministerial colleagues responsible for health, were immediately placed under massive pressure to ensure that the then-diverse national health services would be made much

Box 4.1 The Coalition health team, May 2010

Secretary of State for Health:
  Andrew Lansley
Ministers of State:
  Anne Milton (Conservative, former nurse)
  Simon Burns (Conservative, health minister 1996/7)
  Paul Burstow (former Liberal Democrat health spokesperson)
  Earl Howe (Conservative peer and former opposition health
  spokesperson in the House of Lords)

more responsive to patient need and choice, and would also be affordable.

Within a relatively short time the broad plans for the NHS were introduced in the Coalition's programme for government, *Freedom, Fairness, Responsibility* (2010), and then set out more fully in the White Paper, *Equity and Excellence: Liberating the NHS* (DOH, 2010c). As Lansley put it: 'The NHS is one of this country's great national institutions and we are proud of its values, but it must do better to meet the increasing demand on its services. The Coalition government is committed to increase funding for the NHS but in return, the NHS needs to reform' (DOH 2010b). Efficiency savings of £20 billion were to be made, including a 45 per cent reduction in NHS management costs. It was described as the most radical change in the NHS since its inception, a challenging and far-reaching set of reforms, which would drive cultural changes in the NHS. It was a long-term plan aimed at providing a coherent, stable and enduring framework for quality and improvement, no longer about structures and processes, but about priorities and progress in health for all. The four key themes for reform encompassed the following:

1 Putting the patients and public first – providing them with more information and choice about their care; in future, all activity to be underpinned by the mantra of 'no decisions to be made about them without them'.
2 Focusing on improvements in quality and healthcare outcomes – with the aim of providing care services which are among the best in the world.
3 Autonomy, accountability and democratic legitimacy – the reforms were aimed at empowering professionals and providers of care, to give them autonomy in practice and to increase their accountability for the results they achieve. General practitioners working with other clinicians were to be empowered and enabled to deliver results, making them responsible for commissioning decisions about services which would best meet the needs of their local people and which would lead to improved health outcomes.
4 The removal of unnecessary bureaucracy, cutting of waste and making the NHS more efficient.

It was stated that the government would be very clear about what *should* be achieved by the NHS, but that it would not prescribe the means. Such activities were to be passed to more autonomous NHS institutions and professionals, with greater freedoms, clearer duties and obligations for transparency in their relationships with and responsibilities to the patients. It was all about freeing NHS staff from political micro-management, increasing democratic participation in the NHS and making it more accountable to the patients it served.

As Lansley explained, the NHS would see significant change if these proposals were fully implemented. He believed that only by putting patients first and trusting professionals would standards be driven up, better value for money be delivered and a healthier nation created (DOH, 2010b). The whole strategy was underpinned by the need for good integrated partnership working across the whole of the NHS, joining up services to deliver the right care, in the right place and at the right time.

The White Paper, like others before it, provided the initial bones of the expected changes. Many of the commitments were going to require primary legislation and parliamentary approval during the first parliamentary session of 2010/11. Feedback comments and suggestions for the implementation of the proposals were welcomed prior to the introduction of a health bill in the House of Commons, with the Chief Nurse and Health Minister, Anne Milton, encouraging nurses to become involved in the process at that early stage and to make their voices heard (Snow, 2010b; Milton, 2010d) – an example of how all nurses can influence policy and are clearly encouraged to become involved. As Drake (2010a) reminded us: 'It can be tempting to keep one's head down and hope that it will all go away. But nurses who do so will miss a unique opportunity to shape patient care.'

🗒 Activity: discuss with your fellow students or colleagues

- What were initial reactions by nurses to the health White Paper, *Equity and Excellence* (DOH, 2010c)? It might be helpful to have a look back at articles in the nursing press to remind yourself of all the issues raised.
- Do you think there have been many changes made to nursing and healthcare services since then? If so, what are they?
- Are you and your patients seeing the proposed benefits taking shape and coming through within your local health community?

Initial discussions

The key themes were lightly fleshed out within the White Paper and then considered more fully by the media and professional commentators. Let us do the same, and in turn reflect on the benefits (or otherwise) to date for our own patients and for ourselves as nurses. First, we will note some of the proposed changes.

> *We will give patients more information and choice about their care – in*
> *future 'there will be no decisions about me without me' (DOH, 2010c:*
> *3) – patients will have more comprehensive information about the NHS*
> *services that are available and will share in decisions about their care.*

Making patients central to the NHS was to be about further improving their experience and the quality of care they would receive. There was to be a so-called 'information revolution', which was aimed at giving all patients greater choice in services and, in turn, greater control. From April 2011, the comprehensive information to be provided would help patients to choose which provider, consultant-led team (subject to clinical appropriateness) or GP they wished to access for their care.

The targets and tick-boxing activities of previous years were to be replaced by ratings on how people felt about their care experience and how well they had recovered – something like the consumer feedback sought after a car service or obtaining computer help from an internet provider. The information gleaned would be made available so that people could compare and contrast healthcare experiences, and then make choices as to where they might go next or to source a better treatment.

The providers, in turn, would have to become much more business-focused. They would need to be proactive in offering, delivering and providing evidence of a high-quality service with good outcomes. Also, they would have to be very aware and responsive to the potential movements and preferences of their patients, as, for example, in the retail and hospitality sectors – or go out of business.

A new consumer champion called HealthWatch would be created to help strengthen the patient voice. It would be based nationally within the new-style Care Quality Commission (CQC). The previous Local Involvement Networks (LINKs) were to become the local HealthWatch teams, creating a strong local infrastructure aimed at enhancing the role of local authorities in promoting choice and complaints advocacy. Local HealthWatch groups would have the power to recommend that poor services be investigated – it was hoped to avoid another mid-Staffordshire experience, where patient and staff concerns were continually overlooked and the poor quality of care went unchecked (Francis, 2010).

📋 Activity: discuss with your fellow students or colleagues

- Have the patients with whom you work been given more opportunities to have their say about their care and services?
- Are they becoming more involved in the formal decision-making around their healthcare services and choices? If so, in what ways?
- 'At its best the NHS is world class, full of talented and dedicated people. But compared to other countries, the NHS has achieved relatively poor

outcomes. Some of our mortality rates for illnesses such as stroke and lung disease have been among the worst in the developed world. Our ambition is for health outcomes and quality health services that are among the best in the world. We are confident the NHS can meet this challenge because of the talent of our staff, clinicians and scientists' (DOH, 2010c). Do you agree with this statement?

It was said that the Labour government's targets and top-down control of activities had disempowered doctors and managers, creating many perverse situations in practice. These had diverted the focus away from delivering quality care, increased safety, reductions in mortality and morbidity, an improvement in the patient experience and better health outcomes. For the future, the NHS would be held to account in terms of clinically credible and evidence-based outcome measures, and not in terms of process targets (Sprinks, 2010b).

The new NHS Outcomes Framework national goals were to be chosen by the Secretary of State following consultation with relevant bodies. The first framework was to be available in April 2011, with full implementation expected the following year. It was going to encompass the domains of quality, safety and patient experience. All providers of care would be rewarded according to their performance in this respect, with pay reflecting outcomes achieved and not just activity. It was believed that this would be an incentive for providing better-quality care.

📋 Activity: discuss with your fellow students or colleagues

- Do you think your patients are having a good, high-quality experience of healthcare?
- In answering this question you might like to reflect on the following question: would you like your own family to be treated in this way?

We will hand back power to patients and the NHS professionals who treat them: We will empower doctors to deliver results – putting them in charge of what services best meet the needs of local people . . . the headquarters will be in the consulting room and clinic.

The White Paper set out proposals to 'liberate' the NHS from excessive bureaucracy and political control. The aim was to set professionals free to be innovative and to make decisions based on clinical judgement and the assessed needs of patients. Budgets and commissioning-for-care responsibilities were to be devolved to groups of GP practices (consortia), away from government control, and enabled to shape services appropriate to their local communities. However, they would have 'a duty to provide choice' and would be expected to 'contract with as many potential providers as possible', including the private and third sectors.

The public health agenda was to be strengthened by a new relationship between the NHS and local authorities (LAs), the details of which were fully set out in a subsequent health White Paper, *Healthy Lives, Healthy People* (DOH, 2010d). The LAs were to take on the responsibility for local health improvement, which until that point had been the remit of the primary care trusts (PCTs). This move was aimed at increasing the ability of local councillors to ensure that the health and social care needs of local people were being met. For patients, this would mean a better integration of services across health and social care – for example, for those with long-term conditions (LTCs) and for the safeguarding services for children and older adults.

Further to this, all NHS trusts were to become or be part of a foundation trust by 2013. The idea was that their managers would have increased freedom from central control and national targets to develop new, innovative and improved services. Trusts would compete with each other for business, with the best flourishing to the benefit of patient care. Pay bargaining and decisions around the required content of contracted work by their professional and non-professional employees would become a local activity, determined by each individual employer organization. It was argued that local trusts were best placed to assess the health needs of their communities and had to have freedom to deploy staff in the most appropriate ways for local conditions and to make relevant changes and developments as needed.

📋 Activity: discuss with your fellow students or colleagues

Reforms in the White Paper *Equity and Excellence* promised freedom to develop innovative and improved services based on clinical judgement and as a response to locally assessed health needs.

- Have nurses been freed to work in this way?
- What, if any, new services are now available to your patients?
- 'We will remove unnecessary bureaucracy, cut waste and make the NHS more efficient.' Have these measures been achieved?

The government stated that it valued and wanted to keep the professional talent within the NHS and was determined to remove all the unnecessary bureaucracy that had been holding back the freedom to innovate in practice. It intended to review a number of arm's length bodies, abolishing those that did not need to exist (Dean, 2010b, 2010c), and streamlining those that would be needed. The 10 strategic health authorities (STAs) and 150 PCTs were to be abolished and would not exist beyond 2012/13. It was said that money saved by these and other means would be put back into frontline services.

The new streamlined bodies and responsibilities included:

- An NHS Commissioning Board: this would allocate and account for NHS resources, lead on quality improvement and promote patient involvement and choice.

- Monitor: to be developed into an economic regulator, taking responsibility for NHS providers from 2013 irrespective of status, across both health and social care.
- Care Quality Commission (CQC): to act as a quality and safety inspectorate across health and social care.

Future providers would need to have a two-part licence to practise, overseen by both Monitor and the CQC to ensure that services provided the required levels of safety and quality, that essential services were not lost and that agreed budgets were met. In the spirit of developing further patient choice, 'any willing provider' who was able to deliver these required standards would be able to provide NHS care. Finally, Lansley commended the 'ambitious' plan as set out fully within this first health White Paper from the Coalition government. He believed it would make the NHS a truly world-class service that put patients at its heart and offered care that was safe, of the highest quality and able to withstand the funding pressures of the future.

Initial responses

While many of the proposed new developments seemed to be a continuation of the many routes already taken by the previous Labour government, the actual destination being pursued by the Coalition was far from clear, but, to say the least, remained worrying (Carter, 2010a; Duffin, 2010). Promises that the dismantling, even privatization, of healthcare services was not a long-term agenda for the government failed to quell concerns felt by many involved (see Dean, 2011a; Snow, 2011a). The breakneck speed of the proposed reforms and the seemingly relentless daily reports of cuts in public expenditure did not make for comfortable reading, nor augur well for the maintenance of a well-integrated, diversity-sensitive, inequality-reducing NHS (Ham, 2011).

Toynbee (2010) described the proposed reforms as 'an experiment, a game, a folly on a grand scale', believing the changes heralded the demolition of the NHS. Others referred to 'a huge experiment' (Crumbie, 2010), an 'expensive experiment' (Drake, 2010a), a 'botched job' (Karim, 2010), a 'field day for private operators' (Booth et al., 2010a), and argued that it might lead to cracks in the system, with NHS services and patient care suffering (Jebb, 2010). As Ramesh (2011) put it: 'Letting market forces overrun this system may make it more efficient, but every taxpayer pound will come at a cost of job security, the [further] rationing of healthcare and parts of taxpayer-funded medicine [and nursing care] abandoned on the basis of cost.'

The RCN (Royal College of Nursing) was by turn both constructive and critical. It welcomed the focus on quality, the centrality of patients and the stated empowerment of professionals. However, like others, it was concerned at the significant risks to the NHS in terms of the scale and pace of the reforms. While much was said about the power and contribution of clinicians and about meeting the needs of the patients, a worrying silence around nursing's contribution was palpable – and at times appeared to be something of an afterthought. As Cole (2010) noted, nothing in the White Paper suggested that nurses on the front-line would be exempt from budget squeezes and skill-mix dilution. Indeed, nurses were only mentioned twice.

By contrast, the noisy influx of private sector interests, well developed and eager to take on commissioning provision and administrative services right across health and social care, reflected loudly its enthusiasm for 'the clarity it had seen in the government's programme', and the business opportunities and openings clearly available (Booth et al., 2010). This private sector boom came amid the toughest financial climate for public services in a generation, and despite continued assurances from all health ministers that the reforms to the health service were aimed at achieving greater value for money and improved efficiencies – not to dismantle or privatize the service.

However, the proposal to increase the choice of any 'willing provider bodies' and thus competition for service licences did not sit well with the notion of 'shared access to collective health care and a shared responsibility to use resources effectively to deliver better health care' (Catton, 2010); surely the very basis for a *national* health service, and important too for the promised continued delivery of the NHS Constitution.

📋 Activity: discuss with your fellow students or colleagues

- Policy and its implementation develop day by day. Have a look at the commentaries on all the new developments provided daily on news programmes, within the press or via one of the online healthcare commentators, for example the King's Fund.
- Relate this developing knowledge to your current experience as a nurse and to that of your patients.

General issues

Wright (2010) expressed concern at the apparent chopping away of tranches of employees to save money – not least those who contribute in many different ways to the delivery of an 'in-the-round' NHS. He referred to the importance of having the support of professional managers, sound financial advisers, secretarial and administrative support, receptionists, cooks, porters, cleaners, etc. The experience of industrial action and general discontent in the 1980s demonstrated the importance of having a complete, fully engaged team of differently skilled support staff so as to enable doctors and nurses to deliver high-quality care in a clean and safe environment.

The continuing news of redundancies and cutbacks in the NHS at large, against a mantra of the introduction of innovative ways of working and the need for ever greater 'flexibilities', has caused much concern, not least for those whose jobs were most likely to be 'on the line' and at risk of redundancy (Catton, 2010). The subsequent reality of these fears has been truly felt across all parts of the UK NHS workforce – in Northern Ireland (Dean and Kendall-Raynor, 2011), in Scotland (Dean, 2010c; Fyffe, 2010), in Wales (Dean 2011c) and in England (Cole, 2011).

Bailey (2010) was unsure as to why the scale of the proposed upheaval in services or structures was either necessary or sensible in light of the economic problems. As the think-tank Civitas noted, previous NHS reorganizations had been followed by reduced productivity for up to a year in terms of quality of service and use of resources (see Bailey, 2010). It remained unclear as to who would manage or indeed carry through the change effectively when there was a commitment to a 45 per cent cut in management costs and efficiency savings being sought of £20 billion. Indeed, the right-wing Conservative group, the Bow Group, expressed concern at the lack of specific detail on how these reductions would be achieved. Interestingly, it highlighted the importance of keeping staff on side for the changes to take place effectively. NHS staff could ultimately make or break the government's ambitious NHS vision (Bow Group, 2010).

Nursing issues

The changes proposed were neither comfortable nor clear for nurses, whether in hospitals or the community. For example, the previous government's policy, Transforming Community Services (DOH, 2009g), had, as we know, already begun a major restructuring process. Services were to be provided by social enterprises, community foundation trusts or by vertical integration and merger with an acute trust. PCTs had been ordered to separate their provider and commissioning arms, and work on this was already well under way. Broadly, the previous Labour health team had already done much of the spadework for transforming the community services. The incoming Coalition government was, therefore, easily able to take over the reins and introduce its own reforms, not least with the proposed abolition of the PCTs and SHAs and with very strong support for an influx of social enterprise and private sector providers across the whole of the NHS (Lansley, 2010; Milton 2010c).

These moves clearly left many thousands of district nurses, health visitors, school nurses, community matrons and other professionals wondering who their future employers might be. Possibilities raised included foundation trusts, local councils, the new GP commissioning consortia, social enterprises or the private sector in its many different forms. Unsurprisingly, the required achievement of the £20 billion savings left many concerned not just for their future roles and employers, but also for their continued employment prospects (Duffin, 2010). The reported influx of private healthcare companies looking for business, together with the commissioning and purchasing powers of the new GP consortia, all combined to provide a very unsettling environment.

Drake (2010b) and Duffin (2010) both argued strongly that community nurses would be a valuable resource for any type of commissioner or provider body because of their experience and knowledge. As Amadi (2010) put it, there was a good case for strengthening the community-nursing contribution in the future and not risking reductions to save money. The trend towards an ever-growing workload for community nurses was going to continue as a result of more services being transferred from hospital to community settings, the increasing numbers of people with long-term conditions and the continued emphasis on health promotion and illness prevention (DOH, 2010c; 2010d; Duffin, 2010). The 2010 National Audit Office report on addressing health inequalities had, for example, noted the importance of having a good understanding of population needs and a greater investment in prevention activities (NAO, 2010) – potentially all good news for community nurses if that advice was heeded.

Concerns were also felt about the apparent diversification of healthcare providers and the increased potential for the acceleration of the privatization of a wide variety of services. It was suggested this would fragment both service provision and continuity of care and, in turn, make access for the most vulnerable – such as older people, those with long-term conditions (Muscular Dystrophy Campaign, 2010) and other marginalized groups – much more difficult. This of course would not help in the government's stated focus on reducing health inequalities – a complex activity which requires effective and well-coordinated 'joined-up solutions' (DOH, 2010d; Marmot, 2010). As Scott (2010c) helpfully reminded us, there was nothing wrong in encouraging trusts and others to develop new and innovative approaches to patient care. There was a need, however, to remember that the NHS was not a supermarket competing for market share, but an organization funded by the taxpayers to keep them healthy and to make them better.

Drake (2010a) was similarly concerned that the well-established systems for NHS care delivery, whether in the community or in the acute sector, would be destabilized and staff subsequently demoralized as the changes progressed and competition increased. New and different providers competing for business might lead to variations in service provision and standards across the country, creating a 'postcode lottery' for patients – a situation we saw happen in the 1990s with the introduction of the internal healthcare market. This situation, Drake believed, would necessarily lead neither to cost savings nor indeed to improved health outcomes for patients. It might prove to be once again an expensive experiment, rather than a solution to the financial challenges that face the NHS.

Catton (2010), speaking on behalf of the RCN, reiterated support for innovative and radical ways of providing care to improve services and to use budgets wisely in the difficult financial times. Support was not however given for making savings quickly by just cutting services and staff. Wards and services were already being targeted for closure as pressure grew for the NHS to save money.

It was noted that many specialist nurse roles were being cut or reduced, in spite of the proven benefit to patients, and that those nurses were being moved over to general duties to save money (Kendall-Raynor, 2010b). The DOH response to this concern was that local trusts were best placed to assess the health needs of their communities and must have freedom to deploy staff in ways appropriate for local conditions – a response which did not necessarily bode well for future local pay bargaining, good terms and conditions of service or indeed for a strong future for professional nurses.

Activity: discuss with your fellow students or colleagues

- Has professional nurse practice been enhanced or reduced over the past year or so? It would be interesting to raise this question within your current nursing or multidisciplinary team. In addition to this, explore the topics nurses have been writing and talking about in the nursing press.
- Do you feel your patients are receiving all the professional nurse care and services they need and want? If not, what is happening? Is care being provided by other non-professionals?

GPs and the responsibility of being both commissioner and provider in the new NHS

The proposed centrality of general practice within the government's vision for the NHS also raised many unanswered questions and concerns. Some queried the notion of GPs spending more time on dealing with contracts and finances and, in effect, less time with patients. Halstead (2010) believed that most doctors would rather spend time dealing with patients' medical problems than wrestling with 'the latest number-crunching exercise'.

Roberts (2010) similarly noted that although doctors are highly trained and highly paid to be clinicians, they are trained neither as administrators nor even as supervisors of administrators. Even if, by some mysterious process, training in the mysteries of the human body and its ailments somehow also made them into good administrators, it would still make better sense for them spend their time on what they were trained for rather than on running the NHS. While it was accepted that some doctors would and could commission care and manage budgets with more enthusiasm and skill than others, there was the fear that the system could potentially become divisive.

In a similar vein, the apparent enthusiasm for the introduction of private sector services to help both in GP consortia commissioning and in providing community services posed worries. Some feared that the acceleration of privatization could make access more difficult for the most vulnerable, such as older people and those with long-term conditions, and that the new-style GP fundholding through the consortium mechanism would be likely to increase the postcode lottery for services (Cole, 2010) This sounded like a return to the problems of budget-holding practices in the 1980s and 1990s, which we discussed in Chapter 3. The government did, however, acknowledge this issue and said that it had learnt lessons from that period and would not be making the same mistakes again.

Other commentators stressed the importance of the varied and specialist skills required to assess patient needs in order to be able effectively to commission and manage the appropriate services (Bailey, 2010). There was a generally expressed belief that many GPs would not want the job and do not have the requisite skills to take on the work of spending £80 billion of public money. Further to this was doubt as to their breadth of knowledge to spend correctly on acute services, community services, social care, mental health, learning disabilities, ambulance trusts and other specialist services. The suggestion that others would have the skills to take on this role on their behalf raised further problems.

The proposed importation of the private sector to carry out the commissioning function, for example, could distance GPs from patient choice and commissioning decisions – the very opposite of the proposed intention of using GPs' knowledge of their patients to deliver a more patient-led organization. In turn, this whole process might end up destabilizing hospitals and other provider bodies, because of others making less-knowledgeable decisions based on budgets and desktop information rather than on patient choice or professional understanding of what was needed to meet the diverse health needs of varied communities and individuals (Muscular Dystrophy Campaign, 2010).

Further related concerns around commissioning power resting with GPs was the perceived lack of clarity on the involvement of hospital consultants, nurses, pharmacists and allied health professionals. Chief Nursing Officer Christine Beasley and Lynn Young (RCN) were, of course, adamant about the importance of the contribution of nursing to commissioning (see Snow 2010b; Duffin, 2010), in spite of the lack of focus given to it, both in the White Paper (DOH, 2010c) and in post-publication discussions with the DOH (Dean, 2010b). While Lansley asserted that GPs knew what their patients needed for commissioning purposes, there was also the required focus on those wider groups and individuals in the population who did not come anywhere near doctors in general practice settings.

Professionals other than GPs, who work with the broader population, would surely be required to help with commissioning in order to meet the wider agenda of health promotion and the reduction in health inequalities. The practicalities of this were not made clear in terms of general care in the community, although it was self-evident that community nurses and others would need to play a significant role if the government were serious in taking this particular agenda forward – a view held by the NHS Alliance (see Snow, 2011b) and the RCN (2010a, 2010b).

The Health Minister, Anne Milton, speaks to nurses and asks for their help

In the late summer of 2010 it was confirmed that a public health White Paper would be published in the autumn. Anne Milton (Conservative Health Minister and a former nurse) said that she wished to see a concerted effort to improve public health. She believed that prevention and early intervention needed to become a greater part of the general nursing mindset (Milton, 2010b, 2010d). She noted that nurses work with a wide range of partners and have very good access to sectors of the population that other professionals do not reach. She referred specifically to health visitors, school nurses and occupational health nurses, who, she noted, all made significant contributions to the health of the public.

Milton was also very positive about the contributions of nurses and other primary care practitioners to the developing consortia agenda, describing practice nurses, community nurse partners and other practitioners as playing a crucial part in the new consortia. In turn, the consortia would need to work with all clinical professions to design services that provide high-quality care and improve the health of the local population (Knight, 2010b).

In further support for other nursing contributions, Milton parried many previously expressed concerns. She stated her absolute intention of building a service which was patient centred, professionally led and responsible for a reformed social care system. She looked for an active and developing role for nurses in commissioning, education and leadership. She wanted new models of care, with nurses working outside the NHS, 'stepping outside the currently known system' and, for example, running a wider network of social enterprises.

Box 4.2 Central Surrey Health (CSH)

- a social enterprise created in 2006;
- the first nurse-led social enterprise;
- provides community nursing and therapy services to a population of 280,000;
- positives: employee-owned, 'fleet-of-foot' initiatives possible, and able to do things differently;
- benefits: increased efficiencies, reduced waste, and improved patient experiences.

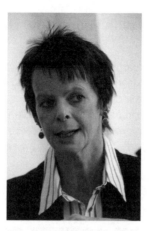

4.2 Conservative Healthcare Minister Anne Milton played a role in debates surrounding the influential 2010 White Paper, *Equity and Excellence: Liberating the NHS.*

By August 2010, a nurse-led social enterprise, Central Surrey Health (CSH), had been chosen to mentor staff who were looking to run health services. CSH had been selected to support 12 fledgling social enterprise projects, and was a response to Andrew Lansley's pledge in July 2010 to create a 'vibrant' culture of social enterprises in the NHS.

Health outcomes revisited

The development of the new health-outcome measures to be applied to all provider bodies was under way, and the measures were being drawn up in partnership with professionals, patients and their carers. Nurses already involved in this work included nurse consultants in learning disability, and mental health nurse directors. Milton believed that this new focus on outcomes rather than processes would remove the unintended consequences and pressures of achieving all the targets that had littered the previous government's programme for the NHS (Sprinks, 2010b).

Emphasis was placed on the importance of strengthening the relationship between community and acute nursing services. It was hoped that new ways of working together would streamline access to acute care and make effective, timely and supported discharge and admission possible, not least by involving patients and their carers more fully in the planning and decision-making process. As Milton explained, the government wanted to cut through the barriers that stop nurses from improving care in either the community or acute settings, but they needed to hear the profession's ideas on how to go about it (Milton, 2010c). In the meantime, she thanked all nurses for the work they do everyday – from mental healthcare to learning disability, from midwifery to community nursing, and across the nursing spectrum.

📋 Activity: discuss with your fellow students or colleagues

- Have you been able to contribute professionally as you would wish to do as a nurse in the reforming health services? You may need to consider this question within your own nursing team.
- Have you been able to influence the commissioning process by advising or reporting nursing information to your local consortium?
- Have any of the concerns expressed about the reforms come to fruition or were they scaremongering?
- Are your patients receiving a good service?
- Have services improved or deteriorated?

Conclusion

As we now move forwards through the second decade of the twenty-first century and face the work of implementing the health policy agendas set by the Conservative–Liberal Democrat Coalition government, it is sometimes easy to forget the lessons of history. We have glanced back briefly at the creation of the NHS and then, on a whirlwind trip, explored how it has been changed and developed by successive governments and by ourselves as nurses, as we have implemented the changes over time at practice level.

This is the inevitable pattern of NHS life, and of course one in which we, as the majority in the NHS workforce, have the power and knowledge to play an influential role. Part of this important role and responsibility is to learn the lessons of the history of the NHS and to seek to avoid things that did not work and to promote those which were effective and relevant. Questions we now face and that need answers may include:

- Have the Coalition government's changes improved the work I am doing with the patients?
- Are the changes helping to reduce health inequalities and improve the health of the whole population?
- Are the multidisciplinary, multi-sector, collaborative-care ventures delivering care that is effective for the population with whom I work?
- Are the patients and their carers really the central focus for care, and are their voices being heard and listened to in both care commissioning and delivery?
- Do I have the necessary technological support to deliver high-quality care?
- Is there clear room for me to develop my professional nurse practice in the currently developing NHS or are there problems?

These questions should undoubtedly be part of the political debate and our activity around the success or otherwise of any proposed health agendas. All these issues are fundamentally relevant for professional nurses, as they shape and, it is be hoped, provide the context in which the shared and communal values of nursing can be implemented effectively and developed at practice level. It is hoped that the discussions in the chapters that follow will go some way towards clarifying the present position of nursing and towards ensuring a strong, successful, professional future in the NHS of the second decade of the twenty-first century.

Learning outcomes

- an overview of the Conservative–Liberal Democrat Coalition's programme for the NHS;
- some reflections and food for thought on the potential impacts of the currently developing reforms for the patients, the service and for nurses.

Further reading

Try to read a daily newspaper, the nursing press and a health service-related journal and follow the fate of the NHS and nursing as the reforms unfold.

5 Working in Partnership and the Policy Agenda

Aims

- to promote the importance of effective integrated working for both implementing and creating new policy agendas in the currently ever-changing NHS;
- to reflect on the importance of working in partnership with the currently widening community of healthcare providers in the public, private and third sectors;
- to consider the implications of this challenging agenda for both nurses and their patients.

The NHS as a workplace is a large, complex and rapidly changing environment. By definition, many of the issues addressed in the working lives of all nurses inevitably involve multiple professionals, non-professionals and many organizations across health and social care, in the public, private and third sectors. As Glasby and Dickinson (2008) remind us, if you are going to make a positive and practical difference to the patients and service users you face, it will involve working well with other professions, other sectors and organizations and, of course, with your communities, your patients and their families and friends (i.e., the informal carers).

Current national and local health policy calls for enhanced and effective partnership working – a theme which reverberates from all previous governments' periods in office. Then and now, there are many strongly worded policy documents reflecting a serious commitment to the concept of partnership working. It is not an option for anyone working within the NHS to ignore, but a given and expected approach. While caring professionals mostly learn their trade in individual disciplines (Goodman and Clemow, 2010), their real-life work situations are much more complex, and the requirement to work collaboratively is a skill of great importance to learn, develop and apply – not least to ensure a joined-up, caring and effective service which meets the needs of the patients and their families and does not add to their worries or concerns.

📋 Activity: discuss with your fellow students or colleagues

- Think about the family's experience as described below by parents Olive and Peter and reflect on the importance of good teamwork and organization in healthcare delivery.
- Do you know what all the roles involve? If not, try to find out. An understanding of what others do is fundamental to good team working.

'We have twin girls aged five, both have moderate learning disability. Jenny also has autism. We're totally confused with all the different professionals and agencies we have to deal with. The following are some of the people we deal with on a regular basis: GP, counselling nurse, occupational therapist, psychiatrist, psychologist, teacher, classroom assistant, ophthalmologist, audiologist and administrators, to name but a few. We're so confused sometimes. We don't understand the different roles and have so many appointments that clash. Can nobody or no system sort it out?' (Integrated Care Network, 2004).

What is partnership working?

Partnership working as a concept is succinctly defined as organizations or individuals working together or acting jointly (Ovretveit, 1997a). For nurses, it is about working with other people, be they professionals, non-professionals, patients, clients, families or children (Goodman, 2008). Glasby and Dickinson (2008) also emphasize a whole range of potential partnerships between the public, private and voluntary sectors, not just between services, but also between professionals and people who use the services. This may involve collaborative working with organizations and personnel involved with employment services, the retail sector, transport, leisure, education and criminal justice. As Jelphs and Dickinson tell us:

> Whether it be gun crime, substance misuse, prostitution, social exclusion, regeneration, third world debt, teenage pregnancy or public health, the issues at stake are often so complex that no one agency (or professional group) working by itself could ever hope to provide a definitive solution (or even understand the problem in its entirety). (2008: xi)

NHS healthcare today relies increasingly on effective teamwork; with the development of multi-sectoral teams working not only in hospital and primary care settings, but across all the traditional boundaries of health and social care and indeed beyond (DOH, 2010c). It is an important part of everyday practice in all fields of care (McCray, 2009) and will continue to be so, because the concept of partnership working has been, and remains, an important theme underpinning all current policy activity (Darzi, 2009a; DOH, 2010c; 2010d).

While noting, however, that the changing contexts of healthcare organizations continue to support collaborative team working, McCallin (2001: 419) and others (Glasby and Dickinson, 2008: 27) remind us that there is little empirical evidence to suggest or prove that *effective* interdisciplinary, multi-sectoral teams improve patient outcomes. On the other hand, of course, there is plenty of evidence to show that *ineffective* team working can and does cause poor (as noted by Olive and Peter in the case study), if not disastrous, outcomes for those involved – child deaths (Munro, 2010), the neglect of older adults (Care Quality Commission, 2011; Parliamentary and Health Service Ombudsman, 2011) and the mismanagement and abuse of people with a learning disability (Mencap, 2004).

🗒 Activity: discuss with your fellow students or colleagues

- Think of a patient or patient group with whom you are working at the moment.
- List all the different professionals, non-professionals and other organizations that are involved in the assessment, planning and delivery of their care.
- Do you think you and your team work effectively with this 'mixed economy'* of care providers?
- Do you think the patients and their families and friends (the informal carers) are happy with the service they receive from you and your team?

a variety of care providers from different sectors – public, private, voluntary, mixed – providing healthcare and other services to the population

Who is required to work together?

The ownership and delivery of the current government's health strategy is clearly predicated on meaningful working relationships between the DOH, the patients, their representative groups and the public; NHS staff and their representative and professional bodies; local government; and the voluntary, social enterprise and independent sectors (DOH, 2010c). These are all key stakeholders in delivering healthcare today and, as such, need to work together.

Lansley described this required partnership culture in the NHS as one which was integral to David Cameron's notion of a 'Big Society', reflecting the social solidarity of shared access to collective healthcare, and a shared responsibility to use resources effectively to deliver better health and effective healthcare (Hetherington, 2010; DOH, 2010b). This 'Big Society' concept, introduced in 2010, currently underpins the Coalition's legislative programme (see Box 5.1). The aim is to create a cultural climate that empowers and encourages local people and communities to take much greater responsibility for their own lives – not

> ### Box 5.1 The core ideas of the Big Society
>
> 'We know that the best ideas come from the ground up, not the top down' (David Cameron, Prime Minister, BBC News, 18 May 2010).
>
> - approach based on encouraging greater personal and family responsibility and community activism;
> - to give communities power to stop post-office or pub closures;
> - to train community organizations;
> - to encourage volunteering;
> - to create a Big Society Bank to fund social enterprises;
> - to give people access to government data and to review local government finance.

least by taking on active roles and volunteerism. Its priorities include greater executive power for local communities, with a transfer of power away from central to local government. In addition, it supports the growth of cooperative groups, mutuals, charities and social enterprises to encourage locally funded innovative services and activities which fit the specific needs and choices of each locality and community. The idea is supported by a national Big Society network which exists to generate, develop and showcase new ideas to help people come together in their neighbourhoods 'to do good things' (*Financial Times*, 2010).

Concerns, however, have been expressed by many as to the implications of the programme set against the current retrenchment in public spending across the UK. While there may well be positives in encouraging people to play an active role in their own community and to take greater responsibility more generally for their own health and well-being, there are obvious downsides for those who really do need 'helping to health'.

The initial public expenditure cuts of spring 2010 took a serious toll on a wide variety of projects and financial benefits, which, until then, had provided support for some of the most vulnerable in society. These included Sure Start services, domestic violence centres, HIV prevention schemes, help for women with postnatal depression, a work scheme for the blind, day centres for street drinkers, refugee advice centres, a work project for those with a learning disability, debt advice services, mobility benefits for those with disabilities, family support centres, a clinical music centre for young people with severe learning difficulties and a rape crisis centre – to name but a few (Gentleman, 2011). It is very difficult to see how removing these services will encourage those who need such help suddenly to become the active citizens and volunteers as envisaged by the Big Society movement. Instead, many nurses are likely to find themselves dealing with potentially more difficult workloads and health agendas as such fragile individuals look for help elsewhere, slowly become more unwell and have greater needs – a situation which does not bode well for the stated attempts by the government to reduce health inequalities or, indeed, to promote better health across the whole population (DOH, 2010c; 2010d).

Delivering healthcare – it's not just about professionals ▮

While many government health and social care documents often tend to refer only to professionals working together, in reality there are many other important 'stakeholders' who are also involved, and who are vital for effective healthcare delivery – within whichever sector (see Box 5.2). Such contributions, however, were noted in *The NHS Plan* (DOH, 2000b), in *Patient and Public Involvement in the NHS* (DOH, 2007c) and by the government in 2010 in its programme for health. The list of those to be considered include the patients and their families, informal carers, porters, cleaners, housekeepers, administrative staff, professions allied to medicine, IT and technical support, radiographers, education and training staff, and secretaries.

Box 5.2 Definition of stakeholder

- a person or group with a direct interest, involvement or investment in something – e.g., the employees, shareholders and customers of a business concern; in a healthcare organization this means the staff who organize and deliver care, as well as the users of the service;
- those people who have a stake in the outcome of any service delivery – their inputs may be the physical work they do, the education they provide, the management of the finances or the way they organize delivery;
- those who are affected by how the organization works.
(http//uk.encarta.msn.com/dictionary)

🗒 Activity: discuss with your fellow students or colleagues

- List all the stakeholders with whom you and your nursing team work.
- Do you know exactly what they all do? If not, find out, so that their care contribution is clear and appropriately applied in making your patients' experiences effective and safe. It will also help to improve your partnership-working experience.

Partnership working – an ever-developing and popular theme in health policy ▮▮▮▮▮▮▮▮

The development of partnership working across diverse health and social care fields has been widely researched and analysed (Leathard, 2004; Glasby and Dickinson, 2008; Jelphs and Dickinson, 2008). It has also become a major policy theme for all recent governments in their pursuit of healthcare that is cost-effective, cost-efficient and provides value for money.

Reasons given for its developing popularity in policy initiatives over time reflect a growth in professional specialization and subsequent complexity of health and welfare services with a need to manage the different teams and team working arrangements, not least with the increasing presence and diversity of care provision from the statutory, private and third sectors. All governments have stressed the policy intention of delivering a more effective, integrated and supportive service for patients, with multidisciplinary teamwork as a core theme, linked to a need to rationalize resources and to reduce the duplication of care services and providers.

The health and social care policies of today embody all the reasons given above in some way or other, providing focus, impetus and practical frameworks for multi-agency teams to consult and collaborate closely, as they aim to deliver care together. This is not always easy to achieve in practice, in spite of the best intentions of the individuals and agencies involved.

📋 Activity: discuss with your fellow students or colleagues

- Have a look at current policy documents related to your area of practice. Find out where they refer to partnership working and see what sorts of ideas are raised to help you work in this way.
- Reflect on your experiences of trying to work with others from different organizations. Think about both positive and negative issues and consider how things might be improved.
- Do your patients like a multidisciplinary team being involved in their care? Or are they concerned that too many people know about their lives and health status?

Reflections on government support for partnership working within the NHS

During the past decades, health and social carers from all sectors have faced many difficult dilemmas as they have tried to implement and deliver the proposed partnership policy agendas as proposed by the DOH. At the same time, they have had to focus on their own organizational needs and wants and, importantly, to keep within budgets.

We can see how this happened in the 1980s and 1990s with the development of an internal healthcare market in the NHS. On the one hand, there were exhortations to collaborate with other providers in order to give an eclectic and appropriately broad response to assessed health needs. On the other, the formation of a more business-like NHS, with its environment of competition and secrecy between care providers, in order to raise standards of care and to become cost-sensitive, did not necessarily create an environment conducive to effective multi-agency partnerships.

A quote from this period should sound a warning for today's eclectic and very similar developments in all fields of care within and beyond the NHS. As Flynn et al. (1996) concluded, coordination of care and effective team working were made more difficult with the commercializing cultural change, the introduction of a variety of new services from other sectors and the subsequent complexity of health and social care services being provided by the mid-1990s, following the reforms set out in the White Paper, *Working for Patients* (DOH, 1989c).

However, the Conservative government of the day did not accept such problems: 'We need constructive co-operation between different parts of the NHS as well as the beneficial impact of competition. Improving health care is not a question of balancing one or the other. We have to find the appropriate balance between the two' (NHSME, 1994). A similar belief permeates the current government's economic and health agendas. It clearly acknowledges the difficulties now facing the UK, but has made its view very clear. As Lansley said:

> The massive deficit and growing debt means there are some difficult decisions to make. The NHS is not immune to these challenges. But far from that being reason to abandon reform, it demands that we accelerate it. Only by putting patients first and trusting professionals will we drive up standards, deliver better value for money and create a healthier nation. (DOH, 2010b; DOH, 2010c)

As we now move on into the second decade of the twenty-first century, it is helpful and appropriate to heed words of concern from the past, to try to learn from that experience and to achieve a more effective response within today's similarly competitive, financially focused and rapidly diversifying health and social care environment. The achievement of an 'appropriate balance' may not, however, be secured easily.

Nocon (1994) noted that the process of working together in such changing times is a difficult one, and the rewards are sometimes uncertain, with different organizations often having their own agendas and other priorities. These may well be financially led, and this alone may not necessarily make for success in either multi-sectoral partnership working or in providing high-quality healthcare services.

There is much reliance being placed currently on the effective working of the NHS Commissioning Board, which, together with Monitor, is overseeing NHS activities. While these bodies are playing a broader controlling role over care delivery and NHS finance on behalf of the Coalition government, it is up to all professional and non-professional carers to protect and to challenge any adverse outcomes in standards of care provision and poor partnership working within and between local health teams across the UK.

It is worth remembering at this point that more than 300,000 people from all walks of life joined together in a major demonstration (March for the Alternative) in London in March 2011 to show their concern about the radical changes being made to the NHS and the imposition of wide-ranging cuts to important projects and benefits which had supported the most vulnerable in society (Gentleman, 2011). As discussed in Chapter 2, there are many ways and opportunities to make your voice heard and to influence policy. Joining a march in partnership with others may not be your choice, and may not necessarily achieve what people want – exemplified by the earlier anti-Iraq war and anti-foxhunting rallies. It is, however, a means of expressing your concerns with others at current developments – the point being to influence a change in the direction of policy.

🗒 Activity: discuss with your fellow students or colleagues

- Go back through some of the copies of the nursing press published in the first few months of 2011 and reflect on the different views and opinions around the changes to the NHS, to nursing practice and to the effects on patients.
- What was said about the demonstration? Do you think it helped to influence change?

Moving on

We will now consider a number of issues that are pertinent to our discussion of the importance of effective partnership working and that may elucidate and develop some of the points already raised – of course, with your help and reflections on practice. These include: the concept of partnership working; the potential advantages and disadvantages of multidisciplinary care teams; attributes of effective team working and partnerships in care; current policy imperatives – commercialization, diversity and fragmentation of providers; the creation of low-trust and high-trust relationships; changes needed in structure and organization; professional development and support.

The concept of partnership working

Ovretveit's succinct definition, cited above, pulls together a multitude of interpretations and terms used to discuss and explain the practice of working and caring together within teams. Glasby and Dickinson (2008), Leathard (2004), McCray (2009), McKimm and Phillips (2009), Payne (2000) and Wallace and Davies (2009), amongst many others, explore the terminology and its application in practice in great detail. For our purposes, we need to note that national and local health policy requirements call for ever more effective partnership working with the patients, and the mantra 'no decision about me without me' clearly permeates all policy documents (DOH, 2010c).

Glasby and Dickinson (2008) noted the 'growing importance' of the statutory duty of public bodies to work in this way, as set out in official parliamentary records. The word 'partnership' was used 38 times in 1989 (Jupp, 2000: 7), 6,197 times in 1999, 17,912 in 2006, and currently in much higher numbers. Glasby and Dickinson also note the importance of 'strongly worded statements' by governments around beliefs and guiding principles for policy implementation. As they remind us, 'the fact remains that partnership working is no longer an option, but a core part of all public services and all public service professions' (2008: xv).

There is clearly continuing policy pressure for professionals to work with a large number of stakeholder groups and to listen and respond to a variety of voices, putting patients at the heart of all activity. It goes without saying that, for nurses, this should be second nature. *The Code* (NMC, 2008) is based on the principles of partnership working. It refers to:

- working with others to protect and promote the health and well-being of those in your care;
- collaborating with those in your care;
- sharing information with colleagues;
- working effectively as a team.

The potential advantages of working collaboratively are many, not least the development of a better understanding of each others' roles, foci and contributions. According to Stephen Covey, in his best-selling book *The Seven Habits of Highly Effective People* (1989), an effective team is likely to demonstrate a number of important attributes: an agreement on leadership, group goals, direction or mission, clear roles, effective communication, and respect for team members and for the resources made available to deliver good care. Finally and importantly, this team will have a sense of humour – a prerequisite for work enjoyment in the challenging environments of healthcare today.

While all nurses would hope to work like this within their teams, it may still prove to be a challenge in practice – it is not an easy process to achieve well. There are clearly many pitfalls and disadvantages of multidisciplinary partnership working, which may easily come into play, not least when partners belong to different sectors or groups, or work at a distance from each other (see Table 5.1).

📋 Activity: discuss with your fellow students or colleagues

- Relate the pros and cons list given in Table 5.1 to your team.
- What is good? What is alright? What is bad?
- Is your team stuck in a rut and resistant to change?
- What do you think you need to do to improve or maintain the effectiveness of your team?

Table 5.1 Advantages and disadvantages of working collaboratively

Advantages	Disadvantages
Care by a group may be better than care by one individual	It can be time consuming
	Administrative and communication costs
	Differing leadership styles
Special skills can be appropriately and effectively used within a well-managed and diversely skilled team.	Inappropriate leadership
	Language/jargon differences
	Poor communication
	Attitudinal problems and differences
Work can be shared out and be more efficient in delivery	Different values between individuals and groups
	Rivalries between professions
Activities can be better coordinated	Individual professional and personal concerns and insecurities
Promotes continuity of care	Professional-group insecurities and feelings of threat from other groups or sectors
Knowledge, skills, equipment and facilities can be shared	Inequalities in status and pay
	Conflicting professional and non-professional boundaries and loyalties
Standards of care are likely to be raised because of peer presence and attention	Lack of clarity about roles
	Negative mutual perceptions and latent prejudices
Job satisfaction	Personality clashes
Responsibility is shared	

Current policy imperatives – commercialization, diversity and fragmentation of providers

In chapters 3 and 4, it was argued that the process of reform in the past decades has slowly added a commercial dimension to the culture of the NHS. While for some this has opened up many new ventures and opportunities, for others it has created a climate of uncertainty, suspicion, confusion and low morale – feelings experienced and expressed by many in the internal healthcare market environment of the 1980s and 1990s (Fatchett, 1996; Rillands, 1997) and again today.

During earlier decades, this response clearly erected a barrier to effective collaborative partnerships in care. Denise Platt referred to the continuing difficulty of getting people in the health service away from thinking about the market and competition, and thinking more of coherent planning and collaboration (Healy 1997). It seemed that for many the changes were not necessarily conducive to the creation of high-quality care environments, underpinned by trusting and smooth-working collaborative relationships between a wide range of professionals, organizations, sectors, patients, users and carers. The quasi-commercializing environment at that stage, for example, created metaphorical demarcation lines between the fragmented provider units. In turn, many health service employees felt unable, or indeed were forbidden, to collaborate externally in any truly meaningful way. Commercial secrecy between competitive provider units bidding against each other for contracts became a central theme (Best and Brazil,1997). Collaboration with other competitors, whether internal or external to the NHS, whatever the depth of previous relationships before the start of the internal healthcare market, appeared to take a back seat. As Kurtz and Nicholl (1992) described it: 'Where there was collaboration, there was now invoicing; where there was give and take, there were now accountants bent on capturing items of service.'

Flynn et al. (1996) concluded that central government instruction to promote contestability, accountability and value for money ultimately came to dominate their (professional) commissioning and contracting approach. The effect was all too often to corrode rather than nurture common values and commitments, to create an atmosphere of mistrust and to exacerbate problems of uncertainty in the contracting process. Collaborative partnerships and openness were clearly not central to this activity.

In today's increasingly complex and diverse healthcare provider world, in which the NHS is being joined rapidly by the private and third sectors, we do need to learn lessons from what happened just two decades ago. Indeed, in many respects the successive Conservative governments' attempts in the 1980s and 1990s to inject a sharper financial edge to delivering healthcare were only just the softball forerunners of the developments and changes that were introduced by successive Labour governments under Tony Blair and Gordon Brown from 1997 to 2010. While apparently promoting a new environment of partnership working in delivering healthcare, with a move away from the sharp downsides of competition of the previous decades, the reality was the opposite. Labour's policy agenda was clearly underwritten by the push to open up healthcare delivery to the vagaries of the marketplace, a diversity of providers and even sharper competition.

The structures, processes and organizations that were developed under Labour are now being nurtured to further fruition by the current Coalition government. The overt search for value for money, cost-effectiveness and efficiency, set against a backcloth of competition, are now major themes and part of the raft of reforms being applied to the NHS structure, organization and personnel. As such, remembering the difficulties of partnership working in a more commercialized organization as noted earlier (chapter 3), there is much work to do today if we are to deliver the proposed new agendas with others outside the traditional NHS family of carers.

🖹 Activity: discuss with your fellow students or colleagues

- Are you now working with other sectors outside the NHS – e.g., the private, voluntary or social enterprise sectors?
- What are relationships like with these non-NHS organizations?
- Reflect on the issues which relate to delivering value for money and cost-effective care while budgets are being tightened and reduced.
- Are there any constraints or difficulties in providing the care needed by your patients?

While you may recognize some difficulties in partnership working posed by the organizational and structural changes currently going on around you and your patients, it would surely be unfair to blame these alone. As Trevillion (1995) reminds us, 'collaboration is as much about an organizational culture as well as practitioner culture'. Although an increasingly commercialized and competitive environment in the NHS is no doubt sharpening up the organizational culture, all professionals within this context contribute their own practitioner culture too. The fact should not be ignored that, over time, professional groups have perpetuated a 'Berlin Wall of secrecy', a lack of willingness to collaborate with others, not only outside their own organization, but, sadly, even within it and certainly with patients. Hugman (1995) referred to those who are inward-looking and too defensive of established practice to be able to work with others.

While that may well have been true for many, Ross and Mackenzie (1996) offered a broader and more eclectic explanation for professional difficulties in partnership working. They believe it is a reflection of the complex conceptual, structural and professional issues that lie at its roots, which have resulted in the slow progress of understanding, interpretation and implementation in practice. This may also reflect the historically very separate educational and training routes pursued by all the different people involved in healthcare services. McCray described how this occurs:

> During professional education, socialisation through a combination of a series of activities and the ongoing process of learning, results in the development of a particular professional identity. For example, nurses may feel this when they are fitted for uniforms for the first time, while doctors entering medical school may experience a similar feeling of belonging when they get their basic medical kit, just as social workers in their first module in university explore values in social work practice. This orientation continues as professionals qualify and continue into new roles. (2009: 147)

It has been argued that current methods of healthcare professional and non-professional education and training encourage 'silo working' and do not prepare students of different health disciplines to work together and form effective teams once qualified. They relate to dealing with entrenched cultures, administrative challenges, curriculum requirements linked to registration, licensing and certification, and the need for institutional and governmental leadership and support to make it become a reality (Health Policy Digest, 2010).

Many others have also analysed the concept of partnership working within health and social care and considered solutions to the many other challenges it clearly poses. The fact that the process has been examined from diverse theoretical perspectives, including psychology, sociology, social policy, economics, organizational management, government and social administration, suggests that effective collaboration in care is not easily achieved – because it is a difficult and complex activity. Nor are there any easy answers to the problems of ineffective collaboration. While this observation is no doubt true, the almost in-built and historical professional antipathy towards multi-disciplinary partnership working has clearly not helped the situation to develop in as constructive and as positive a manner as might have been possible.

Current policy developments, however, require all of us to revisit our professional roles and ways of working, and to challenge the arrogance of long-held views of the perceived greater or lesser value given to others' contributions to healthcare delivery. We may need to conclude at this stage that any blame for shortcomings in successful partnership working lies both with professionals themselves and with organizational structures for delivery of care.

The reality is that a great deal of individual work and goodwill is needed to make it happen well, combined with a reciprocal and supportive stance from the policy-makers who design and redesign health service provision in this country. An understanding of its nature, by both professional and policy-maker alike, needs to move beyond the easy and often-stated acknowledgement that partnership working is a good thing and needs to take place if effective care services are to be provided. According to Hudson (1997), although the centre can create a legal, administrative and financial framework that facilitates such collaboration, these are not characteristics that can be conjured up by administrative fiat. The real issue – whether at professional or organizational level – is whether or not there is a willingness to align decisions. This is a question of politics, personalities and culture, rather than one of legislation and finance.

Hudson's conclusion perhaps reflects the old saying: where there's a will, there's a way. That said, apparently insuperable barriers to collaboration, as noted earlier, have confounded many in practice. While collaboration between agencies can help to ensure that the totality of people's needs is both recognized and met, fragmentation of organizations and the more commercialized approach to care can and has hindered the effective delivery of many important policy developments requiring multidisciplinary partnerships.

Currently, then, the developing competitive character of contemporary health service provision, with its conflicting policy perspectives, multi-sectoral involvement, pay differentials, status and budgetary concerns, are tending to perpetuate role separation, to fragment the delivery of care and ultimately to inhibit effective partnerships. So what might be a solution? This will perhaps involve two responses:

1   The development of an organizational structure and culture which actively promotes working together, rather than being in directly competitive relationships.
2   Greater professional understanding of, and enthusiasm for, the concept and process of collaborative working.

An immediate question may be: will this happen in the foreseeable future? A positive response at this stage may suggest to you a large degree of hope over experience. The Coalition government is in the relatively early days of its tenure and its healthcare agenda is only now taking shape. It remains obvious, however, that the health policy agendas and developments currently under way can only achieve the success desired if the collaborative principles underpinning them are also addressed in equally serious measure.

Professional and public support all need to be harnessed into collective and collaborative effort and will. It is not sufficient to tell or to ask people to work together, or even to pretend that they are when they are not. In turn, supportive structures and organizations and, of course, a positive financial environment are all needed so that people can work together and feel supported in doing so. That said, even if some serious and meaningful effort is put into the collaborative agenda by the Coalition government, the legacy of negative experiences of previous years is likely to have a continuing stultifying effect on the many multidisciplinary programmes currently being proposed.

📋 Activity: discuss with your fellow students or colleagues

- Consider some of the new policy agendas that you are being required to address within your practice.
- What are your experiences of working with other agencies or professionals in order to deliver new policy goals?
- Do any issues of costing or financial stringency come into play, either in helping developments or reducing or stopping them?

The developing environment and perceived impacts on working with others

The current policy developments and reforms within the NHS are slowly but surely creating a very complex and challenging environment for care, one which is not of itself always conducive to effective collaboration with all the other, currently expanding, external sectors and services. In many situations, NHS professionals feel too preoccupied in delivering the policy imperatives of their own organizations, or indeed in preserving their own employment, to reach out immediately and enthusiastically to work in partnership with others. The recurrent waves of new and ever-developing changes and, importantly, the need to demonstrate financial effectiveness and efficiency are keeping all professionals metaphorically on their toes. Currently, attracting, competing for and keeping consortia interest in buying services from one's own organization, group or team is a central fact of life.

As noted, in earlier decades positive statements in support of a collaborative approach by the policy-makers appeared to gloss over the many real difficulties practitioners faced in trying to fashion such an agenda in an environment apparently more intent on pursuing financial objectives. During that period, and seemingly now, while partnership working is much promoted, it may well be secondary to the task of keeping within budgets and the pursuit of financial objectives. As Ross and Mackenzie (1996) remind us, conflicts can arise and other apparently less important pleasantries are put on the back burner when the main motive or focus in work is geared towards competition and the winning and securing of business and contracts.

Hunter (1997) expressed similar concerns that are worth remembering today. He reflected on several telling pointers to the apparent lack of effective, professionally led multidisciplinary or multi-sectoral collaborative projects. Admittedly, a number of controversial workforce developments and changes at that stage (fragmentation of care provision, short-term contracts, casualization and skill mixing) engendered individual feelings of employment instability and insecurity – feelings which resonate again today for many in the NHS. More generally, Hunter referred to the overarching and sharper commercialized environment which seemed to have eroded the qualitative niceties and complexities of multidisciplinary care partnerships in favour of the more easily manageable and measurable. For example, the claimed special and professional nature of the professional nurse contribution was challenged on many occasions.

Arguments were made that nursing could and should be carried out just as effectively, and certainly more cheaply, by non-professional carers – a theme which is very much alive today. The outcome of this was the development of 'low-trust' relationships between many different individuals, professional and non-professional alike, both within and outside the NHS – the very opposite of the reciprocal feelings needed for effective working partnerships. Some deeper understanding of this concept of 'low trust' may help us to understand and to develop better solutions for some of the problems we face in working with others in our practice today.

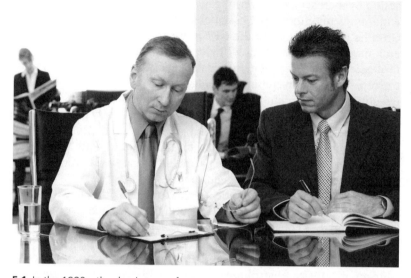

5.1 In the 1980s, the dominance of a more corporatist agenda within the NHS led to a constrained environment in which collaborative work was inhibited.

Low-trust relationships and lessons for today

The work of Flynn et al. (1996) on the effects of contract arrangements in the provision of community health services provided a detailed and interesting critical commentary on how markets and networks evolve within a purchaser/provider framework for healthcare delivery. Specifically for our discussion, there is an analysis of workplace relationships, both high and low trust, engendered by the contracting process.

The work of Fox (1974) on authority/employee relationships and the differing degrees of trust created by economic exchanges and environments was used as a model for this analysis. Flynn et al. discussed the 'complex dialectic of trust/distrust which affects all relationships, but is especially manifested in all forms of economic exchange and contractual behaviour' (1996: ch. 1). There is a qualitative change in the way people relate to each other once there is a cash nexus or a relationship of 'money changing hands' between people or organizations.

We might consider this statement in relation to health and social care professional behaviours as the general management and internal market reforms began to develop in the 1980s. Many professionals became increasingly distrustful of each other, whether colleague or manager, because of the professionally constraining environment created by the more corporatist NHS agenda and style. The importance of competing for, winning and holding contracts encouraged a climate of enforced secrecy and confidentiality within and between individual providers.

Alongside this, professional voices and choices were effectively stifled by increasingly powerful general management executives. The apparently unfettered professional discretion, which, according to Griffiths (1983) existed in the NHS prior to the introduction of general management, came under tight financial and functional control. Professionals in a very general sense began to feel that they were not trusted, that their discretion and judgement around care activity were effectively being circumscribed and reduced in both content and flexibility. It is easy to see how relationships between many professionals, non-professionals and managers changed and soured into one of 'low trust'. In turn, with such feelings around, it is not difficult to see why attempts to develop collaborative partnerships in care delivery services were often unsuccessful or, indeed, at times impossible.

Fox (1974) offered a theoretical explanation for this negative and potentially destructive situation. He found that if work activity was formalized and thus constrained between individuals and groups within a commercialized environment, then the low-trust relationship created between worker and authority figures would create a number of significant attitudes and attributes, which would make working together difficult. He believed that low-trust relationships in work situations created participants who:

- had divergent goals and interests;
- had explicit expectations which had to be reciprocated through balanced exchanges – a favour given had to be returned;
- carefully calculate the costs and benefits of any concessions made;
- restrict and screen communications in their own separate interests;
- attempt to minimize their dependence on others' discretion;
- are suspicious about mistakes and failures by others, attributing them to ill will or default, leading them to invoke sanctions.

All or some of these aspects may reflect to some degree or other the reasons why many professionals and others involved in healthcare delivery in the 1980s onwards felt unable to collaborate with others, either seriously or effectively. Personal, professional and structural barriers created by the internal market reforms, in combination, discouraged collaborative activity or made it more difficult. The commercialized and contractual nature of NHS relationships, both within and without the organization, seemingly replaced its altruistic nature (surely a necessary attribute for collaboration and interprofessional trust) with that of a cash nexus. As Fox (1974) concluded, 'the keen calculative specificity of reciprocation which characterises purely market transactions is a contradiction in terms to high discretion relations'.

Hadley and Clough (1996) commented on such difficulties faced by local authority social carers trying to work effectively with NHS colleagues. Johnson (1994) highlighted the constraints of the similarly commercializing community care environment of the 1980s, including the problem of collaboration across the fragmented and increasingly pluralized agencies on both sides of the health and social care divide. Without a doubt, the ever-increasing breadth and diversity of organization and carer – both professional and non-professional, statutory and non-statutory, all with differing aims and employer allegiance – made joint working and shared responsibility nearly impossible at times. Ovretveit (1997a) appeared to arrive at a similar conclusion:

> Neither market nor bureaucratic modes of organization facilitate collaboration; co-ordination is more difficult to obtain where the actors' interests and issues are divergent, and where they have different objectives. Associational or network approaches are preferred as most likely to secure more effective co-ordination, but these are weakened by the impact of market competition.

He looked to the creation of a more appropriate networking environment, one that required and promoted a different set of relationships, which were not about competition or contractual straitjackets, but which emphasized trust, warmth, flexibility and sharing. Such attributes would encourage altruism and not self-interested individualism in care. In effect, he argued for a need to replace the low-trust scenario with one of high trust, to emphasize a real belief in professionals' ability to make appropriate choices, to take risks and to use their discretion and knowledge together in meeting patient needs.

With this in mind, it is useful to reflect on your current collaborative experiences and to see whether you can recognize any high-trust or low-trust environments. While the previous discussion has harked back to the 1980s and 1990s, there are surely lessons to be learned for today's health services, the patients and ourselves as professional nurses. The NHS environment today, in terms of structure, focus and organization, has developed and is developing further into a more commercialized body. It also continues to face many of the barriers and difficulties already described. Having said that, if we wish to pursue some 'appropriate balance' between competition and collaboration and, indeed, to enjoy a more high-trust environment, we do need to clarify our understanding of the concept of high trust so that our goal is quite clear – however difficult that might be to achieve.

The creation of a high-trust environment and collaborative potential

We need to return briefly to the analysis by Fox (1974), who refers to the creation of high-trust relationships at work. The attributes he describes would suggest a perspective on life and work which are likely to be supportive of the sort of collaborative environment proposed by Ovretveit (1997a). High-trust participants seem to exemplify the converse picture and package of attributes surrounding the low-trust participants. For ourselves as nurses, it is worth considering whether our own current experiences at work and of colleague behaviour match up in any way to the following positive description of high-trust relationships:

- people share or have similar ends and values;
- people have a diffuse sense of long-term obligation;
- people offer support to each other without calculating the cost or expecting an immediate return;
- people communicate freely and openly with each other;
- people are prepared to trust each other and to take risks and rely upon others;
- people give the benefit of the doubt to others in relation to motives and goodwill if problems or mistakes are made.

📋 Activity: discuss with your fellow students or colleagues

- Do the 'high-trust' attributes listed above fit with your current experiences at work?
- Are you experiencing any 'low-trust' relationships?
- How could these be improved?

Fox's perspectives on the creation of high- and low-trust relationships in the working environment offer us a model of attributes and attitudes, ranging through a continuum of low-trust to high-trust perspectives. In real life, of course, this ideal typical model, portrayed as the opposing ends of a continuum, is not totally reflective of individuals' positions in practice. In reality, we probably all move and shift along this continuum, depending on time, place, circumstance and need. As already suggested, the structure and organization of the internal healthcare market in the 1980s and 1990s tended to push professionals and others towards the low-trust end of the continuum. In the main, the tightened market-like structure and more corporate agenda were not overly encouraging of flexible and collaborative ventures.

At the same time, Trevillion's (1995) comment, noted above, on the effects of practitioner culture on collaborative effort should not be ignored. While no doubt professional barriers did come into play, the required pursuit at that stage of economic aims and objectives did not necessarily help to harness the collective will and enthusiasm of professional participants. As such, it appeared to create a low-trust competitive environment in which multidisciplinary, multi-sectoral team working was very much a secondary agenda.

As noted before, Platt (1997) criticized NHS personnel from the perspective of a social services employee. Reference was made to their being stuck in an internalized mind-set of short-term competition and, as such, almost unable to think about long-term planning and collaboration in care. Smith et al. (1993) and Wistow (1992), for example, noted the lacklustre attempts at that time by NHS professionals to work with the voluntary sector. And, while any ventures between the statutory and voluntary sectors were described as limited, bland and non-committal, efforts made to work with the users and their carers were even less propitious. The centrality and value of their contribution to the success of health and social care delivery were barely recognized, and their views often ignored in care planning – an issue raised by Griffiths and his team in their inquiry into NHS management in 1983, and in subsequent health White Papers (DOH, 1989a).

Sadly, then, the long-erected professional barriers to collaborative working seemed to have been consolidated rather than broken down during that period of internal market reform. So currently, we have every reason to be concerned and to explore what may be happening today in what appears to be a very similarly developing scenario – indeed, for some commentators, one which has gone many steps further in the development of an even-more competitive and commercialized environment for healthcare delivery than hitherto (Lister, 2008; Pollock, 2011).

After 1997, with the subsequent election of three Labour governments, the NHS world changed and developed almost out of all recognition. Many of the more commercialized and competitive changes that had been proposed and introduced by the Conservatives in the 1980s and 1990s, and challenged strongly at that time by Labour parliamentarians in opposition, became an almost everyday policy reality under Prime Ministers Blair and Brown. The Coalition, in turn, has easily been able to continue and expand a great many of Labour's health developments and ideas. Crucial steps in the replacement of the NHS as an integrated public service by a healthcare market, in which a multiplicity of 'willing providers' can now play a steadily growing role, had already been taken by the previous Labour governments.

The current environment is now extremely competitive and business-like. That said, the ever-developing push for patient centredness and a

---

Box 5.3 Private sector provision introduced to the NHS by Labour governments, 1997–2010

- NHS treatment centres;
- Independent-sector treatment centres (ISTCs);
- clinical-assessment and treatment-service centres (CATS);
- private walk-in centres;
- out-of-hours (OOH) services for general practices;
- some completely private general practices;
- surgical teams from abroad to boost NHS surgical capacity;
- diagnostic and treatment centres;
- the extended choice network of private providers;
- private-sector opportunities in primary and community care – health centres and polyclinics.

(Player and Leys, 2008)

diversity of healthcare providers from all sectors is underpinned by the need for very effective partnership working. However, is a low-trust environment as described by Fox, and implicit within a commercialized setting as in the current NHS, likely to hinder the collaborative potential and positive outcomes, as proposed in current government thinking for delivering healthcare?

📋 Activity: discuss with your fellow students or colleagues

- Revisit the question of whether or not there is high or low trust in your working relationships with other teams or care sectors.
- What experience do you have of high-trust working?
- What experience of low-trust working?
- Are finances determining what you can do or cannot do with others?

Delivering the government's current policy agenda

The concept of partnership working underpins all the current policy changes and developments. The proposals can work only if collaboration in care is pursued with some seriousness by all participants – the public, the professionals and the politicians. The notion of partnership is thus broad and all-inclusive. Rather than health professionals 'doing' and 'deciding' for others within care relationships, the emphasis is on transparent reciprocal partnerships and relationships and an ability to demonstrate these very clearly, as needed along any whole care trajectory.

Importantly, the success of delivering care in this way is absolutely dependent on the professionals involved playing their part, and accepting and promoting others' contributions, whether professional or not. Also, the proposed potential for low-trust feelings and actions in the current economic climate needs to be addressed, and strategies for positive partnership working created. This will involve two broad areas: (i) changes in structure and organization; (ii) professional development and support.

Changes in structure and organization

In the discussion so far it has been argued that, while partnerships in care delivery have always been beset with difficulties and barriers, the health policy reforms of the previous decade demonstrated how external factors could (and did) make this situation worse rather than better. The introduction of general management, a corporate-style agenda and the development of an internal market-like organizational structure made joint working and responsibility sharing much more difficult. This was also confounded by the slowly growing, complex and fragmented network of health and social care providers. Boarden

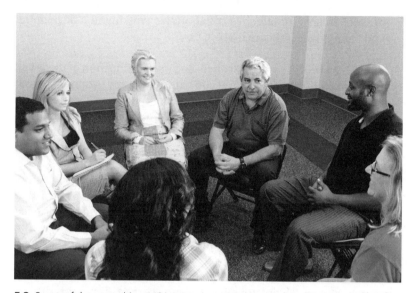

5.2 Successful partnership working involves giving a voice to all interested parties, whether professionals or not.

and Rillands (1997) noted that 'if integration of provision and shared professional activity are to be the hallmarks of future care . . . existing structures will need to be swept away. Unless this is changed, managers will face a heavy burden in trying to secure interactions between different agencies and professional and non-professional staff.'

Lewis (1997) examined the potential for change in both organizations and human resources, which he believed needed to be considered in order that a more effective and complex healthcare delivery environment could be attained in the future – one in which a mixed economy of providers could be helped to work together in partnership. Clarity about what needed to be done, who should do it, and how it might be provided and paid for would be essential factors. A decade or so on, we are now in Lewis's 'future' and face the challenges he noted. So what did he want clarified?

1 The parameters of the NHS – what is and what is not to be made universally available and free at the point of need.
2 The priority of services – overt decisions made on priorities and rationing.
3 The sources of funding – how are these to be found and from where?
4 Organizational structures – how these are to be developed and multidisciplinary collaboration encouraged, and how the users' and carers' voices are to be enhanced in care planning, delivery and evaluation.
5 The use of human resources – how increased legitimacy is to be given to collaboration, including authority, development of trust, time and resources for educational support, and the development

of mechanisms for effective collaborative working in a developing and changing healthcare market.

Points 1–3 are of great significance, because clarification of these will demonstrate the political will and commitment to any proposed health agenda. We noted in our discussion on policy-making in Chapter 2 that a very specific focus on certain programmes provided status and priority over other agendas – and, it is to be hoped, the financial back-up. Educational development in the skills of collaborative working, for example, will not be a cheap option, whether at unqualified or post-qualification levels. Those currently working in the NHS will require support for continuing professional development or other learning opportunities. The unqualified, new students and learners will need to learn together about each others' roles, techniques to use within 'real-world' teams, effective communication and listening skills and methods for conflict resolution.

Points 4–5, those of organizational structures and the use of human resources, very much link together and are also relevant to this discussion in terms of providing clarity for activity and enthusiasm about working with others in partnership, irrespective of differences and organizations. Currently, the specifics of all these issues need to be made clear. There needs to be a structure and process for pulling together all the very disparate providers of care, coupled with the appropriate legitimacy, resources and time for the development of any effective and well-managed collaborative approach.

According to Lewis (1997), the key resource of the NHS is its staff and any government needs their full support and enthusiasm, not least in the collaborative effort. He proposed that staff at all levels should be involved in the debates around the redevelopment of the NHS – a notion addressed and supported in the earlier discussion on nurse involvement in the policy-making process. By doing this, it may be possible to create the necessary shared vision for now and for the future.

The potential for the development of an increasingly low-trust environment as the currently proposed policy changes bite could be reversed, and even become a positive high-trust affair. This is unlikely to happen easily or speedily. It requires the contextual changes and financial commitment already discussed above. Also, and very importantly, there need to be changes in professional behaviour and motives. As Rodgers (1994) noted: 'To pursue and achieve interprofessional collaboration, professionals [nurses] need to value their sense of worth and to relinquish defensiveness' – or indeed sometimes subservience – as well as developing their own self-esteem and a belief in the value of their professional care contribution, together with a belief in their ability to influence policy. They will need to see evidence of others also viewing them in this light. Policy-makers and authority figures need to demonstrate very clearly that they do intend to harness and praise professional nurse skills and knowledge, rather than forever challenging the level of care they offer and providing more and more hoops through which to jump.

It is evident that, for all concerned, there is much to be learnt on how to work together more effectively. Continuing education, resources and time all need to be made available specifically for the development of skills and an understanding of the nature of the concept of collaboration. At the same time there is a need for professionals themselves to acknowledge the necessity to work hard with others in achieving effective partnerships. It does not just happen by itself.

All stakeholders have to value and develop a shared understanding of concepts and remits, and acknowledge and create strategies to develop new ways of working together. Without this effort and enthusiasm, progress will prove difficult. It will be of little use if professionals and other participants are ambivalent, opposed or even prevented from doing the work needed to develop shared care approaches and good teamwork.

On a positive note, Gregson et al. (1991) reminded us of the value of focusing on the concept of collaboration in a meaningful way – the greater the understanding gained, the greater the potential for much improved joint working and a raised standard of care. They referred to the importance of clarifying the differing perceptions, values, expectations, assumptions, behaviours and structures which colour and shape the nature of collaboration in and across health and social care settings. This will, by definition, require major changes in organization, culture, professional education and training, and inspection and quality-assurance processes (Glasby and Dickinson 2008).

Biggs (1993), and others have supported such developments. They have challenged interprofessional work for its tendency to exclude users. Biggs argued that it was vital to look at the interface between user and provider in order to refocus attention on new pathways and methods of care provision. A reinvigoration of interest in, and efforts to look again at, the concept of collaboration in practice, specifically with the patients, would offer such an opportunity.

In 2010 the Nuffield Trust gave support to the establishment of policies and systems for both collaboration and competition to exist side by side within the current NHS. By these means they hoped to create an integrated NHS, one which effectively engaged the patients and the public and at the same time tightened up activities, removed distracting bureaucracy and allowed the benefits of competition and also collaboration to reflect proportionate importance and influence on service and team delivery, depending upon time, place and circumstance in each local community.

The Nuffield Trust examined the experience of integrated working in five areas of England: Cumbria, Nottingham, Redbridge, Torbay and Trafford. Important factors for moving forwards in this respect broadly included: the removal of unsustainable acute services; the development of better care models for people with long-term conditions;

better partnership working between primary, community and social care services; developing networks of GP practices; learning from international experiences of integration; having effective clinical leadership; integrating and sharing patient information; effectively engaging the public; and implementing new forms of organization and governance to run the service. By these means, they proposed that a new integrated environment could be created in the NHS, within which partnerships in care could begin to flourish and institutions reflect a competitive edge in providing only those services that are sustainable as well as needed.

Conclusion

A serious desire to achieve success in partnership working on the part of policy-makers, professionals and the public could change dramatically the currently complex environment of health and social care delivery. In turn, the many proposed policy developments for the NHS, if well implemented, should offer opportunities to enlarge and enrich professional care roles, and to improve the standards of care offered. Most important of all is an acknowledgement that complex health needs require an effective multidisciplinary response if a degree of success is to be achieved.

All healthcare professionals, including nurses, who claim the centrality of client need as the focus of their care agendas, clearly have much work to do in removing the continuing barriers to effective partnerships in care. As an earlier, but still relevant, Green Paper put it: 'Connected problems require joined up solutions. While people on their own can find it hard to make a difference, when individuals, local agencies, communities and the Government work together, deep seated problems can be tackled' (DOH, 1998d). Good partnership working would seem to be the way forward to implementing the policy imperatives of the current government and to promoting the good health of the population. That said, it remains to be seen whether such an important goal will be achieved in the foreseeable future.

Learning outcomes

- an understanding of the importance of effective integrated working for both implementing and creating new policy agendas in the currently ever-changing NHS;
- an understanding of the importance of working in partnership with the currently widening community of healthcare providers in the public, private and third sectors;
- an understanding of the implications of this challenging agenda, both for nurses and for their patients.

Further reading

Glasby, J. and Dickinson, H. (2008) *Partnership Working in Health and Social Care.* Policy Press.

Goodman, B. and Clemow, R. (2010) *Nursing and Collaborative Practice.* Learning Matters Ltd.

Jelphs, K. and Dickinson, H. (2008) *Working in Teams.* Policy Press.

McCray, J. (ed.) (2009) *Nursing and Multi-professional Practice.* Sage.

Wallace, C. and Davies, M. (2009) *Sharing Assessment in Health and Social Care – A Practical Handbook for Interprofessional Working.* Sage.

6 Policy and Technology: A Developing Relationship in the NHS

Aims

- to reflect on the historical and parallel development of the relationship between health policy and technology within the NHS;
- to discuss the importance of technology, both for information and communication and also as an enabler in modern healthcare delivery;
- to consider the practicalities, responsibilities and difficulties of nurse professionals working within an increasingly high-technology NHS environment;
- to encourage professional-nurse engagement in the current technological developments in order to tackle the complicated and often dichotomous pull of current health-policy imperatives.

'The opportunity to translate basic and clinical research into local, national and global therapeutic and healthcare benefits, and to link information from a wide range of medical and non-medical sources using electronic patient records to ensure better treatments, improve patient safety and advance medical [and nursing] research are opportunities not to be squandered.'

(Langlands, 2008: 106)

'Today's nurses must embrace the technological revolution if they want to provide the best care for their patients.'

(Hamer, 2010)

Modern nursing practice and healthcare are driven relentlessly by changing policy demands and expectations and the search for care services that are cost-effective, efficient and user-led – something which Florence Nightingale acknowledged was needed in the nineteenth century (Bostridge, 2009). Today, the implementation of such a regime requires information, knowledge, skills, competencies and the effective use and application of the ever-developing benefits of current information systems and technology. According to Walshe (2009), intuition, instinct, personal experience, anecdote and hands-on guesswork are now no longer the acceptable central tenets for proposing or defending decisions on healthcare spending, management and delivery, even though all of these may well come into play in practice in everyday care decision-making, and may well be not far from what mostly takes place (Milligan, 2009). However, as Krotoski (2011) and others (Munro, 2011b) remind us, the delivery of twenty-first-century healthcare in the UK is, and will remain for the future, an information-intensive and highly technological industry.

The availability of well-researched information and the current myriad of modern and developing technologies are vital, providing a major contribution to the achievement of measurable and sustainable improvements within the NHS, for our teams, our patients and communities. Their efficient and effective systemic delivery within and between organizations can help to change the way we analyse health issues, find solutions to the health and social care challenges faced across the UK, and support us in the delivery of high-quality and effective care to our patients. In today's terms, it is all about creating value-for-money services which are innovative, evidence-based and affordable responses to the ever-moving waves of policy direction, national economic movements and changing societal health needs and expectations (DOH, 2010c).

As proposed earlier, we all need to ensure that we are playing our part in this policy-making process, and of course to utilize all the supportive mechanisms available to expedite care which are relevant, successful and responsive to the specific needs of our patients. In tandem, all activity has to be both affordable as well as achievable – an absolute must in today's economic climate. The interwoven complexity of policy objectives is not an easy thing to deliver in practice, but can be assisted by the use of technology – currently described as contributing to 'an information revolution' (DOH, 2010b).

What is technology?

While often initially perceived by many as only relating to information gathering and its use within the field of healthcare, technology adds up to much more than computers, information and communication. It also encompasses a wide variety of developing processes, products, equipment and care-supporting opportunities, described as 'enablers' for healthcare delivery (see Table 6.1). These include, for example, medical devices, biotechnologies and screening facilities.

The continuing advances in medical and nursing knowledge, together with the benefits of these and many other modern technological innovations and communication systems, enable us all as care providers to improve the health outcomes for our patients and community. It aids speedy access to helpful information on which to make better decisions about care, and, at the same time, to focus on the policy imperatives as directed by the government, helping to save time and costs.

The potential benefits are clearly well worth the effort and can result in major improvements, not just for patients and other service users, but for ourselves, our teams and for other contributors in the local care community. The availability of technological information systems, products and processes, whether or not they are good and of

Table 6.1 Technological information and enablers

Medical devices (assistive devices)	From handrails, bathing aids and devices to help people grip items such as hairbrushes, cutlery, socks or shoes, to intelligent walking sticks for the blind, to cochlear implants and hearing aids, to telecare and telemedicine systems providing hands-off care and support to patients away from the hospital and out to homes and other primary and social-care centres.
Biotechnologies	New and less intrusive wound-healing products and drug therapies.
Screening facilities	Diagnostic ability, varied surgical and medical procedures – including both equipment and processes.

proven benefit to us or the patients, may nonetheless be constrained or even denied because of other more pressing policy and financial requirements (Gentleman, 2011; Elliott and Wintour, 2011).

🖉 Activity: discuss with your fellow students or colleagues

- Reflect on the technologies you are currently using in your practice.
- Are these helping you and your patients?
- Are there any technologies you know about, which, if they were available, would enable you to improve the lives and health of your patients?
- Have you any innovative ideas of your own on some technology which would be worth exploring or developing?

Whatever *your* experiences so far, the use of technology is certainly perceived by many as an important asset, not only for improving care, but also for managing the complex and very demanding health-policy agenda set by the current government. Ham (2009) aptly reminded us of the importance of using the excellent intelligence and horizon-scanning functions within the health service to reform and to develop policy, to be able to plan care, both strategically and locally, and to manage and deliver performance to the standards set by the government. The attempt to reconcile technological solutions with complex organizational, professional, individual and community healthcare challenges still, however, remains a fraught, difficult and often controversial issue.

Technology is not the universal panacea for sorting out challenging people issues and policy implementation. It can only play one part – albeit often an important one – in providing helpful data, evidence and a means to find potential solutions (Hamer, 2010; Naish, 2009).

Good decision-making in the health services clearly includes a wider network of potentially conflicting contributors, not least of whom are the patients, offering their own judgements on what is needed and appropriate to meet assessed health needs. At the same time, it is to be hoped that careful consideration will be allied to the stringent financial and other defined imperatives for delivering current health policy (Lansley, 2010)

The pursuit of support for our own specific causes as nurses is clearly a challenge. As in politics more generally, it is all about interested people pursuing the so-called 'art of the possible', with competing players all vying for finances and special attention for their particular agenda from the slowly tightening public expenditure purse. The use and application of technological support and 'smart working' in marshalling our arguments, backed by evidence and statistics, are potentially invaluable, and skills which are needed by every nurse who aspires to deliver high-quality care (Younger, 2010) – for increasing efficiency, flexibility and satisfaction in the face of major workplace changes (Munro, 2011b). Hamer (2010) has argued that individual nurses need to understand the critical importance of technology to their practice. She believes that failing to understand how to access the electronic system in one's patch, for example, is almost as fundamental as not knowing where the fire exits are placed. Healthcare technology in whatever form, whether for information or as an enabler of care, is not an optional extra for nurses, but a tool that is essential for delivering safe, high-quality care.

Progress, policy and technology

The ever-developing need to use modern technology to aid decision-making and effective healthcare delivery in the very complex NHS of today is the inevitable and dramatic cost of progress. The roots of such change can be traced right back to its very beginnings. It is very much about the developing relationships between man, technology and social change. The NHS, like other institutions, has witnessed the shift from a very manual and personal approach to management and administration to an organization which is reliant on the availability of technological information, communication networks, products and processes (Kumar, 2005; Rowntree, 2010).

The users of the service have similarly been affected, and their relationship with the organization has also changed, as part of the developing 'knowledge society of today'. By becoming 'information rich', computer users have become potentially more powerful by being able to access knowledge once held and hidden by professionals. As a result, users are now supposedly better able to challenge practice and organizations, both to lead developments as well as to make better-informed choices (Castells, 2000; Rowntree, 2010). Krotowski (2011) has described this phenomenon as a public increasingly informed about healthcare options and personal well-being, and able to access a trove of health-related content online. Anything someone wishes to know about any symptom is available, accompanied by prognoses, treatments, social support networks and other forums for confirmation. If users wish, they can effectively bypass the doctor or nurse completely by self-diagnosing and self-medicating. Anyone with an interest in their health 20 years ago might have gone to a library and diagnosed their illness with the help of research journals, but nowadays a search engine will deliver a diagnosis and what to do next in an easy printable format.

This may be true, of course, for the many people who can access information and know how to evaluate it, often without the need for further help. But, there are, without a doubt, others who need encouragement, equipment and guidance even to begin to find information – never mind considering service choices or becoming powerful users of the services (Beasley, 2010). According to current research, ten million people in the UK do not have access to the internet, with four million of these amongst the poorest groups in society (Lane Fox, 2010).

The implications of these findings are explored further in our later discussion on patient empowerment and efforts to address the continuing inequalities in healthcare provision and status (NAO, 2010). As we may discover, broad assumptions made about the potential of any health-promoting policy development which seems to work out well for one group may well, in turn, cause or highlight perverse or negative outcomes for another (NHS Confederation, 2010c).

🗒 Activity: discuss with your fellow students or colleagues

- Do any of your patients use technology in the way Krotoski (2011) suggested?
- Have you ever been challenged by a patient who has questioned their treatment or medications as a result of a web search? What happened?
- Do you have patients who do not or cannot use the internet? Does this matter?
- Do you have effective internet access at work to source health information for your own professional use? What sort of things do you explore and why?

Moving on

We will now reflect back on some of the developments that have led to the technological environment in which we all work, and will explore how and why the relationship between the NHS and technology has developed over past decades. As in other discussions so far, it is both interesting and important for us to understand past experiences, to avoid making the mistakes of previous years, to learn lessons, to reflect on the benefits of changes to date and to consider the potential of future plans for the NHS and for our patients.

Technology and the NHS – a growing relationship

The creation of the NHS in 1948 saw the strategic drawing together of a wide variety of care services and personnel, to a great degree still acting within disciplinary siloes and using fragmented information and paper records (the Gutenberg method) – a far cry from current developments in the increasingly complex matrix of technological activity required to deliver twenty-first-century NHS healthcare provision and policy imperatives.

Different UK governments over time have of course changed and developed the early NHS, so that it has grown into a very different organization from that at its birth in 1948. The forces at play have included many social, political and economic drivers, backed up by developing knowledge, skills and technology. There has been a growth in the complexity of professional and non-professional players, both internal to the NHS and externally from other care sectors. These moves have seen the creation of new roles, values and norms in activity within the now very diverse fields of healthcare and, in particular, nursing.

Many different approaches to care delivery have developed as a result of a growth in the complexity of services in both acute and primary care sectors, allied to the expansion in knowledge and applied technology. There has been an increase in specialization with the invention, creation and development of many very specific and supportive products and processes. The developing need to collect, research, analyse, define and refine the use and application of information in updating healthcare delivery has been swept along by an ever-modernizing flow of technological invention and innovation. This increasing complexity and potential for healthcare providers to promote health and extend life has seen Bevan's NHS plan of 1948 move onto planes never envisaged by its creators and now populated by major technological milestones (see Figure 6.1).

As we know, the costs of such progress within the NHS grew and grew 'like Topsy' (Beecher-Stowe, 1852), and challenges to its continued financial viability, and indeed to that of all publicly provided health and social care services, were loud and vociferous during the 1970s. It was argued that the nation could not afford a welfare state because of its relentless pull on the public-expenditure purse – all areas needed to be reviewed, not least the very costly NHS. It was led and managed in the main by health professionals, who did not particularly concern themselves with the financial implications of their work. In addition, technological developments in care provision and

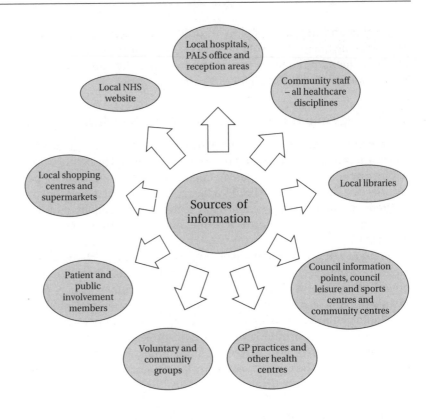

Local hospitals, PALS office and reception areas

Community staff – all healthcare disciplines

Local NHS website

Local libraries

Local shopping centres and supermarkets

Sources of information

Council information points, council leisure and sports centres and community centres

Patient and public involvement members

Voluntary and community groups

GP practices and other health centres

Source: www.bmj.com (2007)

Figure 6.1 Milestones to modernity in the NHS

treatments had not only extended longevity and other possibilities, but, at the same time, had massively pushed up costs. Furthermore, the public's demand for more, newer and better services had grown, outstripping the funds available in the public expenditure envelope to pay for these.

The broad argument was that the health services provided within the NHS were neither quantified nor qualified and were out of control. The gathering of information to aid care planning and delivery was haphazard. The ever-rising costs of the newer and more leading-edge developments meant that public funds were being poured down the proverbial black hole – and it had to stop because the country could not afford to continue on this financial out-of-control NHS roller coaster. This constantly repeated message appealed to the population at large, and in 1979 it voted into power a Conservative government led by Margaret Thatcher. She believed that the financial management of the NHS and other public-service developments and activities should be run on a tightly controlled budget, akin to the practice of good house-keeping (Hughes, 2005).

Information gathering really begins – good housekeeping pursued

The need to take control of expenditure in the NHS was probably the defining driver for a serious attempt at data collection and its use in understanding and determining care activity and spending, with the potential for service and staff rationalization and subsequent cost reduction. A number of early attempts at relevant data collection began the process of defining and analysing what was really happening within the NHS. These included, as we already know, quality initiatives, efficiency reviews, central control of staffing and performance indicators (Holliday, 1995).

In the early days of Margaret Thatcher's new Conservative government, we can see the beginnings of what we now take for granted – a burgeoning information industry within the NHS for collecting and distributing relevant information to managers, professionals, users and politicians. At the same time, however, there was a perceived lack of appropriately qualified and experienced *professional* managers, skilled at using the collected information to help deliver organizational goals and, importantly, who were strong enough to take control of both professional activity and NHS spending. The Griffiths Management Inquiry of 1983 was set up to provide a view on how to move forward in this respect. Unsurprisingly, the inquiry team expressed a number of concerns around the lack of a strong general management focus within the NHS, the crucial issue which they and the government believed needed urgent and special attention – not least to control costs.

What did the inquiry team find?

Health professional groups, all demanding a voice, caused long delays in the management process because of the need to include everyone in discussions. This not only led to 'lowest common denominator decisions' (Davies, 2009), but also made changes slow and incremental. In addition, the inquiry team was concerned that general management and administrative decisions were constantly overridden by professionals, and little information was collected, analysed or used to improve the service and be responsive to the user voice. Griffiths (1983) likened the NHS to a mobile hanging above a baby's cot, which never moved because of the lack of a breeze to make it change direction or to entertain.

The solution according to the Griffiths Inquiry Team

What was needed in the NHS were skilled general managers at every level who could pull the organization together: individuals who knew how to collect and use information for the benefit of their organizations – abilities perceived as clearly missing at that stage from the very

Box 6.1 Skills needed by general managers

- knowledge about quantity, quality and levels of service;
- knowledge of costs and how to meet budgets;
- how to reward productivity;
- knowledge of evaluative mechanisms;
- an ability to use information or research to foster new developments and to purchase products and services which were relevant, research proven and affordable.

(Griffiths, 1983)

powerful leadership of the health professions, in particular the doctors and, especially, the consultants. The Griffiths Inquiry Team report advocated the linking of activity, staffing and finance together through management budgets, and proposed that a general manager should be in charge in every unit and hospital across the country and be held responsible for what happened there. It called for leadership, accountability, clear objectives and measurement – all things that we would take for granted today (Crisp, 2009).

The appointment of general managers across the NHS, from 1984, began to cement a new approach to the management of care delivery based upon the evidence of collated information across the whole field of health and social care (Davies, 2003). There were many reported difficulties in delivering this new-style management approach to informing healthcare and to making financial choices about service provision and product. But there were also many reasons why the use of technology became ever more relevant – indeed necessary for the management of an increasingly complex service.

The growth in technology gathers apace

The need to collect information as a basis for making decisions and spending was a developing fact of economic life in the UK, and the NHS environment could not stand alone or be immune to such developments. Information had often been unavailable or impossible to share between practitioners and organizations, so the possibility provided by the ever-developing communication networks for overcoming these problems was increasingly attractive – even irresistible. Nurses, doctors and other professionals required this ready access to information to help inform their practice in an accessible and speedy way. They also needed information on the updated technological products and services available to improve their care and treatment in line with the growing expectations of the now more knowledgeable patients. They, too, had an interest in all these developments.

In the early days of the NHS the information needed by users of the health services had not always been readily available and the necessary support was often lacking to make choices about where to go for help, advice, treatment or, indeed, to find out about NHS best practice. Importantly, new information systems within the NHS and the growing use of computers by individuals at home was beginning to open up the previously closed doors of health knowledge to the public.

General managers of course needed good access to readily available data and evidence on which to base activity and expenditure decisions. This was important for ensuring the implementation of government policy around the delivery of services and to contain budgets. It was also necessary to track and explore the potential of all the developing technological innovations, both to expedite and improve care services and to obtain value for money.

Activity: discuss with your fellow students or colleagues

- Should general managers manage and control healthcare delivery, determining what can be done and when? Or should decisions on the purchase of technological goods and services be left to health professionals?
- What have been your experiences of working with general managers?
- Are any of your former nursing or medical colleagues now general managers? If so, do they demonstrate a better understanding of the issues you face than colleagues who come from another profession or background?

The next steps

Having established this cadre of general managers right across the NHS, the government moved on to reform its structure, culture and organizational approach (DOH, 1989c). The creation of the internal healthcare market, with a strong competitive remit, completed the winning combination of appropriately qualified professional general managers positioned 'to manage' at every level of the organization, and a purchaser and provider structure for the development of a much more commercialized approach to healthcare delivery. Both of these aspects were important catalysts for the growth in the use of information technology (IT) in aiding decision-making and activity right across the NHS. In turn, this facilitated a tighter and more knowledge-based control over the ever-rising expenditure on the many technological advances in healthcare products, processes and services.

The subsequent changes in governments and prime ministers, the devolution of Scotland, Wales and Northern Ireland, and different health policy foci across the UK have not held back the development of what we now know as a very complex matrix of information systems and new technologies available within the NHS. This has become the inevitable reality of life as we now know it, both for us as nurses and for our patients right across the four countries. There are multiple priorities competing for our time, many changing external pressures, and challenging demands on all staff, whether professional or not. The backing of effective technological resources is and will be invaluable in delivering the policy objectives we all now face in practice as set out by the current Coalition government.

Policy objectives underpinning current practice

- the need to obtain value for money;
- activity which is affordable;
- defined quality and outcome standards;
- care which is based on evidence, is demonstrably effective and of proven high quality;
- care which is integrated across all sectors – statutory, private and voluntary;
- care activity which is predicated on user centrality and choice driven;
- efforts made to reduce health and social-care inequalities;
- IT systems and high-technology interventions to be used to help deliver care in more efficient, effective and speedier ways;
- all activity to involve the pursuit of new, flexible and innovative ways of working. (DOH, 2010c)

The ability to deliver these high-level, wide-ranging and demanding foci in nurse practice today is very much dependent on the environment of care within which we work – or what Butterworth and Bishop (1995) referred to as being in 'the appropriate milieu'. Managers need to lead by example through the skilled use of information, the clear communication and sharing of findings, the encouragement of multidisciplinary discussion and the use of new ideas and ways of working. There needs to be time and support invested in such activities – not just lip service paid or lists ticked (NNRU, 2009a) – and with the computer technology easily accessible and available (Godson, 2010). However, as Stuttle (2006) and others remind us, irrespective of difficulties, we must either embrace technology or it will be imposed on us. We all need to influence what is happening – managers, nurses and patients alike. Nobody is immune.

📋 Activity: discuss with your fellow students or colleagues

- Do you have access to the technological equipment you need to work effectively with your patients? If not, why? What is happening?
- Are you given appropriate support and time for any updating and learning opportunities to get the best out of the technological products with which you are expected to work?

It is, however, acknowledged quite openly that some find using technology very difficult – described variously as 'laggards' (Rogers, 1962), 'digital immigrants' (Prensky, 2005), 'sceptics and traditionalists' (Williams, 2007). Others, who are at ease with technology, have been called 'early adopters and pragmatists' (Williams, 2007), the 'net generation' or 'digital natives' (Bennett et al., 2008). Perhaps we should not dwell too much on names or on which one applies to us. But, to use an old phrase, 'if the cap fits, wear it'. If this means our acknowledging that more learning and effort is needed with respect to technology, then so be it.

The reality is that the technological environment of healthcare is going to continue developing and growing and, as nurses, we have much to offer in ensuring its relevance and application in practice. By standing apart and maintaining both ignorance and disdain for technology, we surely do ourselves and our patients a disservice. Others with perhaps less understanding of healthcare and social need, but who are 'early adopters' of the technological machinery and opportunities, could end up creating a less responsive and less relevant national health service. So we all have a vested interest in becoming informed, involved and, it is to be hoped, technologically dexterous.

The important message to bear in mind, in any event, is that you do not have to be technically minded or skilled to recognize the opportunities that technology offers. More importantly, it is confidence in your own experiences and knowledge of your patients' and community's needs, their specific circumstances, how they feel and cope, how we care for them now and, most crucially, how we want to improve this working partnership in the future. Technology can also play a relevant part in this care equation. But, as in any type of relationship, there has to be a reciprocal and positive effort to make it work well, whether for the short or long haul. We do need to get involved in a meaningful way.

It is necessary, for example, to go beyond the 'given use' of new systems and to be part of their development and use in practice in order to avoid the resentments and concerns felt by many district nurses, school nurses, midwives and health visitors when the Körner statistics collection was introduced in the 1980s (Körner, 1982a; 1982b). Hamer (2010) notes the importance of involving nurses at an early stage in the development of any technological 'enabler' intended for nurse usage or for qualifying and quantifying nurse activity in practice. We need to ensure today that the informatics used by managers, for example, reflect fully and fairly our care contribution and outcomes achieved, together with a clear audit trail of evidence demonstrating that policy is being implemented.

There needs to be an information-gathering system which is fit for the purpose and properly describes both what we do and the outcomes achieved. It should enhance and support patient care, helping us to deliver the required efficiencies safely. Ideally, it can help ensure that current policy is woven into proposed care planning and service developments, and provide a broad oversight of others' agendas to help integrate responses to health needs for the benefit of both individuals and the wider community.

Help for the patients and users of our services

Offering choice in healthcare is a current policy mantra, as is the promotion of personal responsibility (DOH, 2010c). As such, patients need to be given the tools and technology to access help, knowledge, information and the appropriate supports which can help them to live independent lives and to manage their own health and well-being (Rowntree, 2010). Of course, there are already many in the general public who use technology in this way at home to good effect – just like some, if not all, health professionals.

Activity: discuss with your fellow students or colleagues

- Does the example of the technology-rich birth experience outlined in Box 6.2 hold any broad relevance to your own patient group? If not, what are the issues you might need to address?
- Check out any similar informational and/or interactional websites to Mumsnet and note the variety of possibilities for finding and sharing information about health-related issues

Mumsnet is an example, along with other similar focused websites like NHSBabyLifeCheck (Knight, 2010a), of how individuals today can come together and help each other using current technology, having the power to communicate, organize and change healthcare experiences in line with their own needs – a far cry from the professionally determined care and organizational straitjacket of past decades within

Box 6.2 A case study

A pregnant woman, going into labour around Christmas and living in a remote village in the High Peak area of Derbyshire, used technology not only to call for midwifery help, but also to network with her friends on the Mumsnet* website for support as she waited for help to arrive. Her experience as an 'information-rich' and keen computer user included the assistance of the technology-armed Kinder mountain rescue team, a midwife with a mobile telephone and other modern birthing equipment, high-tech hospital monitoring, along with friends and many strangers on Mumsnet, providing continuing messages of support both before and after the birth of her baby. (Jones, 2010)

*Mumsnet (www.mumsnet.com) is a website created by parents for parents. Topics discussed online include conception, pregnancy, babies, toddlers, education, teens, special needs, books, food, travel, politics and safety campaigns.

the NHS. As Shirkey (2008, 2010) observed, the technological revolution has provided the means of unlocking spontaneous civic collective activity. It has also helped to remove barriers to public participation in healthcare delivery and revealed that interested people can create and share experiences of care provision that are relevant to them, rather than being passive consumers of services that the professionals (sometimes wrongly) believe are the most appropriate.

The potential of this sort of development appears exciting. It fits with many of the proposed policy themes around the development of personal responsibility for health, the reduction in health inequalities and the importance of partnership working across all sectors, with the anticipated release of civic efforts to improve the health and well-being of the whole population – the so-called Big Society approach (DOH, 2010c; *Financial Times*, 2010). However, whether such benefits apply to the 10 million people in the UK who currently do not use the internet, for whatever reason, is clearly open to debate (Lane Fox, 2010).

The benefits of information technology for nursing practice

Whatever your thoughts about the use of technology, whether you be a laggard, early adopter, tweeter, twitterer, blogger, Bebo, Facebook or Cloud user, let us now just focus on the specific and potential benefits of IT for us and our patients, and also for meeting the government's health policy requirements in whichever part of the UK we live and work.

Goldacre (2009) for example notes that NHS professionals are very dependent on accurate information in order to accommodate future changes at the lowest possible costs, and in any event have a responsibility to deliver relevant, research-based and effective care. Beasley (2010) reminds nurses of the benefits of the use of IT and its many directories of collated information. She sees the possibilities for informing practice, the creation of new roles and improvements in the quality of

---

Box 6.3 What can information technology do for you?

- IT can enable decision-making on policy implementation by bringing together statistics, information and research findings, together with the views of the public, professionals and politicians.
- IT can maximize efficiency and avoid time wasting.
- IT is able to use, synthesize and relay information about current best practice.
- IT can provide support for decision-making.
- IT can speak seamlessly to partner organizations when relevant.
- IT can provide accurate information for business management and development.
- IT can enable conversations between all interested parties.

care delivered – by reducing inefficiencies, improving patient safety and supporting new and innovative patient/nurse partnerships.

According to the DOH (2008c), evidence shows that high-performing teams are characterized by the use of measurement to support improvements. Investment in clinically relevant IT can lead to dramatic cost savings, in addition to improving quality, reducing mortality and improving efficiency. The provision of such a tool clearly helps us to pull together the myriad policy, professional and organizational agendas that require our attention.

Playing your part

Importantly, Carlisle (2008) reminds us of the importance of everyone acquiring 'data dexterity' in this search for improvements in care. It is not just about having access to banks of useful information, but also about being able to navigate these, to create new knowledge and to make good decisions about care planning and delivery, in partnership with others – foremost, of course, with the users. Ball and Callen (1984) said that the strength of nursing depends on its ability to take advantage of the best that technology can offer and to use the evidence provided to best effect. Field concurs with this view, noting the developing possibilities for expediting and improving care responses and ultimately saving lives and promoting health (see Campbell, 2009a).

Scott (2001) similarly spoke of the need for all nurses to become computer literate in a bid to meet patient needs and to deliver the developing health policy agendas. Her insightful examination of practitioners' understanding and knowledge of the use of computer-provided information and the potential benefits for patient care is persuasive. While acknowledging that there are fears amongst many nurses that computer technology may increasingly interfere or even replace face-to-face care, Scott counters these concerns:

> The use of computers *does* have an impact on the nurse's role and ultimately on the quality and quantity of direct patient care. It seems evident that two important relationships exist in this process, the *nurse–computer relationship* and the *nurse–patient relationship*. The first relationship does *not* take over from the second. When used effectively, it should complement the second, thus allowing more time for nurses to demonstrate all those core human care qualities and competencies that nurses bring with them to what Bernard et al. earlier (1981) aptly termed 'a people-orientated profession'. (2001: 6)

Watt (1987) agreed with this view, noting that computers could not replace interpersonal contact, creativity and the bond between nurse and patient. They could, however, help to assist in attaining the goals of providing cost-effective, high-quality patient care, not least by providing more time for patient contact that is meaningful and well informed.

Further to this, it is taken as a given by the government, and therefore also by NHS management (NHS Confederation, 2010b), that everyone who plays a leading or frontline role in the delivery of high-quality care in today's health service must have an interest in, and a felt need to, keep abreast of IT strategy and developments – of which there are now a great many. All of these affect everyone in the NHS: GPs, nurses, midwives, chief executives, therapists, allied health professionals, managers, hospital doctors, booking clerks and many others who will use the new technology to transform patient care. However, while this complex IT highway provides us with many signs and directions to pursue, busy practitioners need help in applying the broad strategic vision on policy requirement, as well as understanding locally applicable evidence for practice development and change. The partnership agenda is clearly a requirement for success in this respect.

Walshe (2009) looked to those who research, analyse and present findings online for the application and development of policy-focused best practice. They are charged with communicating their findings clearly and imaginatively – not just in turgid, difficult-to-understand and obscure journals, but as briefings, practical toolkits, guidelines, assessment tools and template business plans. Being able to understand the material provided by the information networks within the NHS relies very much on those who input the information, making it accessible, trustworthy and very clear – otherwise there is a risk of its being ignored and redundant.

🖥 Activity: discuss with your fellow students or colleagues

- Do you use IT to aid your decision-making with patients?
- What sort of help do you have in using this technology? Did you receive training?
- Is time made for a journal club, seminars, report discussions and briefings, etc. to share ideas around policy requirements and current information available online?

Current developments

The push to use technology which helps to collate informative data is an invaluable resource for us all, whether manager, practitioner or user. It 'enables' us in a number of ways to focus on what we do, including team and organizational performance, successes or failures. It can provide comparative and cross-referenced clinical and information data, which can help us to focus on the merits of our own delivery against a broader context and background – not least other similar areas or specialities. Such performance data can also help in the provision of high-level data to underpin questions around current activity and make arguments for changes and improvements based on the evidence garnered. Importantly, it enables a comprehensive picture of care to be obtained from a single point of entry.

Improvements in care for our patients should always be the driving force and purpose behind the introduction and use of any technology. But no technology can work in isolation. There is a need to integrate new developments and applications with the continuing policy agenda. The echoing mantras of fairness, freedom, responsibility, quality, innovation, productivity and prevention should be reflected in the current delivery of health and social care (DOH, 2010c). The help of technological services is clearly needed, so that relevant data can be turned into helpful information, that information turned into knowledge, and this knowledge used to inform change and development in practice (Sutherland and Coyle, 2009; Farrar, 2009).

All NHS organizations are signed up to this approach, and creating a more patient-led NHS has been the driving force behind a whole raft of new technologies which have come into the health service – many under the auspices of the NHS National Programme for Information Technology (NPFIT). It has been described as the largest public sector IT programme in the world, affecting everyone working in the NHS and social care right across the UK (III, 2007). Its work is led and developed by NHS Connecting for Health – a body of IT specialists, clinicians, improvement leads and other professionals. In addition to this, many health localities are adapting and creating their own technological services in order to meet the specific needs of their own users and communities.

A word of caution is, however, needed here. The implementation of this very ambitious national project has not been easy, having hit delays and criticisms since its beginning, and it certainly looks as if it will have difficult times ahead, not least because of the current financial situation. The Coalition government partners each expressed their views about it before the general election of May 2010: the Conservatives wanted to make significant reforms to Connecting for Health, and the Liberal Democrats pledged its abolition. Since the election, the government has made it very clear that £20 billion must be saved from NHS budgets (DOH, 2010c), with IT spending heavily scrutinized and subsequent changes announced: the NHS programme is to be scaled back and no longer to be centralized, with hospitals allowed to introduce smaller, more manageable change (NHS Confederation, 2010b).

Cruickshank (2010), an NHS IT consultant, described the programme as having 'grown in scope and lost its clarity of purpose'. However, he did not envisage the whole programme being dismantled, noting the success of NHS Mail, PACS (Picture Archiving and Communication Systems) and Choose and Book. Sweeney (2010), Director of IT at King's College London, believed 'the one size fits all' national technology package, not least for very different acute (and other) care settings, was not helpful, as it had tended to remove the elements of choice and diversity in application, which he believed was important. Flatman (2010), Director of IT at Portsmouth Hospitals Trust, concurred with this, saying that no one model could be a perfect fit for all acute trusts. Instead, he looked to the adoption of more localized arrangements and applications, particularly in light of current budget constraints, with locally specific products and best use of what was available to connect up locally.

The government, along with many in the NHS, was attracted to this more localized approach for information sharing and delivery (DOH, 2010c). Providers of services would be under contractual obligations, with sanctions, in relation to delivering accurate and timely data about their services. They would be expected to agree technical and data standards to promote compatibility between different systems, particularly concerning record keeping, data-sharing capabilities, efficiency of data transfer and data security.

Importantly, the 2010 White Paper was also very clear about its intention to create 'an information revolution', to enable patients and the general public to exercise choice and have easy access to relevant data on their services and standards achieved. The practicalities and breadth of this approach were to be part of a new Health and Social Care Information Centre, with clearer powers across organizations in the health and social care system.

Broadly then, the total dismantling of the Connecting for Health project (if it happened) would potentially have immense repercussions for many services. Perhaps equally worrying is that more localized initiatives might defeat the object of having a 'national communication system' for the health service, and the plurality of providers would surely lead to fragmentation in activity, the sharing of good practice made more difficult, and progress in practice potentially jeopardized or lost. More broadly, it would clearly be a retrograde step for the NHS to step down from a national technology agenda, weakening its position as a national institution in the twenty-first-century world.

Activity: discuss with your fellow students or colleagues

- Do you think a national agenda for IT is the way forward or is a more localized approach of greater relevance?
- Which might provide greater benefits for your patients?
- How has the developing IT agenda, as set out by the government, impacted upon your services at a local level?
- Can your patients use the new systems and are they gaining greater choice of services as a result?

Different types of technology being used in the NHS today

1 *The capturing, storing, and sharing of information*
   - The holding and sharing of electronic patient records.
   - The use of digital technology rather than film to take, store and

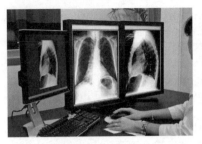

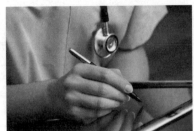

6.1 The digitization of X-ray images has enabled clinicians in multiple locations to view the same images the moment they are taken.

6.2 Clinical notes can now be taken on electronic devices, enabling more reliable storage and maintenance of records.

share x-rays and other clinical images, enabling clinicians at different locations to see the same images as soon as they have been taken – PACS.
- Electronic prescription service.

2 *The better use and sharing of knowledge*
- The Map of Medicine (www.mapofmedicine.co.uk) has been created by health professionals for health professionals and is giving staff swift access to best-practice guidelines on a number of different conditions at the point of care. Users can also access this material and add to the map themselves, using their own expertise and local knowledge of services.
- In Wales a relative-centred information pathway has been developed to improve customer service and provide an opportunity for bereaved relatives to seek further information about the death of a loved one in hospital (Hetherington, 2010). It provides a single point of contact and an opportunity to discuss any concerns and anxieties. The contact card is provided in both Welsh and English and enquiries are logged, then followed up by telephone. This project is part of a major push for 'making connections' and improving citizen and customer centredness, and is being evaluated and developed (WAG, 2007).
- In Scotland an e-library on all health matters (www.knowledge. scot.nhs.uk) supports all healthcare staff in their day-to-day practice, learning and research. It provides evidence, information, e-learning and communication tools.

3 *Technology is now being taken to where to it is needed most*
- Paramedics in some areas are carrying specially adapted and robust laptops on board their ambulances. Touch-screen controls allow crews to use and update the patient's record at the scene.
- Defibrillators are now in many public places – transforming the way people are cared for immediately after a cardiac arrest.
- In Scotland, electronic patient records and emergency care summaries (ECS) provide basic demographic data and life-

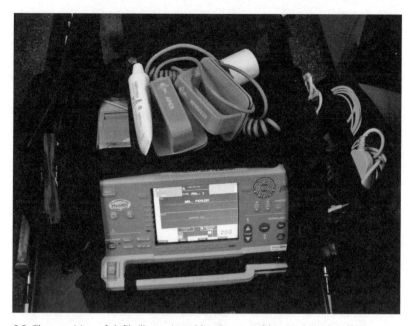

6.3 The provision of defibrillators in public places enables much more efficient treatment of cardiac arrests.

saving information on patients' prescribed medications, both to accident and emergency units and, importantly, to out-of-hours doctors and nurses (Mathieson, 2010).

4 *Technology is being used to improve care, choice and access*
   - Patients with long-term conditions, such as chronic obstructive pulmonary disease (COPD) and diabetes, are being sent a text on their mobile phone by their health teams to remind them about routine check-ups, medications and self testing (Cooper, 2010).
   - Choose and book appointment-booking service (www.choose-andbook.nhs.com) is a national service that combines electronic booking and a choice of place, date and time for first outpatient appointments.
   - The NHS N3 broadband network (www.nhs24.com) supports several government policies and initiatives, including modernizing public services and creating a knowledge economy based on information and communications technology.
   - NHS24 – Scotland's version of NHS Direct (www.nhs24.com) – provides comprehensive up-to-date health information and self-care advice to people in Scotland.
   - NHS Direct and NHS Choices combined provide a 24-hour online information and telephone service to both Wales and England. This includes health advice and information, the promotion of well-being and informed decision-making about healthcare providers (www.nhsdirect.wales.uk, www.nhs.uk).

- Artificial intelligence is being developed to share healthcare workloads and ease patients' anxieties. In the United States scientists have created an empathic virtual nurse counsellor. In the UK developers are working on a less professionally extended robo-nurse – a machine which can mop floors and collect drugs (Naish, 2010).

5 *Technology is being used to help people with disabilities or impairments to stay independent and active in their own homes*

- Patients suffering from head and neck cancers, for instance, can now benefit from electronic speech aids.
- More sophisticated 'intelligent' systems are monitoring the daily activities of vulnerable people in their own homes, generating an alert to the care team if the person's normal routine changes (Munro, 2011b).
- Community matrons are using interactive-video monitors to help patients with chronic obstructive pulmonary disease. The patients measure their own vital signs and input them into a device that can be accessed by the matrons in NHS Central Lancashire. If necessary, nurses can interact with the patients using videoconferencing technology.

These examples are just some of the developments that are currently taking place and are all about improving and making changes to care and meeting the policy imperatives as defined by government.

The implementation of the Ten High Impact Changes for Service Improvement and Delivery (Modernisation Agency, 2004; see Figure 6.2), for example, has been facilitated by the wide use of technology and, as Helen Bevan (2004) has described it, if these changes were adopted across the NHS to the standard already being achieved by some NHS organizations, there would be a quantum leap in improvement in patient and staff experience, clinical outcomes and service delivery. The potential, then, of the development and use of technology within and across the NHS is massive and, in turn, is clearly a very relevant force for improving care and also for transforming the way we nurse, in whatever circumstances, time and place within the UK.

📋 Activity: discuss with your fellow students or colleagues

- Reflect upon the following three passages and the use of technology (taken from Mathieson, 2010).
- Consider the broad relevance to your own experience in practice and that of your patients.

1 GP Sadie Morris in Scotland, who chairs the Emergency Care Summary (ECS) Board, cited a case where the electronic record of a 62-year-old woman saved her life. She had not mentioned on admission to hospital that she needed insulin.

Day surgery (rather than in patient surgery as the norm for elective surgery)	• **IT support** – theatre systems are enabling improved booking and scheduling of theatre resources • **Other technologies** – keyhole-surgery techniques, fibre-optic instruments, rapid acting anaesthetics with fewer after-effects
Improve patient flow across whole NHS system by improving access to key diagnostic tests	• **IT support** – community-wide 'Picture Archiving and Communications Systems' (PACS), making a patient's x-ray and scan images available almost instantly from several different locations • **Other technologies** – instant diagnostic tests in the community / improved compact ECG in GP practices
Manage variation in patient discharge, thereby reducing length of stay	• **IT support** – order communications and results reporting, enabling faster and more accurate diagnosis and earlier treatment • **Other technologies** – automated drug-dispensing systems and patient-medication bags to reduce delay in discharge
Manage variation in patient admission processes	• **IT support** – patient admissions streamlined and clinics managed more effectively as the potential of the choose-and-book system is being maximized • **Other technologies** – pre-surgical assessments in the community using portable equipment and avoiding unnecessary admissions through self-care monitoring devices used in the home
Avoid unnecessary follow-ups for patients and provide necessary follow-ups in the right care setting	• **IT support** – community nurses and other professionals are benefiting from mobile access to care records and assessment data, improving the care they can offer in people's homes • **Other technologies** – self-monitoring technology, including blood pressure, blood sugar and respiratory functions
Increase the reliability of performing therapeutic interventions through a care-bundle package	• **IT support** – electronically enabled Single Assessment Process (e-SAP) supporting a patient-centred care approach for older people and for people with long-term conditions • **Other technologies** – improved drugs management in the home using low-tech reminders and dose organizers (e.g., daily pill boxes)
Apply a systematic approach to care for people with long-term conditions	• **IT support** – patients with mobility and breathing problems being supported in their own homes by telephone monitoring systems that alert community teams if their condition worsens • **Other technologies** – devices to assist in everyday living tasks, such as opening a tin or gripping a pen
Improve patient access to acute care by reducing the number of queues	• **IT support** – better 'patient administration systems' (PAS) improve flow and access to information resulting in more effective management of resources and quicker access to diagnosis and treatment • **Other technologies** – specimen deliveries through pneumatic tubes
Optimize patient flow through service bottlenecks using process templates	• **IT support** – improved PAS systems
Redesign extended roles in line with efficient pathways to attract and retain an effective workforce	• **IT support** – community nurses and pharmacists are able to deliver enhanced prescribing services to patients in the community through the Electronic Prescription Service (EPS) • **Other technologies** – transportable diagnostic equipment, such as respirometers, that community-based staff can use, widening their role in care delivery

Source: List adapted from Modernisation Agency (2004)

Figure 6.2 High-impact changes

2 A 17-year-old unconscious victim of an overdose was admitted to casualty. Staff were able to find out the drug he had used after the father had given them permission to access his son's records. His life was saved.

3 Sadie Morris has little doubt as to the worth of the ECS system in Scotland, particularly for those treating elderly people in psychiatric care. Many people tend to have long lists of medicines they cannot

remember. A major benefit is increasing the safety of medicine reconciliation, and making sure that doctors and nurses have the most up-to-date record of medication and other continuing needs – not least in circumstances outside the regular healthcare environment.

How to be involved

Thomas and Warm (2009), exploring the experiences of nurses in Wales, are very clear of the positive benefits of nurse involvement. They set out three important aspects:

1 A *listening function* – 'capturing the opinion of nurses and midwives on the potential benefits and application of information and communication technology to enhance the provision of care.'
2 An *influencing function* – 'ensuring that the nursing and midwifery profession has the opportunity to shape the design and testing of new technological methods to support care delivery.'
3 An *evaluating function* – 'measuring the effectiveness of the engagement process against desired outcome needs careful managing to ensure meaningful information is collected. The lessons learned from any audit and evaluation work will be used to inform sustainable service improvement.'

In Wales this has included the involvement of general nurses, midwives, specialist nurses and other healthcare professionals in both identifying and assessing the benefits of potential electronic methods of improving outcomes for patients, carers and service users. Clark (2008), Hannah et al. (2006), Stuttle (2007) and Rowntree (2010) would all agree with this, and have said that all those involved in healthcare need to be at the forefront of informatics development and require greater awareness and involvement to ensure that the many benefits of technology are fully realized.

Any 'local-to-you' strategy needs to be fashioned by the information-management and technology (IM&T) team, with input from clinical and managerial colleagues and from other IT partners. This partnership should ideally involve early day discussions and agreement, with the ability to create the appropriate interface and integration with others' systems, so that implementation in practice is beneficial to all participants concerned. It will help to ensure that clinically relevant information is available to all staff involved in delivering care.

One other important consideration is the ability to access information relevant to clinical care at the point where care is given – an important issue in the light of current national policy attempts to provide personalized care closer to home (Darzi, 2009a; Cameron and Clegg, 2010; Mitchell, 2010). In broad terms, then, the IT strategy developed within your local organization should have identified the national core policy messages which need to underpin local care policy strategies and developments.

Developments across the UK

Wales

This approach has been applied in Wales, where IT strategies have been developed in the context of the current and emerging Welsh policy agenda for health and, in particular, its implications for the nursing profession and nursing care. According to Thomas and Warm (2009), the information strategy in Wales (WAG, 2003a; 2004; 2005; 2007) reflects a broad set of policy imperatives. It defines the ways in which new information services will be delivered to support patient care: developing methods to increase collaborative working, removing barriers and eliminating any unnecessary bureaucracy. It sets out several long-term strategic principles and policies relating to healthcare service improvements for the people of Wales, defining the priorities for informing healthcare activities that support these aims. It also describes a political approach to endorsing shared values, common goals and joint aspirations for the people of Wales, offering an agenda for improving the quality of life of people in all communities, especially for the most vulnerable and disadvantaged.

Northern Ireland

The attempt in Wales to marry health policy aspirations and delivery with the support of developed and developing IT systems is not alone. In Northern Ireland, plans were developed to implement a computerization programme for district nurses to collate and analyse information for a multitude of administrative and professional functions in delivering health policy objectives (Scott, 2001).

Scotland

The NHS Knowledge Network, an online database that improves staff access to health and social care information, has been launched in Scotland. The system contains data on clinical practice, patient care and research. More than 100 organizations in the care sector have collaborated to provide more than 11 million entries about research, evidence-based practice and patient care (*Nursing Standard*, 2010b). Aberdeen's Robert Gordon University has invested in a personal response system (PRS) similar to audience-voting technology used on TV game shows. This allows nursing students to be assessed both formatively and summatively, in real time, in relation to questions posed in their lecture presentations. It highlights areas that need revision and those that are not understood (Main, 2010). In effect, this is an important way of educating, checking and supporting the effective development of the nursing workforce in Scotland.

📋 Activity: discuss with your fellow students or colleagues

- What involvement do you have in any of the aspects highlighted above by Thomas and Warm (2009) and others ?
- Does your local IT support system help you to implement required health policy changes? If so, how?
- Is the information provided relevant and helpful to you and the patients and of benefit to your organization?
- Who is responsible for making and influencing changes in the IT resource bank in your organization? If you don't know, why not find out?
- If you are not directly involved, how can you share in developing the IT delivery systems which will help you to deliver better and safer care?

Advice on making progress

Hills (2009) notes that those who are best at delivering care use information well, are assiduous in their approach and are likely to pursue a number of key features which we need to emulate in our own practice, both as professionals and for the benefit of our diverse service users and patients. The issues we are advised to address are varied and invaluable to all nurses trying to deliver high-quality care in today's rapidly changing NHS environment.

It is vital to work in partnership with other care organizations in the community from whatever sector. In this way local bodies can potentially share information, so that decisions, irrespective of who makes them, are based on a common understanding of need and, it is to be hoped, help to ensure an integrated, relevant and affordable response. Useful high-quality resource data and health knowledge needs to be gathered, analysed, shared and disseminated. It is proposed that this process can be used both to stimulate change and to construct challenging questions about local service provision. This is important if it is to lead to action and positive change for the diversity of patients within the current healthcare environment.

It is important to obtain a total picture of health need, both met and unmet, within our local communities, and to use this knowledge to influence and to determine the most appropriate healthcare responses, not least from the powerful general practice consortia groups. As commissioners of services, they need to have a good understanding of formal health data as well as information about a range of social risk factors, such as crime levels, educational attainment and housing quality (all important proxy indicators of health need), backed up by nurse-validated evidence of need gained from real-life practice experience (Marmot, 2010; Hetherington 2010).

All our communities have a range of differing population groups and life expectancies, and the notion that a 'one size fits all' response to health need is likely to be unsuccessful in many ways – as a waste of resources and in attempts to tackle health inequalities. It is important to harness knowledge gained by the third sector, which covers both charities and social enterprises. This sector has extensive experience of working with specific and often hard-to-reach groups. They not only serve as a valuable source of information, but also as potentially effective providers of services – not least in meeting unmet needs and supporting the reduction of health inequalities (Merron, 2010).

The use of readily available, good, local information is an invaluable tool for decision-making on a whole variety of issues, and enables the development of new ways of working and frameworks for care in response to complex and very diverse health and social care needs. Benchmarking information collated online, for example, helps in the identification of individuals, conditions and situations which need to be addressed (Marmot, 2010). The ability to stratify the risk to local people whose condition puts them at medium or high risk of admission into secondary services is another invaluable technological resource. By stratifying the local population according to risk of hospital admission, it is possible to alert primary care services to put in place interventions to keep the patient well and out of hospital. This approach has helped the activities of community matrons, by maximizing their success in stemming the rate of hospital admissions (Gaffney, 2008). However, as we already know, there is still much work to be done to achieve this particular goal (King's Fund, 2010a; Lansley, 2010).

The capturing of all of this material, together with the means to analyse and to share it, is imperative. However, in the developing, financially competitive health arena, this may become an increasingly difficult proposition. Not only does there have to be the will and, indeed, the ability to do this by individuals and by organizations, but also compatible networks need to be available for the sharing of information. Issues around record keeping, data-sharing capabilities, efficiency of data transfer and data security, together with clarification of legal ownership and responsibilities of organizations and people who manage data needs careful clarification, particularly in the now very diverse commissioner and provider health groups.

The use of regularly and currently updated information systems is imperative. These are essential for tracking trends and noting problems which need immediate and timely attention. Online benchmarking, for example, is helpful in encouraging scrutiny of one's own services, and in comparing health outcomes and service effects with other like-for-like situations. This can help in looking for, and finding, the best solutions for similar problems and issues found in one's own community. It is to be hoped that the new diverse NHS environment is both transparent and honest enough in providing such detail. It may, however, be a questionable notion in the competitive market of 'willing providers' who are currently pursuing the available business opportunities.

Ham (2009), in giving advice to any future governments about health policy planning, proposed that leaders should employ excellent intelligence and horizon-scanning functions to help them plan strategically. In the same vein, it has to be argued that nurses should also employ good IT systems to help them plan their care and to navigate their way through the complex network of health-policy imperatives.

The relentless growth in the use of computer and other IT technology to inform, focus and improve care in the most appropriate ways is set to continue to gather pace. It is likely to move on still further as knowledge extends the realms of possibility and policy remit – no doubt streets ahead of what we can imagine today (MacLeod, 2010; Sample, 2010). The bottom line now for nurses, in whatever capacity, is the need to be informed and involved in the ever-developing symbiotic relationship between policy, information gathering and technology

Learning outcomes

- an overview of the historical and parallel development of the relationship between health policy and technology within the NHS;
- an understanding of the importance of technology, both for information and communication and also as an enabler in modern healthcare delivery;
- an appreciation of the practicalities, responsibilities and difficulties of nurse professionals working within an increasingly high-technology NHS environment;
- the importance of nurse engagement in the current technological developments in order to tackle the complicated and often-dichotomous pull of current health policy imperatives.

Further reading

Blake, H. (2008) Innovation in practice: mobile phone technology in patient care. *British Journal of Community Nursing* 13/4: 162–165.

Blake, H. (2008) Using technology in health promotion interventions, in M. R. Blakely and S. M. Timmons (eds), *Life Style and Health Research*. Nova Publishers.

Hannah, K. J., Ball, M. J. and Edwards, M. J. A. (2006) *Introduction to Nursing Informatics*, 3rd edn. Springer.

Liddle, A., Adshead, S. and Burgess, E. (2008) *Technology in the NHS : Transforming the Patient's Experience of Care*. King's Fund, London.

Straughan, T. (2008) Towards world-class quality of information for healthcare: Magic Touch: the revolution in information management. *Health Service Journal* 118 (October supplement): 6126.

7 Empowering Patients and the Public

Aims

- to explore the concept of patient and public empowerment in healthcare;
- to reflect upon different ways in which patients and the public are involved;
- to reflect on the policy developments aimed at making the patients and the public central to the delivery of health services.

'If you want to know about a restaurant you should ask the diners. . . . We all know what we like to eat, but this doesn't mean we have any idea how to run a restaurant.'

(Muijen, in McGowan, 2010)

'The ultimate measure of restaurant is not how well run it is, but whether people enjoy it, return to it and recommend it to others. When applying this to the NHS, we should not forget who our customers are. A well-run service is something patients should expect, not be grateful for.'

(Griffiths, 2010)

'The best user involvement harnesses a passion for making things better.'

(Muijen, in McGowan, 2010)

Since the 1980s sentiments such as those expressed above have been growing throughout the NHS. In think-tank reports, government policy and local services the message has been: get patients and the public involved wherever possible. As such, people whose primary qualification is that they have used health services are now an accepted part of NHS decision-making, recruitment, policy advice, professional education and training. Of course, legally, morally and as taxpayers, the public clearly has a democratic right and certainly a vested interest in how the NHS is run, who will work in it, what services are provided and the standards achieved. As stated in the Coalition government's first Health White Paper: 'There will be no decisions about me, without me' (DOH, 2010c).

Clearly, there are many potential benefits from patient and public involvement (PPI) in healthcare. Everyone has something legitimate to say about waiting times and access to care, poor buildings, uninterested staff, bad attitudes, dirty environments and the like. We can learn what does and does not work. It encourages people to take an active interest in their health and local services and helps identify ways for improvement.

In addition, some patients have been around long enough to have a greater depth of knowledge about their condition and their care needs than many professionals (DOH, 2001b). These 'experts by experience' may wish to buddy up and share their experiences with someone who really understands their situation and are also in a position to represent the views of other similar users who may be less able to express their thoughts. Broadly, then, PPI is about proactively seeking and building continuous and meaningful engagement with the public, to shape and create innovative services and to improve health.

🗒 Activity: discuss with your fellow students or colleagues

- What experience have you had of patient and public involvement in your nursing practice?
- Do you think the patients are listened to and changes made in both services and care? Do you have any examples?

Effective PPI will of course go beyond consultation. It is about ensuring that views expressed by patients and the public are *really used* to make relevant changes and to commission appropriate services. The approach is part and parcel of an open, accountable and responsive NHS, one which recognizes its duty to the community to provide clear explanations for its decisions and activities. These should be well advertised to maximize local community involvement, knowledge and interest.

Importantly, PPI activity recognizes and shows respect for the diverse communities and individuals it is tasked to serve. It is all about valuing people, ensuring their representation and inclusion, about good communication and working in partnership with all local health services. It is about being open and accountable for the services provided, making improvements which are appropriate, responsive and supportive. In reality, of course, there are many limitations and challenges to this being a successful process. Professional power and a knowledge base make for a potentially unbalanced relationship with patients and this may not always support discussions and decision-making in a supposedly reciprocal relationship. There may well be organizational and structural constraints, resource limitations and conflicts of interest in delivering proposed changes.

It may be very difficult to involve hard-to-reach and marginalized groups and to know what they feel or think about the service. There is also a potential for exploitation if, for example, willing patients and their carers are overused. It can also be difficult if less-productive contributions come into play. This may, for example, include individuals

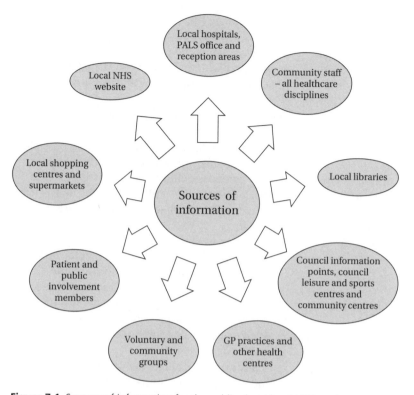

Figure 7.1 Sources of information for the public about local NHS services

who only want to talk about their own issues and are obstructive in discussing other wider health matters.

McGowan (2010) expressed concern that the insistence on PPI seems to be based on potentially unfair assumptions that NHS staff lack passion and the will to challenge poor or inappropriate practice, which then needs to be challenged by the public at every turn. Also, one particular user's understanding of difficulties may not *ipso facto* be the same as another's in similar circumstances. Just by using a service or having a lay opinion does not then necessarily confer expertise in how to improve that service. Sometimes people who are uninformed and driven by personal agendas can bring into play inappropriate frustrations from all parts of their lives and, by turn, make discussion, service delivery and change very difficult.

The reality is that it may not be comfortable for some professionals to listen to, 'hear', accept, agree with or be able to respond to the views and wishes of patients or the wider public, not least if they seem to be or are irrelevant, or perhaps ill thought through. The difficulty is how to deal with this situation. If it is not possible to debate honestly, knowledgeably and critically with patients and the public, there is a potential for the process to become merely a tick-box exercise and of little value, with proposed ideas tabled and aired, but ignored.

Table 7.1 The five core elements of PPI

An embedding of PPI across each organization	Effective systems and processes in place. A workforce with the capacity and capability to achieve this, with training and support as necessary. A true willingness to learn from each other. A commitment to work together. Clarity about what level of involvement is possible – so as not to overburden any PPI contributor.
Commissioning and providing	Robust commissioning and provider approaches which demonstrate and are informed and influenced by the views and opinions of local people.
Service provision	Any changes to services are made as a result of what people have identified and that the impact of the changes are improvements from the perspective of patients as well as the clinicians.
Consultation	A clear understanding by everyone of the duty to involve and consult patients and the public when planning, developing proposals and making decisions. A clearly expressed aim to deliver user-centred and high-quality customer services and strengthened democratic governance and accountability; to provide a fresh perspective on issues, services and policies; to identify the needs of users, reveal problems, concerns and issues; to improve the culture of services and lend authority to decisions made by overtly reflecting and reporting on the PPI contributions.
Partnerships and stakeholders	A clear effort to involve all stakeholders at an early stage in developing proposals for involvement and consultation. In turn regular feedback on processes and opportunities is given, with all chances both to influence and contribute.

On the other hand, if potential PPI people need to fit a job speci-fication, have a set way of behaving or provide evidence of certain knowledge and skills to contribute, then this in turn would begin to defeat and devalue the object of pursuing such lay involvement. That said, patients can be, and are, involved in many significant ways. If their contribution is to have any real meaning, there needs to be a frank debate on these issues. In turn, the process itself needs to be strongly embedded across the whole organization. This should involve five core elements (see Table 7.1).

Encouraging patient and public involvement

There are many different ways in which patients and the public can play their part in an effective PPI agenda within our workplaces, one of which is to encourage them to join a local involvement network – currently Healthwatch (DOH, 2010c, 2010d). Activities might include attendance at public meetings and events, workshops and special interest groups as a patient representative or member of a patient panel. It could involve helping in the recruitment, interviewing and induction of new staff, and relaying experiences of health services in staff training sessions. It could also be about reviewing the documents of the organization, patient-information leaflets or the completion of surveys and questionnaires as a means of gathering views and opinions.

📋 Activity

- Try to attend some public meetings concerned with local health service changes and developments and listen to the discussions.
- Find out what interests people in your locality.
- Explore how members of the public become involved in their local NHS services.

Meeting the needs of a diverse community and population

PPI also needs to reflect the diversity of situation, race, culture, age, gender and sexuality among the patient voice, ensuring that it is representative of the whole community. This will include people who may be isolated: young parents, single parents, people from ethnic minorities, people who are unemployed, older people or people with disabilities. There will be those who experience barriers to communication: people who do not speak English as a first language, people with learning difficulties and people with low educational attainment. Others, for example, may be apathetic and do not believe they can make a difference or that they are valued by society – the unemployed, ex-prisoners, people on long-term sick leave from work, homeless people, drug abusers and people with alcohol problems.

Opportunities for hearing the views of all such people should be advertised in different ways and in appropriate languages, by leafleting, via television, radio and online, with information events held in culturally and religiously sensitive ways, and in places where they meet, or work and live. Encouraging and supporting their active involvement requires a proactive approach, which may involve practical support (transport), financial help (expenses), learning opportunities (training and information) and individual support (confidence building and encouragement).

It is essential to thank people for their contributions and to demonstrate that what people are saying really does make a difference to their healthcare services. The reporting back and communication of news about any responsive change is extremely important. This should be done via press releases, website announcements, newsletters, leaflets, events and public meetings, reports and follow-up visits to relevant patient and community groups.

📋 Activity: discuss with your fellow students or colleagues

- What do you do to involve patients and the public?
- What works? What does not work?
- From which groups do you rarely hear? How could you deal with this differently?
- Think of examples from your own work experience on the following:
  - providing information for informed choice
  - getting information from patients and the public
  - participation activities
  - partnerships
  - patient or public-led activities

The policy push for PPI

The stated purpose of NHS reforms in recent decades has been to provide patients with better-quality healthcare and a wider choice of services that more appropriately reflects their preferences and needs (DOH, 1989c, 1997, 2010c). It has been clearly set out in successive government White Papers that all proposals have been designed to put the needs of the patients and users first. This has been reflected in ever-strengthening attempts to involve them in both challenging and developing the services, the provision of better information to educate and to inform, combined with the backcloth shift towards a more commercialized approach to healthcare delivery in the NHS.

This specific change has been developed in an attempt both to increase and to diversify provider services and to offer a wider variety of choice. The underpinning thrust for a more business-like agenda has led to an increase in competition between providers of services for patients and, it is argued, has created a force for raised standards of care and greater user responsiveness. Patients supposedly are developing into consumers, apparently keen and able to shop around for the best and most appropriate services to meet their healthcare needs (DOH, 2010c).

Empowered consumers or patients?

These now-popular concepts of consumerism and empowerment continue to permeate today's ever-developing healthcare agenda –

'patients will be in charge of making decisions about their care' (DOH, 2010c). Having acknowledged this, it is worthwhile to ponder on the difficulty either of defining these concepts in absolute terms or of making them a reality in practice. It would seem that politicians, policy-makers, healthcare professionals, managers and the public alike latch onto interpretations which reflect their understanding or, indeed, which best suit their purpose. Whether or not the users of the health services have in reality become active consumers, or even become further empowered over the past decades, clearly depends very much on subjective assessment. There is substantial scope for debate.

While some have argued that the internal healthcare market of the 1990s, for example, resulted in a greatly increased consumer perspective, others referred to the creation of an illusion of power, to a 'supermarket' model of consumerism (Winkler, 1987) and to the frills and trappings of ostensible patient power (Fatchett, 1998). This argument continues unabated in today's NHS (Tudor-Hart, 2010). Because of this, some initial comment must be made about the nature of consumerism, and in particular its appropriateness and, indeed, applicability to healthcare delivery and to the patients and users with whom we all currently work.

The debate continues

The first part of what follows will deal with whether the concepts of consumerism and healthcare are actually compatible. This will lead into a number of discussions, which will examine the thesis of enhanced consumer choice within health services. We will then reflect on the policy developments and headline themes introduced over time by governments to empower the varied users of our many different healthcare services, both in hospital and community settings.

As we consider the evidence and the arguments, we may be led to conclude that the system created as a result of the changes within the NHS has not necessarily empowered either consumers or professional nurses. We may also conclude that a distributive system which is based upon a vicarious relationship between individuals and providers cannot, in itself, be guaranteed to add to consumer power or choice. Finally, and against this background, we will look at the consumer empowerment argument and at the changes that have taken place, and at how these relate to the experience and role of professional nurses, not least in their quest over the past two decades to empower both the patients and themselves.

Consumerism and healthcare: compatible concepts?

First, we need to question the basic assumption that health and healthcare are like any other commodity, to be bought and sold in the marketplace or, even, in the supermarket. Every individual is seen as a powerful consumer, because he or she has money to spend on the services on offer. Linked to this is the notion that the potential user of health services can, and should, be expected to play the role of active consumer, and, in effect, 'go shopping' to buy healthcare as and when the need arises.

Unsurprisingly, many have strongly criticized the use of the term 'consumer' in relation to healthcare delivery (Klein, 1980; Winkler, 1987; Normand, 1991; Fatchett 1994, 1998). Abel-Smith (1976), for example, concluded in his analysis that there are few fields of consumer expenditure where the consumer is as ill equipped to exercise this theoretical sovereignty as in the health services. So what 'equipment' might be needed by a true consumer in a free market model of healthcare? Consumer needs could be summarized as:

- adequate information;
- a practical range of alternative services and interventions;
- an ability to make a rational choice;
- the opportunity to select from a variety of options;
- the ability and knowledge to compare the quality of one service or intervention with another;
- legal protection;
- the ability to obtain a refund;
- the ability to take action to seek redress or compensation if a product, treatment or intervention failed to work, was inappropriate or did not reach the quality or standard offered, promised or expected.

While it is easy to see how some of these requirements would be easy, relevant, appropriate and indeed possible for many individuals – perhaps the fittest, the most articulate and the financially solvent – there would surely still be problems for many less fortunate individuals that are worth considering. As Normand (1991) stated: 'Where health is bought and sold as a commodity, it fails on several counts – and not least, if one believes in the principle that care should be given to those in need, and that some equitable approach should apply in its delivery.'

It would appear that the free market is also seen as poor at allocating resources in a fair way to those who are 'less able' and perhaps have more need of healthcare services than others who are better educated and have both the skills and the finance to pursue the necessary health and lifestyle objectives and services available. Having said that, others will equally argue that the same problem applies to the current centrally controlled distribution of NHS resources. Research has demonstrated time after time that the 'inverse care law' and subsequent health inequality continues to apply (Black 1980; Marmot, 2010). In this situation, those who need the most help to be healthy, often the poorest in society, appear to gain the least from the healthcare resources made available, whatever the method of distribution.

Linked to this is the issue of illness and poor health being correlated with low socio-economic status and poverty (Graham, 2007;

Marmot. 2010). Those who suffer ill health and fall into this category may be unable to afford to buy much-needed services and help, even though these are available in the market. The better off and more articulate are, by contrast, better able to access a very broad remit of health-promoting activities and services and, in turn, to achieve and maintain a better health status and greater longevity than those who lack such attributes and opportunities. To compound the issue further, the commercial judgement of those who insure against the cost of ill health, and who also fund private healthcare, will be to charge high-risk groups much higher premiums than low-risk groups, or even to refuse them insurance cover altogether because of the possibility of their developing very costly illnesses in either the short or the long term.

Another important point to consider is that a free market in healthcare services cannot, and does not, aspire to meet the overarching and general health needs of the whole population or community, rich and poor alike. There is a tendency to offer care to meet specific health needs only and to provide these services within areas of appropriate consumer prosperity. Poorer areas of the population are less likely to offer commercially attractive sites or, indeed, sources of potential income. As a result, many of the worse-off consumers in both these and other more affluent areas may have little or no choice of healthcare provision, because it may not exist in or nearby their own area, or may be irrelevant because of an inability to be able to afford or to purchase services wherever they may exist.

While this situation may be broadly satisfactory or acceptable in relation to buying biscuits or designer clothes, in healthcare this may mean the difference between a long life, an early death or long-term disability and discomfort, depending upon individual financial and social situations. As such, many will argue that healthcare is a different and special good or commodity, and that it should, therefore, be made available on the basis of need, rather than on an ability to pay. The creation of the NHS in 1948 was a prime example of such a view, with access to healthcare seen as a collective societal responsibility.

It is also worth considering the belief that an individual consumer of healthcare in a free market situation is more powerful than a patient in a publicly funded and centrally directed organization. This may well be a misplaced belief even in today's consumer-focused NHS (DOH, 2010c). Individuals looking for healthcare, whatever or wherever the setting, may lack information and expertise in health matters. It is the professional providers of care who have the monopoly of knowledge and skills; why else would people seek out their help if they could 'heal themselves' without recourse to professional advice?

Health professionals clearly have greater power than the consumers because of their special understanding and knowledge. If this is abused for commercial gain, for example, it can and does lead to exploitation of the consumers or an oversupply of some more lucrative services at the expense of a broader more all-embracing menu – something which is probably likely to be of greater relevance to the health of the whole population, for example an effective public health programme to reduce the current obesity crisis (DOH, 2010d).

In conclusion, the free market may theoretically offer the opportunity, finance permitting, for any individual consumer to be treated when, where and how they would like. That person will, however, then be reliant upon the provider to determine the degree, type and quality of care deemed appropriate and necessary. The theoretical idea of the active consumer being the more powerful player in the client/provider relationship is thus open to debate, and will surely depend on an individual's ability, knowledge and financial resources.

For the majority of the population seeking healthcare, the power relationship will be weighted in favour of the provider who has the experience and knowledge being sought. This of course will apply whether in the private or the public sector. It begins to become apparent, then, that both sectors may have interests which overlap.

Potter (1988) proposed that a number of convenient principles implicit within a free market could be readily applied to a centrally directed health sector such as the NHS:

- access;
- choice;
- information;
- redress;
- participation.

Interestingly, these are themes that are currently being applied in the NHS of today (DOH, 2010c). The interpretation and appreciation of these principles in practice will reflect the philosophy or ideology underpinning the policy and legislative programmes of any particular government. What is clear, however, is that different governments with opposing views may create differing policy responses to what is apparently the same problem. As noted in the earlier discussions on policy-making, policy activity is not value-free, but reflects a particular ideological perspective. In the 1940s, for example, the Labour government's welfare state was a broad policy response to the health and social care needs of the population of the time, and reflected that government's political views and judgements.

In turn, the Conservative governments of the 1980s, 1990s and to date have argued that their health reforms are focused on empowering the users of the services. They have worked openly to minimize public sector involvement in healthcare, and to release the energies and quality-enhancing competitive aspects of a free market environment. At the same time they have promoted and tried to maximize personal and individual responsibility for health and healthcare choices, thereby empowering the consumer. The principles, as set out by Potter (1988), have continued to flavour successive governments' health policy since the 1990s, and are very much in vogue today (DOH, 1997; DOH, 2010c) – 'no decisions about me without me'.

📋 Activity: discuss with your fellow students or colleagues

- Are your patients able to be powerful consumers of healthcare services?
- If not, why not?
- If yes, how do you know? What examples can you give?

Why do we need to think about these issues ?

A discussion of the ever-strengthening interest in user centrality and responsiveness implicit within current NHS policy developments is both worthwhile and relevant for all NHS employees. For over three decades, NHS reforms have been underpinned by an emphasis on the wishes of the individual users of health services. This clearly reflects a faith in the ability of people to choose between competing health service options, and the power to force the providers of healthcare to become responsive to their needs and wishes. The veracity of these beliefs needs to be examined, not least in relation to the previous discussion. In reality, can this policy imperative ever really be delivered?

Nurses may be somewhat concerned or upset by the criticism implied in the comment of 'needing to put the patient first'. After all, doing just that has surely always been central to nursing. The Code (NMC, 2008), 'our badge of professional integrity' (Kaye, cited in Prandy, 1965), has reaffirmed over time the primacy of patient interests as a dominant theme. Without a doubt, other professions would defend their own long-term position vis-à-vis their clients in a similar way. However, defensive protestations by professionals that they have always put their clients first, and that all the reforms have only reinforced the status quo are perhaps, at best, indiscreet and foolish and, at worst, telling an untruth. It is worth remembering that the NHS has not always been seen as user-responsive and fault-free.

North and Bradshaw (1997) referred to the 'bleak habitat of the would-be consumer'. Klein (1989) wrote of 'ghosts in the NHS machinery'. Pollitt (1989) said professional groups, doctors, nurses and allied health professionals decided who received what, how and when, and the users had little influence or say in the matter. This was a view reiterated by the Griffiths Management Inquiry Team in 1983. The so-called users' voice of the now defunct Community Health Councils (CHCs), created in 1974 (and wound up in 2003), were seen as 'toothless watchdogs' and merely 'throwers of grit 'into the NHS machinery (Klein, 1989).

While the promise of consumer or user centrality has been made on many occasions, it often seems that claims and practice do not in reality go hand in hand – sadly, even today. Tudor-Hart (2010) warned of the potential lack of direct consumer responsiveness if, as expected, the private sector takes over some of the difficult commissioning consortia work on behalf of groups of GPs across the UK. While the White Paper (DOH, 2010c) looked to GPs as being central to commissioning work because they know their patients and communities, the *moving away from* or *hands-off approach to* passing this work to others will effectively put up a barrier to real consumer choice. This harks back to the budget-holding issue of the 1980s and 1990s, in which, as noted earlier, 'consumers' were not empowered by that process, as choices for care were made not by them, but by others on their behalf.

Given that this remains the case, the discussion that follows is of relevance to all nurses who seek to uphold their code of conduct and reaffirm in a serious and meaningful way the primacy of the interests of their patients both within and without today's NHS. For unless we consider the attributes, characteristics, uses, abuses and failures of the efforts intended to empower users prevalent within our practice and organizations, then any desire for truly effective user empowerment is unlikely to be achieved in the foreseeable future.

As suggested earlier, it is useful to reflect back on past policy history to learn from both good and bad experiences. By doing this, we may be able to create a better way forward as we implement today's exhortations to make the patients central to our care delivery. As the Coalition government has reminded us, only by putting the patients first will we drive up standards, deliver better value for money and create a healthier nation (DOH, 2010c, 2010d).

Policy developments leading up to the NHS reforms of the 1990s

British governments of all political persuasions accepted and even promoted without hesitation or question the broad development of the NHS up until the 1980s. From this point onward, however, the developing backcloth of concern about rising government expenditure and criticism of the scale and scope of all arms of the welfare state, and of government interventions in general, began to impact upon the NHS. It became a target for both cost-containment programmes and organizational reform.

Sheldon (1980) and Butler (1992) set out a picture of the NHS which, without a doubt, reflected the beliefs about it held by many in the Conservative Party. It was seen as bureaucratic, totally reliant on government funding, unresponsive, indifferent to the quality of care, providing few incentives for innovation and efficiency, and resistant to change, with appalling industrial relations and restrictive practices by powerful professionals. Very importantly, it was perceived as not encouraging any sense of individual responsibility for health and a marked absence of real consumer choice.

Alongside the critical academic debate, right-wing politicians and much of the tabloid press during the 1980s offered an often derogatory liturgy of accusations against the NHS and other arms of the welfare state. They were described as wasteful organizations which swallowed up the hard-earned contributions of taxpayers. They were accused of providing inappropriate and wasteful services, as well as financial help to people who could, if they really tried, look after themselves and their families instead of relying upon what was called 'the nanny state'.

These sorts of views were widely promoted and, for many, held great appeal. Debates on public spending and all the attendant ills during and after the 1979 election period found a receptive audience in the population at large. The NHS was not immune. As Sheldon (1980) concluded, the NHS does not supply the British people with the best medical care they want, because it prevents them as individual consumers from paying for the services that suit their personal circumstances, requirements and preferences.

The general election of 1979

The Conservative Party's 1979 election promises of reduced public expenditure, decreased direct taxation and, thus, more choice and freedom for individuals to spend their incomes as they wished were clear signs of a new direction for health and spending policy. It was obvious that many of the electorate liked the messages that they heard, and returned a Conservative government to power with a comfortable majority in the House of Commons.

They were given a strong mandate for, among other things, the creation of a different approach to healthcare organization and delivery which, as we now know, was to have profound implications for the NHS, for all health professionals and, by definition, for all users of health service. Few nurses today, if any, will be unaware of the implications of the changes since that time, with the creation of new organizational structures, the introduction of general management coupled with the language of the marketplace, and the stated purpose of pleasing and satisfying the consumer (DOH, 2010c).

Changing the NHS

The newly elected Conservative government was fully aware of the politically sensitive nature of changing the NHS. Its continuing popularity as a national institution made wholesale privatization, for example, politically impossible (North and Bradshaw, 1997). However, while providing reassurance as to its continuing presence and integrity, the government started on changes that it felt were necessary for the creation of a new-style business-like health service.

They were looking to develop the NHS into an organization which, they believed, would be better equipped and more able to deal with the complex and ever-changing healthcare needs and agendas of the twentieth century. Importantly, they wished to be responsive to the expressed interests of both taxpayer and healthcare consumer alike. The initial introduction of new accounting processes to monitor and control costs and then general management, with all its attendant attributes, were felt to be major steps in the right direction (Holliday, 1995).

The introduction of general management and a more commercialized approach

The government believed that to run a truly consumer-responsive health service, professional managers with business acumen were needed at every level (as in industry or the retail sector) in order to make it happen. The 1983 Griffiths Inquiry team (all business people) believed that the clinically led NHS was suffering from 'institutional stagnation'. While it was felt that business people had a keen sense of how well they were looking after their customers, the Griffiths team doubted that NHS professionals even tried to pretend to have an interest in the expressed needs of either patients or the communities they served.

The NHS was not seen as a consumer-friendly organization. There was a lack of information about services available, little choice of care on offer, no easily identified channel for complaints and little effort to find out about, or to involve, the service users. The team's solution to this lack of consumer care was the introduction of general managers from top to bottom of the NHS. The aim of their task was to ensure that the users of the service were to become central to all activities and that the taxpayers gained best value for money.

Making the users central, Griffiths style

The Griffiths team believed that the users needed to be the central focus of healthcare delivery and, as such, should be well informed, consulted and encouraged to participate in all decision-making – in fact, become active consumers of healthcare rather than remain the passive recipients of professional decisions and choices. As in the private sectors, of business, industry or retail, managers would need to seek the views of the consumers by means of market research, user surveys, meetings to give and receive information, lifestyle questionnaires and other research projects.

Interestingly, the team was dismissive of, and unimpressed by, the activity of the Community Health Councils, describing them as 'labyrinthine and often unproductive'. Created during the 1974 period of NHS reorganization, the CHCs were supposed to increase democracy through 'the representation of the interests of the users of the NHS' (Allsop, 1995). With few resources and little power, however, many commentators had found their contributions to be limited (Shultz and Harrison, 1983).

The Government's response to Griffiths, 1984

The rapid acceptance of this analysis of the failures of the NHS, and particularly in its inability to listen and respond to the users, was no great surprise. The imposition of general management and the rigours of commercial life were immediately accepted as the way forward. The providers of care, including the powerful body of health professionals, would be directly managed and made to respond to both central government strategy and, of course, the direct demands of the patients.

The new commercial style to be adopted, with financial rewards and punishments, was to provide the much-needed push to set the show firmly on the road. Rather than the historically guaranteed source of financial allocations from government, the new approach was to be about payment for proven outcomes and successes – by way of pleasing the users and gaining value for money.

As Flynn et al. (1996) explained, the logic which drove these changes was the axiomatic belief, shared by all mainstream political parties, that markets were the most efficient means of allocating resources and of reflecting consumer preferences and responsibilities. In turn, the market mechanisms would control professionals' budgets, making them more conscious of the costs of meeting the health needs of patients and, by turn, improving their performance. This professed belief in the centrality of the consumer voice in healthcare delivery was to be continued and developed still further by the introduction of the internal healthcare market in April 1991. This, together with the managerial changes which had developed since 1984, created the broad backcloth of reform against which we can begin to judge just how much more power the so-called consumers of healthcare really achieved.

The internal market reforms: more power to the users ?

According to Flynn et al. (1996), a central argument running through the rhetoric of reform had been that greater managerial control over professional work and enhanced provider competition in the provision of services would give consumers more choice and more control. The initial principles underpinning the NHS of 1948 were clearly reaffirmed: those of comprehensiveness, universality and equity, with efficiency and greater choice for patients as additional principles. Some likened the package of reforms to the beginnings of a privatized health system (see Robin Cook's foreword in Fatchett, 1994), not unlike that in the USA (Cairns-Berteau, 1991). Some were excited at the prospect of the organizational overhaul taking place, as the consumers (patients) were to be the central focus for all activity.

That said, others doubted the genuineness of this commitment, and whether the reforms simply represented a clever use of words

Box 7.1 Patient and public concerns in 1989

- fragmentation of health services between hospitals, community and primary care – difficulties expressed about joined-up care;
- poor coordination between health and local authority care made it easy for people to fall between the gaps;
- inequality of access to health services, both in different geographical areas and for many disadvantaged groups, e.g. those with disabilities, the mentally ill, those with learning difficulties, the homeless and problem drug and alcohol users;
- lack of clear processes and safeguards for making complaints and seeking redress;
- lack of encouragement or help from professionals for public and community involvement in decision-making and planning.

obscuring other policy objectives, which were incompatible with true consumer choice. Perhaps a judgement on the success or not of the promised policy focus might be reached by comparing some of the concerns expressed by users of the NHS before the changes (see Box 7.1) with some of the post-reform comments on the success or otherwise of consumer activity. Any reform of the NHS at this time, it was argued, needed to address these problems, but some doubted that this would happen. As in any marketplace, there were likely to be both winners and losers. The losers, it was believed, would be the most vulnerable in the population (Voluntary Organisation, 1989).

Activity: discuss with your fellow students or colleagues

- Consider the concerns outlined above and relate them to the experiences of present-day patients with whom you work.
- Are the same issues live today?

Did the consumers of the 1990s get what they wanted?

As already noted, the then government's intention was to create a more commercialized, consumer-orientated environment in the NHS, in which the users were enabled to demand and expect the sorts and levels of services they desired. Conversely, those healthcare providers who failed to meet these demands would lose out financially, as potential clients went elsewhere in pursuit of other more appropriate and relevant choices on offer in the wider healthcare market.

Despite the early promises of increased individual consumer power, the reality was perceived in different ways. According to the government (NHSME, 1992), the NHS was working better and users were gaining greater benefits than ever before. There were clear improvements in the quality of care, greater responsiveness to individuals' needs and, importantly, even better value-for-money activity through-out the services.

Other commentators disagreed with this analysis. As recounted earlier, this period of NHS life saw the rationalization and cutting of services, with wards and hospitals closed. Surgical activity was slowed down or stopped completely when budgets ran out before the end of the financial year. Services previously free within the NHS attracted charges or were no longer available. For many, such outcomes repre-sented stringent prioritizing and ever more overt rationing, with, as result, a reduction rather than a growth in patient choice. The promise to listen and to respond to user views was also felt to be suspect. Some argued that, far from giving people more say in how their health service was run, the internal market reforms actually gave them less (Plamping and Delamothe, 1991).

The proposed consumerist stance was seen as nothing more than a public relations exercise and not about true consumerism. It lacked a clear framework within which to identify the full range and poten-tial diversity of consumer interests and activity in the field of health (Harrison et al., 1989). Mahon (1992) referred disparagingly to the emphasis given to reducing waiting lists, to the chasing of quality care, reducing costs and to the improvement of information flows. Although important changes in themselves, Mahon was more concerned about the vagueness of these policy initiatives and at how they might translate in practice into greater choice for the users in the long term.

As we noted earlier, it is important that policy initiatives are sup-ported specifically and endorsed, so that commitment and finance are available for delivery. While we consider the outcomes in this way, we need to return again to the implications of an internal healthcare market for the users of the service.

Did the internal healthcare market strengthen the patient voice and influence?

There were clearly differences in opinion in answer to this question, as already noted. For ourselves, we might initially consider the fact that in a true market situation the customer is in a direct relationship in terms of buying a product. This is not true in the NHS. The people who purchase and choose care from the provider bodies are not the patients or would-be consumers, but the purchaser bodies who deter-mine, on behalf of the users, what and who will deliver the services needed.

So, as we can see, the purported consumer had not only not been at the forefront of choice-making and competition, but in reality repre-sented the currency by which improvements in efficiency and financial control of internal healthcare markets were to be achieved. Hospitals and other NHS units were funded for the volume of services they pro-vided, and those hospitals which offered patients the best service and value for money were better rewarded than those which did not; that is, the notion of money following the patient. It may well be that the users did benefit as a result of the changes, but not as a result of being able to influence change directly.

Another point to consider, as had been suggested by some, is that the real intention of the internal market mechanism was to make clinicians work within general management objectives, to keep costs down and to push up productivity, rather than to meet patient preferences (Pollitt, 1989). As Griffiths (1983) had proposed, clinicians needed to participate fully in decisions about priorities in the use of resources – a theme further developed in the 1989 White Paper.

The reforms did set out proposals for striking a proper balance between two legitimate pressures, both of which were focused on patients' interests:

1 The professional responsibility to provide high-quality care and rewards for those individual consultants and their teams who delivered well.
2 The responsibility of managers to ensure that the money available to NHS bodies bought the best possible services for the users.

Again, the benefits of this were seen as improving the service for the patients, but in no way were they directly influencing the amount of NHS monies made available. Rather, patients were seen as recipients of others' decisions and priorities. The organization at that stage (and also now) was a structure not primarily designed to empower them directly (Tudor-Hart, 2010).

If, as it appears, the patients were no more powerful after the changes than they were before, then perhaps we need to consider the inevitability of this outcome. As already described, the NHS came into being in 1948 to overcome the vagaries of failure of a very diverse market provision of healthcare services. When he first introduced the NHS, Aneurin Bevan never believed that it could actually meet all the expressed health needs of all the people (Foot, 1975). So, why should a return to a market-like situation have been any more successful in the 1990s or, indeed, today? The Conservative government of 1989 did not, however, appear to believe or even to acknowledge such an idea. While promising greater choice and power for the users of the service from the reforms introduced to the NHS, they then claimed to empower them further with a well-publicized paperchase of charters.

Activity: discuss with your fellow students or colleagues

- Are we chasing some illusory notion of absolute choice for the users of our twenty-first-century NHS services?
- Can patients really have everything they want or need?

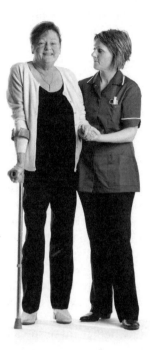

7.1 It has been argued that free market principles do not provide an appropriate framework for services which may make the difference between health and lifelong disability.

Charters: frills and trappings?

The charters were intended to set standards against which the public, the professionals and politicians could check and assess the standards of care and treatment provided by all public bodies. In the foreword to the 1991 Citizen's Charter, for example, the then Prime Minister, John Major, wrote about making public services, including the NHS, more answerable to their users and raising their overall quality. Four key words exemplified his plans to give people more say in how their services were assessed and delivered: quality, standards, choice and value. If the users of the services were not happy with any of these aspects, they could just go elsewhere.

These ideas were reiterated in the Patient's Charter (1991), which was intended to put power in the hands of the public by highlighting their rights within the reformed health service. It created standards by which patients and the public could assess the performance of any provider body. They were described not as legal rights, however, but as major and specific standards which the government expected the NHS to provide as circumstances allowed (DOH, 1992). Interestingly, in the past decade a wide variety of healthcare standards, targets and outcome measures have been set annually, against which all organizations and professionals have been, and are currently being, judged and challenged.

Do charters work?

In the 1990s, some were very dismissive of the power of the charters to ensure better healthcare and choice for consumers (Kargar, 1993). Winkler's (1987) description of such NHS activity as a supermarket model of consumerism fitted exactly with another's description of charters as 'the frills and trappings' of patient power (Editorial, 1991). The various shopping analogies which emerged time after time seem particularly apt. The charters were described as something like the free gifts, leaflets or deals offered by retailers – an encouragement to buy, but not to create, the product on the shelf. Some argued that they just represented a cynical ploy to give the public an illusion of power, but little weight in reality.

A nurse journalist explored the reality of the Patient's Charter with a group of users and concluded that the concept of patients' rights was largely endorsed, but appeared to remain theoretical. There was widespread cynicism about whether these so-called rights were anything other than paper promises, intended more for public show than for real change (*Nursing Times*, 1992).

Indicators and statistics

In a similar vein, the publication of indicators comparing hospital performances was also introduced (Agnew,1995). It was suggested that these would give the public statistical information about which hospital was better than another, and would presumably help them in making choices about where to go for treatment (*Nursing Times*, 1995). These developments, which are commonplace today, were criticized by many.

Moon and Lupton (1995), amongst others, concluded that all these ideas, whether charter, indicator or published statistics, were more about giving information to those directly involved in purchasing and providing care within the internal healthcare market than about empowering the users directly and giving them a real choice. Decisions about choice of hospital and any real response to the standards attained (good or bad) remained with the purchaser bodies, the health authorities and fundholding general practices with budgets.

Complaints: more power to the users?

While it has been argued that the policy reforms of the 1990s may not have empowered NHS users in the various ways proposed by the government, there did potentially exist another avenue in which power could be wielded – that of making complaints. Exploration of this potential was evident, with attempts to improve complaints procedures as part of the government's commitment to taking forward the Patient's Charter and to empower further (in their terms) the users of the service (Wilson, 1994).

As the Wilson report acknowledged, complaining was (and still is) an important way by which the public can make their views known to the NHS (Wilson 1994). However, the report suggested that it was by no means easy to raise concerns, as patients were not in a powerful position and might feel vulnerable when making a complaint. The report recommended that certain principles were necessary to underpin the complaints procedures, and against which NHS managers and others involved in healthcare delivery could check their own professional standards of care delivery – not least in responding to the needs and wishes of the users. These included the need to:

- be accessible;
- be well publicized;
- be simple to understand and use;
- allow speedy handling within reasonable time limits;
- ensure a full and impartial investigation; and
- demonstrate and respect people's wishes for confidentiality.

Subsequent efforts to clarify the procedures, as proposed, potentially strengthened the voice of users, reflected, not least, in a rising level of complaints (DOH, 1995). Nevertheless, although the structures and processes were elucidated at the time, many acknowledged (and still do) the implicit difficulties that were inherent in the system for vulnerable or less-able users – an issue to be considered further in relation to the continuing issue of rising health inequalities, the 'inverse care law' and the continuing problems in providing a diversity-sensitive service.

More efforts and policy promises – the 1997 general election

By the end of 1996 and in preparation for a general election in 1997, the Conservative government published its views on the NHS (DOH, 1996), highlighting its continued focus on the needs and wishes of patients and the public. Its achievements and future aspirations were made clear, by reference to the need for:

- a well-informed public – able to express their needs and make choices;
- a seamless service – well coordinated and free of gaps;
- knowledge-based decision-making – providing treatments which work;

- a highly trained and skilled workforce – continually updating and learning post-qualification;
- a responsive service sensitive to different and diverse needs.

No doubt the Griffiths Inquiry team of a decade earlier would have applauded the essence of its self-analysis and plans for the future, and indeed it would be churlish to ignore the degree of change made in relation to the users of the NHS since 1979.

The incoming Labour government of 1997, however, fundamentally disagreed. It believed the internal healthcare market, general management, charters, indicators and improved complaints procedures had done little to help patients have a greater say in the running of their health service or in decision-making about their care – rather the opposite (Smith, 1996) Labour's new policy imperatives promised to rebuild confidence in the NHS as a public service, to improve its accountability to the public, to be more open in its workings and to be an organization that would be shaped by patient views (DOH, 1997).

Themes and progress under successive Labour governments 1997–2010

The NHS Plan (DOH, 2000b) set out a 10-year programme of reform in the NHS. It reinforced the importance of getting the basics right, listening to the patients and improving their experience of NHS care – to move from a health service that does things *to* and *for* its patients, to one that was patient-led, where the service worked with patients to support them in meeting their health needs.

The creation of a patient-led NHS was all about a commitment to changing the relationship between health professionals and patients. It was to be a move away from patients' feeling a lack of control, perceptions of little openness or accountability and the impression that professionals were doing the patients a favour (Cullum, 2005). The traditional 'doctor knows best' attitude and deference to the medical profession's philosophy in healthcare practice was seen as an outdated notion for a twenty-first-century NHS. Patients wanted to be valued, informed and involved, and to know that changes would take place as a result of their views and that professionals were accountable for their actions (National Consumer Council, 2005).

The government was firmly committed to encourage much greater patient involvement and power. This was to focus on in-depth consultations with patients in order to understand their particular perspectives, listening to their experiences and discussing their preferences, and by giving and expanding patient choice. It was acknowledged that the IT and communication revolution meant that, generally, the public had become much more knowledgeable and increasingly able to challenge professionals in ways that were unthinkable in previous decades. As such, a new adult way of working together needed to be forged.

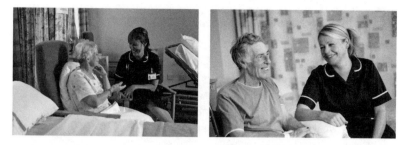

7.2 *The NHS Plan* of 2000 emphasized the importance of the patient experience, calling for a 'patient-led' style of interaction, with improved openness and accountability.

It set out a broad strategy to 'modernize' the NHS with a flow of policy initiatives emphasizing increased involvement of patients in their treatment and care decisions and in the running of the NHS. Three major themes of importance were to be explored in the pursuit of a real say for patients and the public:

1   Patient-informed decision-making about treatment and healthcare.
2   Patient involvement in shaping services more broadly.
3   Citizen involvement in determining how the NHS is run.

Patient-informed decision-making about treatment and healthcare

Professionals were encouraged to expand and develop their roles and activities in new and innovative ways in response to the expressed needs of patients. Nurses, for example, were to become involved in aspects of work previously carried out by doctors – including diagnosis of illness or injury, initiating investigations or treatments, non-medical prescribing, devising management plans and follow-up meetings.

Emphasis was placed on the importance of building on the skilled and effective relationships which nurses had with their patients, not least in being the main catalysts for developing responsive care activities in line with patients' wishes and needs (DOH, 1999b). The National Service Frameworks (NSFs) introduced in 1998 backed up this approach, focusing on promoting the delivery of very specific, user-centred, research-based, high-quality care programmes. These were to involve cross-agency and sector working, pulling together both assessment and delivery of care, with the clear benefit of providing joined-up, better-quality, personalized care experiences for individual patients.

Benchmarking, launched in 2001 by the Modernisation Agency, provided a tool to help any healthcare employee delivering direct patient care take a patient-focused and structured approach to sharing and comparing practice. This reflected the work of patients, professionals and carers working together to agree and describe good-quality care and best practice. The 'expert patient' programme was also aimed at

Box 7.2 *The NHS Improvement Plan* (2004)

- access and waiting times for care and treatment;
- safe, high quality, coordinated care;
- better information and more choice;
- improved communication skills, taking into account individual and social needs, values and preferences, customer care and courtesy;
- clean, comfortable, friendly environments;
- providing care closer to home.

building on individual patients' confidence, knowledge and general motivation, so that they could use their own skills and information to manage their condition more effectively. In turn, it was hoped they could help others in a similar situation – perhaps to give the less articulate a stronger voice and support in gaining a more relevant service from the NHS (DOH, 2001b).

The NHS Improvement Plan (2004f) set out in great detail the many ways in which the NHS needed to change to become truly patient-led, providing a responsive, convenient and personalized service (see Box 7.2). It focused attention on what patients wanted from the service and set out a number of areas for improvement. It also looked at the development of different types of care provision, in particular from the growing independent sector. This potential was seen as helping to meet capacity needs and to provide an increasing choice of services for patients. The diagnosis and treatment provided would be paid for by the NHS, but patients would then have the right to choose from at least four or five different healthcare providers – as long as they met clear NHS standards and were able to give patients what they wanted: very like 'the willing provider' option under current development (DOH, 2010c). This approach was described then (as now) as 'providing incentives for all healthcare providers to ensure care was efficient, responsive, of a high standard and respectful of people's dignity' – a subsequent theme for a major nurse-focused campaign to improve patient responsiveness and dignity-in-care provision (see Figure 7.2).

During this period, the move towards a stronger primary and community-based focus for healthcare, started by the previous Conservative governments, was accelerated (DOH, 2006e). It set the strategic direction for delivering healthcare, with a stronger focus on prevention, on promoting well-being and, importantly, for delivering services in settings that were more convenient to the people who used them – that is, nearer to or at home.

The aim was to deliver a service designed to improve dramatically the quality of care for patients and also to get better value for the money invested in the service. It was about providing a fair service for all, one which treated people as individuals with their own specific needs, to receive personalized, effective and safe care (Ivory, 2010). The primary care trusts, as the 'world class commissioners', were to take up the

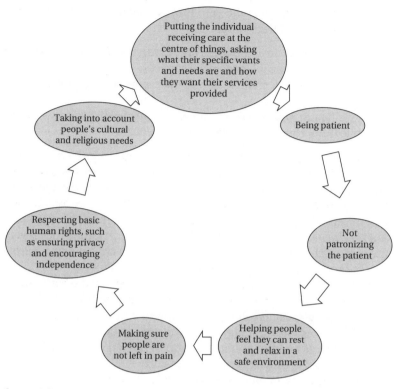

Source: DOH, 2006e

Figure 7.2 How to introduce the dignity-in-care approach

responsibility of working closely with their local patient populations, nurses and clinicians, and other healthcare partners to develop this patient-led agenda.

Patient involvement in shaping services more broadly

Efforts to encourage greater involvement by patients in the broader life and activities of the NHS were pursued in a number of ways. The government said that it would begin to measure itself against the aspirations and experiences of its users. There were to be annual national and local surveys of patient and user experience. The results were to be published and lessons learnt from these findings, so that the users and the public at large would have a voice in shaping the service (DOH, 1997).

Ever greater efforts were also made to promote further patient independence, choice and control, by building on all earlier progress, and developing the patient and public involvement network. The creation of Local Involvement Networks (LINks) in April 2008 came about in an effort to help strengthen the system that enabled patients and communities to influence the care they received (DOH, 2006f; DOH, 2007a). The aims of LINkS were:

- to provide everyone in the community with the chance to have a say about their local health and social services;
- to give everyone a chance to influence how services are planned and run;
- to give health and social care organizations feedback on what the public think about their services. (DOH, 2007c)

As part of this new listening and responding approach, the 2006 White Paper set out an important commitment to implement a single complaints procedure across health and social care. This was a response to the often-stated concerns that making complaints was difficult for patients and the public at large, especially if more than one organization was involved. As Wilson (1994) had noted earlier, the process was unclear, much too complicated and lessons were almost never learnt. Why bother complaining if you were never listened to?

The vision behind the new system was to transform the handling of complaints to become more comprehensive, accessible and patient-focused, using local resolution to respond flexibly and quickly to individual cases. Such an approach was seen as being beneficial not only to patients and the public, but also to the NHS, local authorities and other allied organizations and their staff.

Very broadly, as in care provision, these new arrangements were intended to result in a more patient-led, personalized and accessible experience. A 'one-stop shop' would be created at local level to deal with complaints, and people would be supported through the process by the patient advice and liaison services (PALS; see Box 7.3). It was promised that the new arrangements would help to ensure that complaints would be used to learn lessons, and that these would result in improved and more responsive services.

Box 7.3 Patient Advice and Liaison Services (PALS)

- *NHS Plan* (2000) set out new plan for PPI as part of modernizing programme;
- designed to respond to the 2002 Bristol Royal Inquiry Report;
- provide confidential advice and support to patients, families and carers;
- information on NHS and health-related matters;
- confidential assistance on resolving problems and concerns quickly;
- information on NHS complaints procedures;
- provide a focal point for feedback from patients to inform service developments;
- provide an early warning system for monitoring trends and gaps in services and for reporting these to management.

(www.nationalarchives.gov.uk)

While structures and systems were slowly being engendered by Labour's policy developments, many other means were also used to find out what patients wanted and how they felt about their care experiences within the NHS. Chambers et al. (2009) discussed the value of engaging patients and members of the public in community research. As they explained, patient and public involvement in research was not an added extra; it was good practice (DOH, 1999; DOH, 2000; DOH, 2001; DOH, 2006f). They found that pursuing this process led to:

- an improvement in the quality of the research findings;
- research that was more ethical and respectful of participants;
- users and professionals gaining skills and experience together;
- users feeling more valued, respected and having a voice;
- users bringing energy and enthusiasm to the research.

The potential difficulties and barriers of working with patients and the public, as noted earlier, were all acknowledged. It was difficult to find, involve and engage difficult-to-reach people, and to work with an often diverse range of participants so as to reflect a variety of perspectives. It was necessary to be innovative, flexible and proactive, linking up with local groups and organizations, and in particular the PALS service and LINks.

Another means to improve services and to listen to the patients was that of 'mystery shopping' (see Box 6.4). This idea had been used to improve customer services in the retail sector for many years and was now being used within the NHS. By 2010 services delivered by dentists and pharmacies were being similarly assessed by the Consumers' Association. NHS Direct was also using mystery shoppers to monitor the efficacy of its helplines, and there was a growing awareness that some trusts were using it to monitor patient services in wards, receptions and eating areas.

Sadler (2010) reported on the South Essex Partnership University NHS Foundation Trust, which was using 140 mystery shoppers in a drive to improve their patients' experience. Trained by the Trust's Patient and Public Involvement Group, they monitored direct contact

---

Box 7.4 Work of a trained mystery shopper

- poses as a customer;
- monitors staff for politeness, helpfulness, speed of service;
- enables retailer to improve staff attitudes, the service provided and, consequently, increase sales;
- in health services, appears to take two forms:
  - ❏ volunteers posing as service users or their carers;
  - ❏ service users already undergoing treatment to provide feedback on their experience.

(Sadler, 2010)

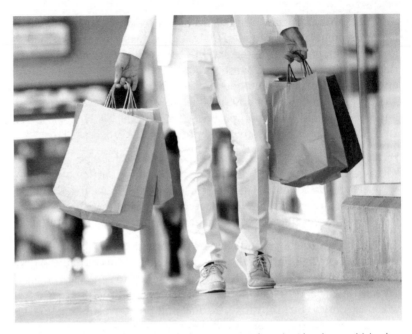

7.3 The introduction of initiatives such as 'mystery shopping' has been criticized insofar as it threatens to turn the NHS into a commercial activity.

with professionals, on wards or in telephone contact experience, the eye contact of staff during discussions of care, involvement in care plans and maintenance of dignity. All the information was collated by the PPI group, with trends noted and feedback returned to staff. This was seen as a helpful process (Sadler, 2010).

However, not everyone viewed mystery shopping in the NHS in such a positive light. Concern was expressed by ethics experts and nurse leaders about the covert methods being used. For example, the late Paul Wainwright, Professor of Nursing at St George and Kingston NHS Trust, said that the term 'mystery shopper' implied that NHS health-care was a commercial activity. He was concerned about such issues as deception, time-wasting and potential confidentiality breaches. Tom Walker, Professor of Ethics at Keele University, argued in a similar vein: that given the high value placed on honesty between clinicians and their NHS patients, carrying out practices that might undermine that trust seemed deeply problematic. Any extension of this approach would need very careful planning and open debate.

Of course, mystery shopping is only one tool for collating patient feedback. There are many different approaches. Chase Farm Hospital in Enfield, north London, for example, introduced patient-experience trackers, star charts and 'message to matron cards'. The Mid Yorkshire Hospitals NHS Trust has used real-time telephone canvassing, following up a percentage of patients after their discharge from the Trust's care.

🖹 Activity: discuss with your fellow students or colleagues

- What are your thoughts on mystery shopping being used to assess your work?
- How do you find out what patients want?
- What methods are used?
- Do you and your colleagues collect feedback and information and share it?
- If not, are you told by others what is needed?
- Have you or your patients been involved in any research exercises?

Citizen involvement in determining how the NHS is run

Attempts at re-energizing public interest and involvement were set out very clearly at the outset in 1997. Any new arrangements needed to be transparent so that they commanded public confidence. The government expected health authorities to play a strong role in communicating with local people and ensuring public involvement in decision-making about their local health services.

The rebuilding of public confidence also required more openness from health bodies, with meetings open to the public and membership on boards more representative of their local communities. The creation of the NHS Appointments Commission in 2001 was instrumental in making appointments to NHS boards a fairer and more transparent process, and in ensuring that contributors selected to serve were representative of local communities, which also added to the balanced package of skills needed around each board table.

The Healthcare Commission, also created in 2001, was made responsible for the new NHS annual health checks and was to assess the progress of organizations in 'getting the basics right' in line with research findings on patient and user views. These findings, coupled with those of the national and local patient survey programmes, were to be fed back to all trusts and PCTs so that they could identify what was needed to improve their services for patients. Linked to this, a body called the Commission for Patient and Public Involvement in Health (CPPIH) was set up to make sure that the public was involved in decision-making concerning all health services, especially in the PPI forum which existed in each NHS trust. The Commission ensured that local people and

Box 7.5 The 'basics' patients said they wanted

- good treatment in a comfortable, caring and safe environment, delivered in a calm and reassuring way;
- information to make choices, to feel confident and to feel in control;
- being talked to and listened to as an equal;
- being treated with honesty, respect and dignity.

(DOH, 2006e)

communities had a say in improving their health services. It collected and collated relevant evidence and information about these activities to share with other health organizations, in order to improve services across the NHS in line with patients' views and experiences.

2010 and onwards

By 2010 and the general election period, many developments had taken place within the NHS to change the way in which services were delivered, and efforts made to respond to patients' needs, wants and choices around NHS services, professional care and attitudes. The King's Fund (2009, 2010a) concluded that public satisfaction had increased steadily over the previous years. The total NHS patient-experience surveys had provided a great deal of helpful information on which to gauge improvements in activity. Most patients reported they had been treated with dignity and respect, but more work was needed around choice, involvement in care and some aspects of the hospital environment, including such issues as single-sex accommodation, help with feeding and the maintenance of good nutrition while in hospital.

Systematic differences in treatment, however, were found according to age, self-rated health status, ethnic group and region. The worst results came from the users of inpatient mental health services, older adults and black and minority ethnic patients. Effort and greater investment would be needed in all organizations to build on the progress to date and to create a complete and true picture of the patient experience in what looked to be growing into a very diverse, fragmented and multi-sector organization.

The analysis above reminds us all of the work that is still needed to be done. A major effort was (and is) necessary in order to encourage everyone in the population to live healthily and to take responsibility for promoting their own health and well-being as well as that of their families. This is set against the current potential of both transforming primary and community care services and the acute sector to deliver more innovative, creative and cost-effective care services in partnership with the ever-growing private and third sector organizations. The clear policy challenge for all of us working within the NHS today is to do more with less, as the financial environment hardens and difficult choices have to be made on what services can be afforded, who can have them and for how long. This debate will no doubt resonate for the foreseeable future.

As Ham (2010) aptly reminded us, the NHS needed to transform itself from a service that not only diagnosed and treated sickness, but also predicted and prevented it. It was vital that professionals and politicians engaged in an honest dialogue with the public about the changes needed and wanted. Following the general election on 6 May 2010, the inherently difficult creation of a patient and public-led NHS was passed into the hands of the new Coalition government, with Andrew Lansley as Secretary of State for Health.

The Coalition's agenda

Building and sustaining a PPI agenda in the NHS has been seen as critical to success by all recent governments in delivery of an effective and relevant service. It is a complex process, clearly requiring a careful balance between ensuring that service improvements are made and value for money achieved, and which also reflects local ownership and engagement.

Support for this agenda was clearly reiterated both in the Coalition's programme for government, *Freedom, Fairness, Responsibility* (HM Government, 2010), and then in much greater detail in its initial White Paper, *Equity and Excellence: Liberating the NHS* (DOH, 2010c). As the White Paper put it: 'It is our privilege to be custodians of the NHS, its values and principles. We believe that the NHS is an integral part of the "Big Society", reflecting the social solidarity of shared access to collective healthcare, and a shared responsibility to use resources effectively to deliver better health' (DOH, 2010c). The Coalition's vision for the NHS (as it had been in all previous governments' health White Papers) restated continued support for care free at the point of delivery, available to everyone based on need and not ability to pay. Specifically for PPI, it looked to a service genuinely centred on patients and carers, and which gave all citizens a greater say in how the NHS was run.

There would be greater efforts to make the NHS more accountable to patients and the public, who would have more choice and control, helped by easy access to the information they needed about the best GPs and hospitals. They would be in charge of making decisions themselves about their own care. Discrimination would be eliminated and inequalities reduced. Success would be measured not according to bureaucratic process targets, but against results that really matter to patients, such as improving cancer and stroke-survival rates Patients would be at the heart of everything that was done, through an 'information revolution', greater choice and control, with shared decision-making becoming the norm.

Information gained from patient and public experiences in the NHS would continue to focus activities. These included Patient Reported Outcome Measures (PROMs), patient-experience data and surveys, real-time feedback, outcome measures and national clinical audits. Comparative peer reviews between staff and an extension of the previous government's quality account system would all be used to encourage competition and provide a clear spur for boards of provider organizations to focus on improving outcomes. Importantly, nationally comparable information was to be published in a way that patients, their families and clinical teams could use to make improvements to services.

Other information would be collected to support patient choice and to increase the accountability of providers for the quality of their services. This data would focus on the following:

- Safety: levels of healthcare-associated infections, serious adverse events and avoidable deaths, broken down by providers and clinical teams.
- Effectiveness: mortality rates, emergency readmission rates and PROMs.
- Experience: information on average and maximum waiting times, opening hours and clinic times, numbers of cancelled operations, diverse measures of patient experience based on feedback from patients, families and carers.

Rights and responsibilities

In future, patients and carers would have far more clout and choice in the system and, as a result, the NHS would become more responsive to their needs and wishes. As was made very clear, however, increasing choice was not a one-way street. In return for greater choice and control, patients had to accept responsibility for the choices they made, be concordant with agreed treatment programmes and responsible for the implications of their chosen lifestyles. The notion of an individual right to care was combined with a reciprocal responsibility to behave healthily.

Extending choice

The 2010 White Paper welcomed a broader and developing remit of 'willing provider' bodies in order to extend choices in care, subject, of course, to meeting required standards and obtaining the required licence to provide care for the UK public as determined by Monitor (the new economic regulator) and also the Care Quality Commission (the quality inspectorate).

The Coalition clearly shaped the argument for patient involvement and set out a full remit of activity, but it could fall apart without full and effective public involvement. In reality, this is often difficult to achieve. The organizational strategies, structures and systems within and around the NHS may preclude the broadening and time-consuming effort required to foster effective patient involvement and a seismic change in the working relationships between professionals and patients. At the same time, the explorations of mystery shoppers and surveys, PROMs, etc., may yield helpful information, but they do not address the imbalance of power in the relationship between care-giver and receiver.

Activity: discuss with your fellow students or colleagues

- In what different ways do you as a nurse involve the patients and the public?
- How do you ensure that your organization listens to the views of all parts of the community?

- What support and resources do you need?
- How does your organization demonstrate that it values the contributions of your patients?
- Do the views of your patients change anything or do others decide what is best for them?

So is the current NHS run by the Coalition government making good progress, and has it learnt from the mistakes made by the previous governments, both Conservative and Labour? In answering this, we do need to remember that the true healthcare consumer needs to have a wide variety of options from which to choose, to be kept fully informed and involved, both in managing their care and also in shaping the services on offer. Have another look at what the user groups over time have wanted and then relate these to your own current experiences and to those patients with whom you work.

Many nurses will of course rightly defend the efforts they have made in recent years to give better care, and to give users a stronger voice in negotiating that care. They will look to developments in both role and practice, and to increasing sensitivity and ability in providing individualized care. They will point to work done and achievements made on quality assurance, as a way of demonstrating genuine concern for patient/user interests and upholding standards of care.

The issue of promoting a true consumerist approach in the NHS must, however, involve a much wider remit than 'window dressing' or 'frills and trappings'. According to Mahon (1992), any new development in user behaviour and expectation is going to take longer than a few years, and to need more than a new name to become in reality something significantly different. This would require a shift away from the notions of user centrality achieved to date, towards alternative models which explore the nature of doctor–nurse–user–patient relationships and embrace the concepts of involvement in healthcare, empowerment and advocacy. Such a shift would require radical changes in the institutional and cultural context of current healthcare provision. Importantly, in addition to this point, Griffiths (2010) reminds us that understanding and responding to user experiences is a continuing challenge that will become ever more vital as the economic challenges deepen.

An agenda for nurses: the challenge for the future

The discussion so far has come to the following broad conclusions. In many respects, all recent governments have made the users of health services central to the NHS agenda. On the one hand, it may be felt that the consumer participation offered to date is limited and, at best, indirect. It is in this contradiction that both a challenge and a risk emerge for nurses. As with 'motherhood and apple pie', everyone is likely to be in favour of increased patient voice and choice. Nurses will be no exception, as professional values and modern practice both point in the same direction of greater negotiation between nurse and user, and ever greater choice from the developing and diversifying health service of today.

If it is accepted, as proposed earlier in this chapter, that the introduction of market values to the NHS may have made access to healthcare socially more unequal, then the agenda of consumer choice today assumes a more radical dimension. Those nurses who argue that there is a link between effective user involvement and adequate resourcing are faced with the task of participating in debates around the sufficiency and redistribution of resources in the NHS. Perhaps that is the only route if you are to speak with strength and conviction on behalf of your clients, and in turn help them to become truly empowered users of the service. This will involve a desire to move into a more sharply defined political agenda. The question remains, however, whether there is sufficient confidence and desire to achieve such an objective.

Learning outcomes

- an understanding of the concept of patient and public empowerment in healthcare;
- an awareness of the different ways in which patients and the public are involved;
- an ability to question policy developments aimed at making patients and the public central to the delivery of health services.

Further reading

Goodman, B. and Clemow, R. (2008) *Nursing and Working With Other People*. Learning Matters Ltd.

Mason-Whitehead, E., McIntosh, A., Bryan, A. and Mason, T. (2008) *Key Concepts in Nursing*. Sage.

Ovretveit, J. (1997b) 'How patient power and client participation affects relations between professions', in Ovretveit, J., Mathias, P. and Thompson, T. (eds), *Interprofessional Working for Health and Social Care*. Palgrave Macmillan.

Williamson, G. R., Jenkinson, T. and Proctor-Childs, T. (2010) *Contexts of Contemporary Nursing*, 2nd edn. Learning Matters Ltd.

8 Health Policy: Building a Healthier Nation and Reducing Health Inequalities

Aims

- to demonstrate the links between policy, the promotion of health and the reduction of health inequalities;
- to discuss the developing policy agendas over time, both to promote the nation's health and to reduce health inequalities;
- to consider the current policy opportunities and challenges;
- to promote nurse involvement in the public-health and inequality agenda.

'Inequalities in health are not a new concern. We stand on the shoulders of giants from the 19th and 20th centuries in seeking solutions to the problem. . . . Doing nothing is not an economic option. The human cost is also enormous.'

(Marmot, 2010: 3)

'The NHS is admired for the equity in access to healthcare it achieves; but not for the consistency of excellence to which we aspire. Our intention is to secure excellence as well as equity.'

(DOH, 2010c)

Introduction

Improving people's health and keeping them healthy is the central work of all nurses and is a continuing major policy and professional challenge. Health as a concept has many definitions (WHO, 1946; Seedhouse, 1986; Black, 1980; Whitehead, 1987; Marmot, 2010). It is a concept with many apparently similar meanings, but the depth of perspective can vary and be viewed and described differently. It can move across a continuum from an individual, disease-focused and medicalized notion to a community and socially varied construction in which health is shaped by the wider structures and influences on our very diverse communities: the economy, the labour market, education, housing, the health services, the benefits system and the environment. The complex policy solutions proposed by succeeding governments for the effective promotion of health are often very differently designed and may or may not have relevance for our particular patients or communities, depending on time, place and circumstances.

Allied to this is the difficult challenge of reducing health inequalities – again, variously interpreted and with different policy solutions given. As a result, the nursing profession is forever faced with the challenge of applying its own defined skills, knowledge and values within the defining context of each new government's policies for the health services and for the health of the public. These policies, in turn, reflect the broader ideological and political goals of those in power, and their pursuit and achievement of 'the art of the possible' during their term of office. The political policy hoops through which we are, therefore, asked to jump may or may not be relevant and effective; they may not only fail to meet the needs of our patients, but in addition they may not meet our own professional needs or values either.

This chapter is therefore going to take us along the multifarious journey of policy efforts made by governments and health professionals over time to promote health and to equalize the opportunities for everyone to achieve a healthy life in whichever country within the UK. It is to be hoped that the lessons we note as we go along will help us:

- to reflect on the efficacy or otherwise of past policies;
- to analyse the currently developing policy focus for health and the reduction in health inequalities;
- to apply the benefit of a broader understanding of these issues for ourselves and for the people who look to professional nursing as their focus for care and support;
- to take up the challenge of promoting health and reducing health inequalities in the newly emerging healthcare environment.

🗒 Activity: discuss with your fellow students or colleagues

- What does being healthy mean for you?
- What does it mean for your patients or your local community?
- Are there people in your community who need extra help to be healthy? Who are they, and why do they need extra help?
- Are you or others able to help these people in ways that are useful?
- Are special provisions or services made available?
- Do people ever fall through the net of help in your community?

To begin at the beginning . . .

Public health has been famously defined as 'the science and art of preventing disease, prolonging life and promoting health through the organized efforts of society' (Acheson Committee, 1988). The definition reflects an emphasis on collective responsibility for health and on the prevention of disease. It recognizes the wider social and environmental causes of ill health and acknowledges the

Box 8.1 A framework to reduce health inequalities

1 Give every child the best start in life.
2 Enable all children, young people and adults to maximize their capabilities and have control over their lives.
3 Create fair employment and good work for all.
4 Ensure a healthy standard of living for all.
5 Create and develop healthy and sustainable places and communities.
6 Strengthen the role and impact of ill-health prevention.
(Marmot, 2010)

challenge of reducing health inequalities. These are seen as the product of often complex interactions between categories of deprivation and, as such, have to be tackled in innovative and 'joined-up ways' (DOH, 1999c).

'Inequalities in health arise because of inequalities in society – in the conditions in which people are born, grow, live, work and age. Taking action to reduce health inequalities does not require a separate health agenda but action across the whole society' (Marmot, 2010: 16). Reducing health inequalities and, indeed, promoting health as a generality require integrated action on six particular policy objectives (see Box 8.1). When Marmot's report was published, it was acknowledged by many that the recommendations for action would be met by protestations of unaffordability in the current economic climate. However, Marmot's response was unsurprisingly robust: 'Inaction cannot be afforded. The economic, and more importantly human costs, are simply too high!'

The stark realities of the inequalities that we face today in the UK remains herculean (*BMJ*, 2010). Marmot's review team painted a very depressing picture of England, one that could be broadly generalized across the other countries in the UK (Marmot, 2010): 'People living in the most deprived neighbourhoods will on average die 17 years earlier than people living in the richest neighbourhoods. People living in poorer areas not only die sooner, but spend more of their lives with disability – an average total difference of 17 years'. The cost implications include productivity losses of up to £33 billion a year, lost taxes and higher welfare payments of up to £32 billion, with additional healthcare costs in excess of £5.5 billion per year.

The incoming Coalition government of May 2010 thus faced the difficult task of calculating an affordable and achievable policy solution to the complex and costly equation of ever-widening health inequalities. The economic situation meant that a myriad of possible actions needed to be moulded together using existing resources and infrastructure, along with the help of voluntary groups and many private sector organizations waiting in the wings, and already very well prepared to take on the business (Booth et al., 2010a, 2010b).

📋 Activity: discuss with your fellow students or colleagues

- Are you now working with a variety of different healthcare providers?
- If so, how is this working for you, your patients and your community?

Whether or not in reality the government's intention of injecting a serious dose of private or third sector medicine into the running of the NHS – and with public health now lodged within local authorities – can make a real difference to the problems of inequality remains to be seen. That said, an exploration of attempts made by previous governments to promote the nation's health and to reduce health inequalities, both successes and failures, may provide us with some helpful reflections on the likelihood of success, or not, for the many developments currently under way (DOH, 2010c; DOH, 2010d).

Reducing health inequalities: a policy challenge for governments

Flynn (1997: 1) noted that the health problems facing the community are too urgent and too large in scale to allow complacency. Every year in Europe millions die prematurely or suffer ill health from serious conditions that could have been prevented. At the same time health systems throughout the [European] Community are coming under increasing strain as a result of the mounting demands being made upon them and the difficult financial situation that member states are facing. The pressures of having to cope with rapidly changing medical technology, with an ageing population, with ever-growing needs for health care and social support, and with people's constantly rising expectations about health services are therefore forcing member states to take sweeping measures to reform their health systems and to control costs.

A decade on, Graham (2007: 161) commented that at both national and international level, the past three decades have seen major developments in public health policy. The traditional concern with improving overall levels of health has given way to a broader policy vision. This broader vision commits national governments and international agencies to tackling health inequalities. For these reasons, the international community has agreed that 'all governments must tackle poor health and inequalities as a matter of urgency' (WHO, 2005: 4).

Marmot (2010) believes that the central ambition is to create the conditions for people to take control over their own lives where people have an equal freedom to flourish.

Over the past decades successive UK governments have not been immune to such concerns and challenges. Policy responses have emphasized a more broadly based public health, community-wide perspective (Greenwood, 2009) This reflects an acknowledgement that (i) attention weighted heavily in favour of secondary and tertiary healthcare services (acute and chronic), as opposed to the primary care sector and health promotion, is a limited and certainly costly way of meeting the increasing complexity and levels of demand created by the ever-growing UK population; and (ii) the promotion of the nation's health can succeed only if proper attention is given to the wider environmental, social, political, economic and individual determinants of health. This needs to be combined with action to increase awareness amongst the population of the impacts on their health, with support to respond and to address any adverse heath outcomes.

As Baggott (1994) put it, 'the many challenges facing health systems and governments require a much broader approach than simply expanding health services'. Adshead and Behan (2007) note also that it is now widely recognized that the health service alone can neither reduce health inequalities nor achieve good public health. Greenwood (2009) concurs with this, arguing that the NHS cannot fund or supply everything, and that we need to work with others to ensure that health promotion becomes everyone's business. Wanless (2002) referred to this as creating a 'fully engaged' scenario. We all have to play our part, both as nurses and citizens.

How we will achieve this fully engaged scenario is clearly a matter for debate – not just for the government and politicians, but for everyone. We are all policy-makers and shapers and we can all make a difference, but it may prove to be a difficult road, already littered with failed ideas and failed policies. As Marmot colourfully put it: 'If you would like the experience of banging your head against a wall I suggest you go out and tell people to behave better' (see Ford, 2010).

This agenda clearly needs a much wider societal response. It needs a listening government, the creation of a serious and wide-ranging policy package, a constructively critical health professional response and a 'fully engaged scenario' within the population. Promoting the nation's health and reducing health inequalities are too important for party politics, professional rivalries and simplistic policy solutions. A right for all to be healthy has to be balanced with a reciprocal responsibility and effort to make it happen. To date, there is still much work to do and many lessons still to be learnt from past experiences.

📋 Activity: discuss with your fellow students or colleagues

- Is the government listening to the views of the nursing profession? What is being said about this in the nursing press?
- Are you able to provide the care which is needed both for your patients and for your community?
- If yes – how do you know?
- If no – what are the barriers?

Historical developments

The promotion of the nation's health as a policy objective in this country is not a modern idea. Considerable progress had been made even before the well-reported sanitary revolution of the nineteenth century. Quarantine facilities and basic programmes to care for the sick within their own communities had been in evidence for a long time (Fraser, 1973). The upheavals of the Industrial Revolution and the creation of immense social problems, however, provided the impetus for a more developed collective approach to caring for the public's health, with the provision over time of clean water, sewage systems, street lighting, better housing and immunization (Ashton et al., 1988; Webster, 2002). If industry, and thus the economic base of the country, were to be thriving and healthy, it was imperative that those who worked to make it happen were fit to play their part. As the Royal Sanitary Commission stated in 1871, 'the constant relation between the health and vigour of the people and the welfare and commercial prosperity of the state requires no argument . . . public health is public wealth' (cited in Fraser, 1973).

It is worth noting that in the 1890s public expenditure in the UK represented less than 10 per cent of gross domestic product (GDP), of which nearly half was for military and war-related expenditure (Le Grand, 1982). As Graham (2007) noted, the government in the nineteenth century played only a minimal role in regulating the workings of the economy and there was little publicly funded welfare provision, either in cash (e.g., welfare benefits and state pensions) or in kind (e.g., healthcare and education) – benefits that are currently available within the UK and which 'consume about a third of public spending, with education and health taking the lion's share' (Sefton, 2002; www.ukpublicspending.co.uk).

It was, however, increasingly accepted by succeeding governments during the nineteenth and early twentieth centuries that there was a growing need for government policy to intervene in people's lives and to enhance individual efforts to be healthy. Without a doubt, the 40 per cent rejection on medical grounds of young male applicants who wished to be recruited for active service in South Africa in the Boer War at the turn of the century helped to initiate the subsequent growth in governmental policy interventions in healthcare (Fraser, 1973) The 1919 Health Act charged the Minister of Health with taking all such steps as were desirable to secure the preparation, effective carrying out and coordination of measures conducive to the health of the people.

Policies introduced by the government emphasized the prevention of illness and the promotion of health. Both themes were clearly of great importance at this stage. Activities introduced ranged widely. We see the creation of infectious disease hospitals, new general hospitals and special services for pregnant women, mothers, babies and schoolchildren (Baly, 1995). There was also extensive involvement in wider environmental factors, including housing and food hygiene which, it was accepted , similarly affected the health of the population (Williamson et al., 2010).

Monitoring, recording, surveillance and generally keeping track of the public's health status had become a major preoccupation for policy-makers (Pike and Forster, 1995). The determinants of health were seen to be complex and multifaceted and, as such, the clear remit and responsibility of an increasingly interested central government. The proportion of public expenditure devoted to welfare benefits and services rose slowly during the early decades. Nevertheless, wide gaps still remained in the provision of health and social care (Baggott, 2007).

Creating the post-war 'fit land for heroes to live in'

After the Second World War, many questions were raised about all previous governments' policies and broken promises, providing the catalyst for a new post-war creation – the welfare state. It reflected a multi-party response to the health and social care needs of the population, and was accepted by many as a necessary and correct focus for government policy. People needed to be helped to health, particularly in the control of those factors over which they could exercise little influence. For example, the high unemployment levels in the 1920s and 1930s and the resultant poverty and ill health were factors which only the development of a healthy economic and industrial base could heal (Webster, 2002). (It was in 1918, at the end of the First World War, that Prime Minister David Lloyd George promised that his government would make Britain 'a fit land for heroes to live in', an emotive phrase that is again being used by the charity Help for Heroes in its efforts to raise money for soldiers and their families involved in the wars in Iraq and Afghanistan.)

The creation of the welfare state

Sir William Beveridge's plan to fight the so-called giants of want, ignorance, disease, idleness and squalor provided a strategy to shape and control those powerful determinants of the health of the public (Beveridge, 1942). Financial benefits, state education, public housing initiatives, employment opportunities and a national health service were collective policy responses aimed at meeting the health needs of the whole population – helping individuals to be healthy and, as a result, creating a healthy nation. This was a clear re-run of the Royal Sanitary Commission's stated aim in 1871 (Fraser, 1973).

This wide-ranging policy response to health and social care needs received much popular support. The National Health Service, along with the other structures of the welfare state, was part of the great collective enterprise made up of several branches across government aimed at equalizing opportunities for all individuals to be healthy. But not everyone was enthusiastic. For example, strong opposition to a national health service came from many members of the medical profession (Foot, 1973). Aneurin Bevan, the Minister for Health, was forced to make political concessions to this very powerful group in order that the plan for the NHS could be implemented in 1948.

As Graham (2007) explained, in spite of dissenting voices there was a general acceptance that such interventionist economic and social policies were unavoidable. The previously unregulated markets had not delivered the employment conditions and the welfare services that rich economies like the UK needed in order to grow, and that their populations needed in order to prosper. More active government control of the economy was, therefore, one part of the consensus; the other was better collective mechanisms to enable people to 'fare well' across their lives – the welfare state would be the means to this end.

As part of this collective public health approach, the new NHS aimed:

- to provide medical care free at the point of need;
- to provide an equitable distribution of healthcare services across the country;
- to provide services accountable to the public and to the nation as a whole;
- to promote a sense of collective purpose or mission;
- to promote the health of the nation.

1948: acute hospital care takes centre stage

Although government policy was focused on a broad public health agenda, exemplified by the creation of the five arms of the welfare state, NHS care appeared to take more of a sickness service than a health service stance. The focus for professional care from that point onwards was shaped by, and pulled into, a narrower, increasingly powerful hospital-based and medically defined illness framework. It was a situation which would continue for many decades.

Public health, primary and community care and general practice were side-lined and clearly viewed as the poor relations at the side of the ever developing, ever more expensive and powerful acute hospital sector. During the 1950s and 1960s care outside hospital acquired a Cinderella-like reputation, reflecting in particular the disproportionate amount of NHS funds spent on increasingly expensive hospital treatments and buildings. The promotion of health and prevention of illness did not appear to be a serious policy agenda and attracted much less attention and financial backing.

This position was to change by the early 1970s, reflecting as it did a response to national economic problems facing the UK. Public spending on welfare came under massive scrutiny, not least for its 25 per cent slice of the public expenditure cake. The Butskellite consensus on welfare spending was now falling apart. The NHS was not immune, and ways of reducing the burden of expenditure on healthcare delivery were being sought right across the service. The shift in focus in favour of a stronger health-promoting policy agenda from central government was one solution amongst many – an agenda which was to grow and develop from that point onwards. It was clearly believed that savings could be made if people took individual responsibility for their own health and, in turn, avoided the need for expensive hospital care and treatments.

The 1970s: a policy for health begins to grow and develop

This decade witnessed a period of economic crisis, and successive governments were forced to re-examine their levels of public expenditure. Orthodoxy determined that efforts be made to reduce public spending, but at the same time to create new ways of providing public services such as healthcare in a politically acceptable and more cost-effective way than hitherto. Baggott (1994) noted the increased recognition that the burden of illness in modern societies required more than a narrow medicalized response. The invigoration of the primary care setting, together with a new agenda for health, offered the government a way forward.

Discussion revolved around the need for each individual to take responsibility for his or her own health, and to play a stronger part in preventing the rising levels of heart disease, accidents, alcoholism, mental illness, smoking, diet- and drug-related diseases (DHSS, 1976). However, the White Paper (Command 7047, 1977) which followed seemed fairly half-hearted in its intention of delivering a new health and primary care-focused shift in policy. While it certainly demonstrated an interest in a strategy for improving health and in encouraging the public to become more responsible for their own health status, it did not appear to want to shift resources away from the curative hospital settings. While the public clearly still loved the NHS, as exemplified by the hospitals and acute care, it was seen as a political minefield to try to reduce or shift resources or focus away to primary care and a real development in public health initiatives.

1979: new agendas for health

By 1979, and with the election of a new Conservative government, previous unwillingness to challenge and change the powerful and increasingly costly hospital sector was put aside. The new government believed that the primary care sector, based around general practice, had the potential – if reformed and sharpened – to reduce the ever-rising cost of hospital services. It was on a serious mission to control and manage professional care, to pursue activities that provided value for money and, most importantly, to increase the public's responsibility for promoting their own health – a theme which continues today.

Developments in the 1980s

The government's continuing need – and, indeed, its desire – to reduce public expenditure across all the boundaries of welfare state provision,

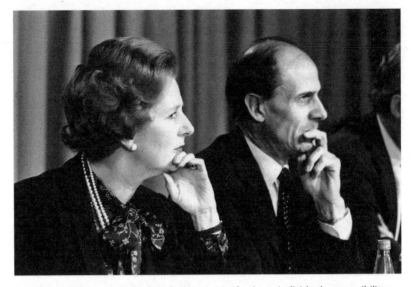

8.1 The 1979 government placed a strong emphasis on individual responsibility – an attitude epitomized by figures such as Norman Tebbit and Margaret Thatcher.

including healthcare, was the prime motive for change during the 1980s. While a more business-like and competitive environment was created in the NHS as a whole, at the same time users and potential users were encouraged more strongly than ever to take greater individual responsibility for their own health.

All practitioners were concerned to promote health education, and they were encouraged to provide the population with sufficient information and advice to pursue healthy lifestyles. Responsibility then rested with each individual to make his or her own health choices, particularly with regard to diet, exercise, smoking, sexual activity and alcohol – even including advice from the then Employment Secretary Norman Tebbit, in response to a question from a Young Conservative, that the unemployed should 'get on their bikes and find a job'.

The Black Report

The Black Report, published in 1980, provided research evidence to show there was a link between inequalities in income and other resources and poor health. It made many recommendations to reduce inequalities and to improve the general standard of health in Britain, including more support for families and young children via tax changes and increased child benefits, a greater emphasis on community care and an improvement in GP services.

The broader social measures called for by the report, rather than specific improvements to the acute health services, infuriated the newly installed Conservative government (Mihill, 1993). Unsurprisingly, it failed to change the government's belief that all individuals could change their lifestyles for the better if they wanted, given enough information – each person was seen as ultimately totally responsible for his or her own health status. The wider determinants of health as proposed in Black's findings were believed to be the responsibility of individuals and their families, and not that of the government.

🖹 Activity: discuss with your fellow students or colleagues

- Is it really possible for everyone to take responsibility for his or her own health if given the right information?
- Can everyone 'get on their bikes and find a job'? What are the positives and negatives of doing this?

Looking to general practice: a new focus for health

During the late 1980s, increasing government interest in reducing public expenditure and in providing more effective and cost-efficient healthcare resulted in a change of focus for healthcare delivery. General practice and the primary healthcare team were favoured (DOH, 1987), perceived as a less costly option than hospital care, and also as providing an opportunity (if its gatekeeper role were sharpened up) to reduce public expenditure on healthcare even further. Combined with this was the role to be played by GPs in encouraging health promotion. A new contract for general practitioners (DOH, 1989c) included the requirement to provide this, as well as to continue to work with the secondary and tertiary services.

A cost-cutting move or a serious attempt at promoting health?

The apparent empowerment of general practice at this stage, together with support for a more positive health agenda than hitherto, was, on the face of it, suggestive of a fresh look by government in response to the developing health problems in the UK of the 1980s (NAO, 1989). However, although the trend towards a more health-promotional policy agenda seemed to be pointing in the right direction, some reached a different conclusion: that this response was both economically and ideologically driven and actually reflected other goals (Soothill et al., 1992; Gough et al., 1994; Hart, 1994). For these critics, the intended impact of the managerial and structural reforms of the NHS during this period was to limit rather than to expand NHS activities, responsibilities and expenditure. The extra attention seemingly being given to general practice and to health-promotional activity were means to other ends, namely:

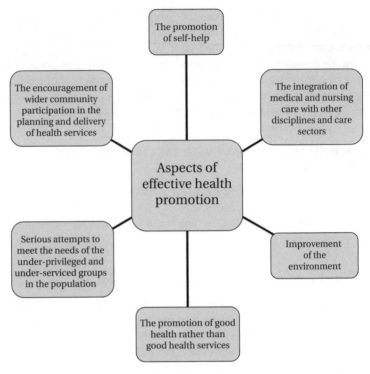

Source: WHO, 1978

Figure 8.1 Fundamental aspects of effective health promotion

- to reduce the power of the hospital sector and implicitly that of the professional bodies, especially the medical profession;
- a developing attempt to reduce public expenditure and slowly remove the state's responsibility for providing healthcare services;
- to reinforce the intention of making the public increasingly responsible for its own health and well-being – not least by emphasizing the importance of individual choice and implying a sort of consumer-style relationship in using and accessing healthcare.

Many concluded that these potentially negative forces at play underpinning the government's apparently new-found interest in public health were clearly reflected in the limited nature of its understanding of the received wisdom about the concepts of health promotion and primary care. Ashton and Seymour (1988), for example, outlined the expected breadth of activity as defined by the World Health Organization (WHO, 1978). The policy agenda of the government did not at that stage encompass all these facets (see Figure 8.1), although it certainly provided a starting point to the activities which are now commonplace (if not always successful) in today's primary care environment.

It was argued by many critical observers that the government's policy did not reflect an appropriate or serious response to reducing health inequalities and to those who had the least resources, as had been emphasized by the 1980 Black report. Instead, it emphasized self-help and seemed less interested in collective responses to health needs. Its proposed strategy for implementation appeared to fail to recognize the formal and informal care roles of other professionals, organizations and individuals working outside the NHS. The notion of multidisciplinary working across a broad multi-sectoral network of providers across the community still had a long way to go. As Baggott (1994: 210) described it: 'The government's primary care reforms have concentrated on the NHS, and in particular on the family practitioner services, as the principal means of improving primary care.' In spite of government protestations to the contrary, it did seem that the policy ignored important aspects of the World Health Organization view of what was needed to implement a broad, relevant and achievable vision for primary care activity: 'The key to solving many health problems lies outside the health sector or in the hands of people themselves – in order to meet contemporary challenges to health, it is necessary for all elements of society to contribute' (WHO, 1978) – a theme that is currently widely promoted (DOH, 2010c, 2010d).

📋 Activity: discuss with your fellow students or colleagues

- What progress has been made to date in delivering the health-promoting primary care agenda as defined by the World Health Organization?
- Do many of the health problems you and your patients face lie outside your professional remit?
- Are you involved in promotional health activity with other professionals and sectors outside the NHS?

Barriers to change

While government policy suggested a new focus for the promotion of public health, the powerful reality of the acute hospital sector still remained a political barrier to change. It needed to be further challenged and made to conform – in particular, the medical profession itself. The earlier introduction of general management in 1984 following the Griffiths Management Inquiry of 1983 had made some inroads at last into the medically led bastions of the acute hospital sector. However, further reform would be needed to push the balance more strongly in favour of primary care and general practice.

The NHS in the 1980s continued to stress secondary and tertiary interventions at the expense of a true public health approach. The promotion of health still remained a relative sideshow to the developing business of NHS hospital care organization, provision and general management. This was not really a surprise. After all, high-tech medical interventions in a 'white-hot' hospital setting had, since the beginning of the NHS, been perceived by the public, professionals and politicians alike as evidence and proof of a successful health service, fit for a highly developed society and nation. Forty years of NHS policy and several different governments had reinforced a structure, organization and culture which was illness-based and costly.

The NHS post-1989: illness or health promoter?

The first review of the NHS for 40 years (DOH, 1989c), coupled with that of community care (DOH, 1989a), led to the enactment of the NHS and Community Care Act in June 1990. The reforms involved, as noted elsewhere in this book, profound changes in the structure, organization and management of the NHS. While the government claimed that these changes provided the chance 'to focus on health as much as healthcare', others disagreed. Some argued that the government had not been concerned to explore and respond seriously to broader heath and social care needs, or indeed to harness other sector care activities in an effort to respond to health needs and inequalities.

The review was about hospitals, general practice and ill people, and not about a positive health agenda and all that this might imply. The review's conclusions were thus seen as a partial diagnosis and prescription and a lost chance for promoting a seriously positive effort to deal with the increasingly widening health gap between richer and poorer individuals in society. As Harrison et al. (1989) explained: 'The diagnosis, it can be argued, is rather narrow and pays scant regard to wider issues including the persistence of health inequalities and the level of preventable illness.' Others argued that the review continued to see the NHS as a national hospital and illness service with its title, *Working for Patients*, reflecting semantically and, in reality, a lack of commitment to health promotion and preventative activity (Community Outlook, 1989). Goodwin (1989) believed the review was not 'much interested in health as such; health promotion was only mentioned once in passing as one of the responsibilities of health authorities, but with no clue as to how that responsibility would be expressed in service terms'. Community care was not discussed, and public health was referred to only briefly.

The Royal College of Nursing said the government in its policy review 'was looking up the wrong end of a telescope, and should be concentrating its attention not on acute care, but on services for the large and rising numbers of elderly people and on the promotion of good health' (Editorial, 1989) Accusations flew around and dismay was expressed because the NHS continued to be equated with hospital care and general practice. The total focus appeared to be on illness and treatment, while other positive health agendas and efforts to ensure that everyone in the population 'fared well' (Graham, 2007) were seemingly ignored.

Large groups in the population, for example the elderly and those with learning and physical difficulties, appeared not to merit special mention. No overtly positive health agenda was addressed, presumably because it was not seen as the business of the NHS at that time. The apparent emphasis appeared to be on directing resources to services for ill people, rather than at true health-promotional work and the reduction in health inequality.

The NHS review and subsequent Act (DOH, 1989c) created new market-like structures and business-like aims and objectives, and further reinforced the limited medicalized concept of health which had underpinned much NHS activity over time. Far from opening up into the wider fields of social and environmental health, the NHS appeared to be pulled back more than ever into a medical and illness service. While some of the descriptive language in the White Paper emphasized the opposite, the detail within it and the subsequent working papers (DOH, 1989b) probably provided a truer picture of policy intentions.

Doctors, acute medical services and hospitals were placed centre stage, with nurses and a wider positive public health agenda essentially ignored. Nurses working within the NHS, and potentially involved in health-promotional work, were limited to those aspects that were seen as within the scope of their nursing roles. The need for nurse managers both to qualify and to quantify allowable activities, linked to budget constraints, often precluded more innovative and expansive activity within the wider care community. This was irrespective of the degree of demonstrated relevance or necessity of reducing health inequalities or of promoting health (Fatchett, 1994). Spending on the more conservative and easily measurable aspects of healthcare delivery and outcome was clearly preferable to, for example, spending on traveller and gypsy healthcare or work with the unemployed. It is against this particular backcloth that we can now briefly look at yet another White Paper – *The Health of the Nation* (Command 1986, 1992), supposedly another serious attempt at promoting the nation's health.

The Health of the Nation, 1992

The publication of this health White Paper was, according to the government minister, a landmark for the NHS and the next logical step in the healthcare reforms which the government had introduced in the 1980s. Many commentators again welcomed the new stress on the promotion of health and, although acknowledging the importance of working at the five key target areas for action – cancer, heart disease and stroke, mental illness, HIV/AIDS and sexual diseases, and accidents – were disappointed that the emphasis was on preventing specific illnesses, rather than addressing the broader determinants of health. Concern was expressed at the failure to address the important issues of poverty, inequality, unemployment and poor housing. As one critic said, the White Paper was based on simplistic ill-health targets (albeit important), but did not address the underlying issues of poverty and deprivation (Kearney, in Mihill, 1992).

The White Paper appeared to offload the responsibility for controlling the wider social determinants of health onto others, many of whom did not work with or under the NHS umbrella. While accepting then that health-promotion activity belonged to many other areas and personnel, the policy strategy could never bring about all the improvements it said it wanted, without a commitment from all other government departments to tackle the complex and wider issues of poverty and inequality – including the requisite financial support.

As Buttigieg said, 'to make real progress we need an economy based on employment, proper childcare, good housing and support for single parents' (cited in Mason 1993). However, the continuing emphasis by the government on individual, as opposed to collective, action and its clear monetarist approach to healthcare did not bode well in this respect. Sir Douglas Black, chairman of the 1980 report on health inequalities, referred stingingly to the government's policies as a deliberate and reckless route back to the 'social evils of the thirties' (Black, 1980).

The health strategy, although presented in very glossy and attractive packaging, lacked real details for action, specific and clear financial backing and thus, in effect, any really serious intent for delivery (Butler, 1997). The policy push for a health-promotional framework for NHS activity seemed to remain as a relative sideshow to other more pressing policy imperatives around the vagaries, failures and continuing emphasis on illness services.

Rather than providing a positive health policy backcloth to the internal market reforms, it was described as a fig-leaf behind which a dismantling of the NHS was slowly beginning to take place, to become an even more limited medical illness service (Black, 1980; Fatchett, 1998). In addition, the apparent diminution in role, decreased training opportunities and increased experience of redundancy for many with traditional health-promoting roles – school nurses, health visitors, learning disability and mental health nurses – all gave cause for concern.

The government's view

Within the UK in the 1980s and 1990s, the Conservative governments' health policy concerns had broadly revolved around management and organizational reform, underpinned, they argued, by the creation of a policy for health. This claim was reiterated by the Conservative government in all subsequent health policy initiatives. It argued that the successful delivery of healthcare required a vision for healthcare services clearly placed in a wider context. Health policy was not to be just about delivering an illness service, but also about improving the nation's health in the very broadest sense.

In spite of the many accusations to the contrary, the government claimed that the 1992 White Paper, *The Health of the Nation*, had set out a strategy which adopted a much broader vision for improving the population's health than that of the acute hospital and allied settings. The NHS was to be at the centre of the strategy, but other organizations, every department in Whitehall, private companies and voluntary bodies, local authorities, health authorities, employers, trades unions and individuals of every age were encouraged to become involved. The aim was to provide new opportunities to raise sights beyond the acute provision of healthcare – important though it was – to the pursuit of health. The priorities for promoting health set out in the 1992 White Paper needed to become everybody's business and not just that of the NHS

According to many, however, by the time Labour took over from the Conservatives in 1997, a large group of people were 'needing to be helped to health' (Brindle, 1997; Chadda, 1998). There was still much work to do, not least in reducing health inequalities. While useful attention had been focused on key areas for service improvement, these had had little impact on service delivery or general health (Williamson et al., 2010).

Changes in structure and organization and a developing policy interest in diversifying and developing a health-focused agenda for the population in order to reduce health inequalities was to become the responsibility of the new government in May 1997. Sadly, these would remain a thorn in the side of New Labour, first under Tony Blair and then, much later, under Gordon Brown.

Another look at public health?

After 18 years in opposition, Prime Minister Tony Blair's speech to the Labour Party Conference at Brighton in October 1997 set out his vision for government. The constant repetition of certain words provided us with a flavour of policies to come: Britain, British, country, nation, people, modernize, change, reform, hard choices, duty, vision, compassion, giving. As one editor put it, Blair was for compassion, but compassion with a hard edge. 'Hard choices' was a barely concealed code for cuts and a shift from public to private provision, from funding provision of services to organizing services. There were to be no magic wands or instant answers (Editorial, 1997). The need to live within budget was all about delivering an affordable vision. The Department of Health, like other public spending departments, was in for a very firm financial ride.

By 1998 emphasis was again being placed on the importance of health promotion and public health (DOH, 1998b). It was acknowledged that although health generally had improved, far too many people were still falling ill and dying sooner than they should. The importance of the NHS acute sector was acknowledged as vital in

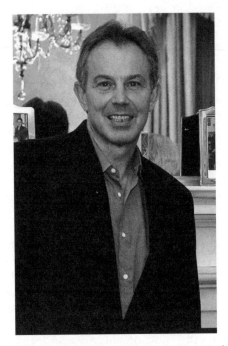

8.2 From 1997, Tony Blair's New Labour government attempted to shift the agenda towards the reduction of health inequalities.

providing much-needed treatment and care for people when ill, but it was perceived as providing only a partial response in meeting the very complex health needs of the population.

More effort was needed to stop people becoming ill in the first place and to tackle the root causes of avoidable illness. This was to include a change in individual lifestyles, combined with government action on those things which damaged people's health, but were often outside their control: air pollution, poverty, low wages, unemployment, poor housing, and crime and disorder. In a sense, the government was emphasizing and proposing a policy for health, rather than a policy for further expanding the acute health sector and an illness agenda.

This apparent shift in health policy towards a much broader public health response was welcomed by many nurses, not least because it appeared to support a much more balanced approach, by combining health-promotion activity with both secondary and tertiary care. At the same time, there was also a degree of cynicism. As noted earlier, if any policy is to be implemented in a serious manner, it needs the financial backing to make it happen and the appropriate people available to carry it through (Butler, 1997). The earlier experiences of school nurses, health visitors, mental health and learning disability nurses of role constraint, diminution and loss in previous years had not left people's memories – and should not do so today either.

Would New Labour do any better?

The New Labour government of 1997 gave all the appearances of revitalizing the policy commitment to a strong public health agenda and to a reduction in health inequalities. Soon after its electoral success, New Labour established the Independent Inquiry into Inequalities in Health (1988) chaired by Sir Donald Acheson. Following this work, there were many subsequent policy initiatives around the promotion of health and the reduction of inequalities. Early policy proposals were set out in a consultation paper, *Our Healthier Nation* (DOH, 1998b). Its two stated main aims were:

1 To improve the health of the population as a whole, by increasing the length of people's lives and the number of years people spend free from illness.
2 To improve the health of the worst off in society and to narrow the health gap, to reduce the well-evidenced inverse care law (Dorling, 2010) and to reduce the persistent and widening health inequalities between rich and poor within the population.

New Labour's 'Third Way'

In order to fulfil these important aims, the government announced a new approach to the delivery of health policy. It wished to pursue what it called 'a third way'. On the one hand, it wished to avoid the difficulties faced by individuals if they were left to take total responsibility for their own health. This had been impossible for many, as was found in pre-NHS times. On the other hand, New Labour wished to avoid the situation whereby the NHS took over people's lives and health, becoming the so-called 'nanny-state' provider.

The 'third way' involved the creation of a national contract for better health, which was set out in the later White Paper, *Saving Lives: Our Healthier Nation* (DOH, 1999d). It was the first government health strategy document to acknowledge a link between poverty and ill health – well-evidenced knowledge, of course, that could have been acted upon much earlier if the Conservative government had implemented the recommendations of the Black Report back in 1980.

Under New Labour's 'third way' contract, the government, local communities and individuals were required to become active partners in improving the nation's health. It promised a broad and pan-government departmental response, so that the breadth of the proposed vision for health could be realized (DOH, 2003b). Activities for its successful implementation would involve a number of important contributions:

• the government would help assess the risks to health and provide information to people which would be accurate, understandable and credible;

- health authorities would have a key role in pursuing and leading local alliances to develop programmes for health improvement;
- local authorities would have a duty to promote the economic, social and environmental well-being of their area;
- private sector businesses would be responsible for improving the health and safety of their employees;
- voluntary bodies were to act as advocates to give a powerful voice for local people;
- individuals would take much greater responsibility for their own health.

Three settings for action were outlined to focus and to develop the health contract in a structured way:

1 In schools: to focus on children and young people.
2 In workplaces: to focus on adults.
3 In neighbourhoods: to focus on older people.

In this way, attention would be given across the entire age range, from childhood to older adulthood. According to the government, 'if individuals do their bit by following a healthy lifestyle, employers promote healthier workforces, and the NHS and town halls provide more equal services and better housing, the government will tackle unemployment and other causes of social exclusion and inequality' (DOH, 2003b).

At the same time, the aim was to reduce mortality rates from the major killer diseases by 2010. Four priority illness areas were selected for action, setting clear targets for improvement year by year up to 2010:

- heart disease and stroke;
- accidents;
- cancer;
- mental ill health – to reduce the death rate from suicide and undetermined injury.

It was argued that rather than have a long list of ill-health targets, as in earlier policy documents, this strategy would be simpler. In this way, all local healthcare agencies would be encouraged to set their own targets, reflecting more specifically the assessed health needs of their own localities.

The 'third way'

The main theme underpinning the 'third way' approach to improving the public's health was a reduction in the persistent health inequality gap between the rich and poor (DOH, 1999c; Nazroo, 2009). As noted by Boseley (1998), policy was pledged to tackle big social issues – poverty, bad housing, unemployment and other forms of deprivation – all factors acknowledged to be at the root of inequalities in health. Indeed, the policy was aimed at helping to improve the health of the most deprived at a rate faster than the overall national rate of improvement in health (DOH, 1999a). It promised a broad and pan-government departmental response so that the breadth of the proposed vision for health could be realized (DOH, 2003b).

Local authorities, for example, were required to work in partnership with the NHS to plan for health improvement by the creation of Health Action Zones, Health Improvement Programmes and also Healthy Living Centres (*Nursing Times,* 1999). The themes, targets and focus on health, and the reduction in health inequalities were again further developed in other subsequent government papers: *The NHS Plan* (2000), *Tackling Health Inequalities: A Programme for Action* (2003) and *Choosing Health: Making Healthier Choices Easier* (2004). The 2004 Public Health White Paper aimed to build on all the previous initiatives. It was based on the principle that the NHS should improve health and prevent disease, not just provide treatment for those who are ill. It acknowledged that a far greater effort was still needed to refocus NHS sights on tackling the wider causes of ill-health and inequalities.

Consultations with the public had found that people did want to take responsibility for their own health, but that they expected the government to help them in making their choices . . . not to make decisions for them, but to provide them with clear information. They wanted personalized help which was tailored to individual needs and circumstances, and was provided flexibly and conveniently. It was understood that individual responses to making progress in improving public health were important, but insufficient in the round. Real progress depended on the development of effective partnerships across communities (see Figure 8.2). People looked to government to lead, coordinate and promote these partnerships and had an expectation that all players would take their health and the health of their families seriously and would be prepared to engage constructively in a shared effort (DOH, 2004f).

Subsequent actions proposed and developed

Efforts were made to encourage whole local economy working to ensure that public health messages would become part of the day-to-day experience of all users of health and social care services. A number of programmes reflected this approach across many communities:

1   The integrated planning and delivery of public health messages in schools through an enhanced school nursing service. This was to include the universal delivery of the National Healthy Schools project combined with the use of personal health guides for young people, and accessible information and support for teaching staff, parents and carers (DOH, 2004f).
2   A change in the focus of health visiting and other child health services through Sure Start children's centre activities, Healthy Home

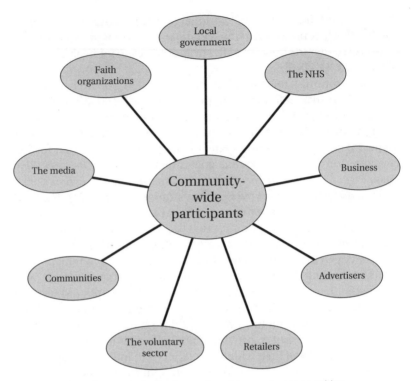

Figure 8.2 Development of effective partnerships across communities

Start programmes, home volunteer visiting programmes for families under stress (HM Government, 2004).

3   Building local community health capacity through health development activities (Fatchett, 2000).

4   Ensuring that pockets of deprivation were considered when practice-led and other commissioning decisions were being developed and implemented.

5   The implementation of the recommendations of the *Improving Working Lives Standards* (DOH, 2000a) as a focus for enhancing staff well-being. This reflected a developing recognition that better public health involves promoting the health of NHS staff through improved occupational health activities.

6   A wide-ranging agenda for good nutrition and healthy eating was developed, especially in response to the growing epidemic of obesity:

  •   Health Direct: to provide easily accessible and confidential information on healthy food choices, diets and good nutrition.
  •   Healthy Start: from 2005 a scheme to provide disadvantaged pregnant women and mothers of young children with vouchers for fresh food and vegetables, milk and infant formula.
  •   Partnerships with industry, e.g. with the food producers and retail sectors: these included encouragement to contribute to

the funding of national healthy-eating campaigns and initiatives to promote positive health information and education around nutritional issues.

- Information supplied to the media by the NHS so that health messages reached a wider audience via television, radio, journals, websites and the press.

Underpinning this attempt both to diversify the public-health messages and also to encourage partnership working were a number of other important developments. The collection of health information and evidence was aimed to achieve real-time health surveillance. New public health 'observatories' were to develop and implement a comprehensive public health information and intelligence strategy (Donaldson, 2010). This was to be used to provide the information and research evidence to support cost-effective interventions to improve health, inform commissioning of services, and improve the practice of frontline staff. Increased funding was made available for public health research and NICE appointed an Executive Director for Health Improvement to provide professional leadership in delivering public health right across the NHS and partner organizations.

📋 Activity: do this with your fellow students or colleagues

- Check out your local Health Observatory and see what current health information is available about your community.
- Is there any helpful health promotional material which you might use with your patients?

The public health White Paper was described as a landmark document. It acknowledged that the NHS could be only part of a programme to improve public health and could not solve all health-related problems. It had set out a genuine cross-governmental, multi-sectoral approach to public health, pushing it towards the top of priorities across the whole spectrum of government. It reflected an understanding and acceptance that the origins of most poor health lie deep within society, and that there was a need for these to be tackled through broad-based strategies predicated on strong and effective partnerships across whole communities. It was described as the next step in tackling health inequalities and 'the beginning of a journey to build health into Government policy and ensure health is everybody's business' (DOH, 2004a).

A positive development for nurses?

As Billingham (1989) put it, this new focus would ensure that public health was firmly embedded within the fundamentals of good nursing practice. The success of the White Paper's goals was dependent upon the commitment of all nursing and midwifery professionals. They were expected to maximize their contacts with patients, clients and local communities to create health-promoting opportunities wherever they worked, be it in acute care, mental health, homes, surgeries or hospitals. The aim would be to make improving health a core part of all nurse and midwifery everyday practice – a fundamental part of care. New training and professional development modules were to support effective practice to develop public health capacity right across all nursing and midwifery disciplines.

📋 Activity: discuss with your fellow students or colleagues

- Are wider public health activities of relevance to your professional work?
- Is your current work imbued with a health-promoting focus?
- Are you encouraged and supported to introduce health-promoting activity into your daily work? If so, how?
- Do you think it is making a difference?

Subsequent Labour government health policy continued and developed the wider themes of public health and reduction in health inequalities, and also set out the clear intention for community services to take centre stage in the health and social care system of the future. It was accepted that people would always want a good hospital service, but that this resource should not continue to be used as the focus for routine NHS care in the future. The NHS juggernaut was being carefully steered towards general practice, a much stronger public health approach and care closer to home. The 2006 White Paper (*Our Health, Our Care, Our Say*) emphasized all these themes and set out its policy expectations. What was needed included:

- a shift of care out of hospital to appropriate care closer to home where the overwhelming majority of contacts with the health service would take place;
- the provision of services that fitted around the lives people wanted to lead and that were fair to all, with 'more choice and a stronger voice' for individuals and communities;
- care in environments that supported each individual's physical and mental well-being;
- frontline local services to continue to develop good, well-evidenced preventative services and to help people to make healthy lifestyle choices;
- an increase in opportunities for partnerships between local authorities, the NHS, and the third sector to support new approaches to care;
- support for independence and quality of life for the growing number of people with long-term needs living at home;

• more help for the people who need support most, with the expansion of services in poorer communities.

These proposed developments were revisited and reaffirmed in all subsequent Labour health policy intentions for the health service. In spite of many important and positive changes in health status for many in the population, inequalities still persisted. Darzi (2008) described these as 'striking'. He noted that the poorest communities in the UK continued to experience the worst health outcomes: a boy born in the city of Manchester was likely to die almost 10 years earlier than a boy born in the Royal Borough of Kensington and Chelsea – sadly this disparity in life and longevity still stands (Marmot, 2010).

Lord Darzi's review of the NHS highlighted the continuing need for a shift in emphasis from a curative approach in healthcare to a model that viewed health promotion as a key priority. In promoting this, Darzi outlined the requirement for PCTs to commission and provide comprehensive health-promotion services that were aligned to the specific needs of their local population. Community nurses were seen as very appropriate to this task, because of their professional abilities in assessing the health-promotion requirements of their local communities. In turn, they were viewed as skilled in providing culturally sensitive interventions to meet the diversity of need in their local communities.

A year on from the launch of the Darzi review some good progress had been made, with growth in the variety of health-promoting activities across all UK communities (Darzi, 2009a). However, there remained a huge distance still to travel in terms of reducing health inequalities. Free golf rounds, the availability of more fruit and vegetables and the appointment of champions for dance and physical exercise were good in themselves (Burnham, 2009a, 2009b; Phillips, 2009; West, 2009), but the serious policy agenda needed to reduce health inequalities required a much wider collaborative contribution from many sectors and personnel – and economic support.

Tackling health inequalities would always be a mixture of dealing with the underlying causes, supporting healthier lifestyle choices and ensuring that good-quality services are available for all. As research would show in 2010, inequalities in health and opportunity had continued to rise and widen (Marmot, 2010; Hills, 2010). The determinants of the differences in income and subsequent life and health chances between groups and individuals were both shocking and deep-seated. These factors faced the incoming Coalition government in May 2010.

Boldly and healthily into a new future?

All new governments arrive in office with their own distinctive ideological policy priorities and style. On becoming Prime Minister in 1979, Margaret Thatcher made very clear her absolute determination to reduce public spending on health and welfare and to control the profligacy of healthcare professional activity. Tony Blair in 1997 and Gordon Brown in 2007 offered a 'seemingly' gentler softly-softly style, but nonetheless pursued a strictly managed market approach to healthcare delivery – with rules, standards, targets and the centralized strategic planning of provision.

In turn, David Cameron and Nick Clegg, as heads of a relatively novel form of coalition government for the UK, produced a programme for health set against the difficult backcloth of a financial and economic crisis and underwritten by the ideologically driven desire to devolve responsibility for health down to each and every individual (DOH, 2010c). As Lansley (2010) explained, the government's view is that society, government and individuals share collective responsibility for public health and the new public health system will encourage all to play their part in improving and protecting the nation's health and well-being – a 'Big Society' view, whereby people are encouraged and trusted to make their own balanced decisions on how they and their families live their lives and make relevant healthy choices (Hetherington, 2010).

The government's public health programme, *Healthy Lives, Healthy People* (DOH, 2010d), was described as transforming public health and, for the first time, as creating a 'wellness' service – Public Health England – to meet all the health challenges and to tackle health inequalities. Directors of public health employed by local authorities and jointly appointed with Public Health England are to lead on driving health improvement in their localities and to deploy resources to improve health and well-being using ring-fenced health-improvement budgets allocated by the Department of Health. Health Minister Ann Milton proposed that school nurses, health visitors and other primary care nurses had a wonderful opportunity to be key players in the government's bid to reduce health inequality and to promote healthy lifestyles (Milton, 2010d).

📋 Activity: discuss with your fellow students or colleagues

- What, if any, opportunities have you had to play a part in any new health-promoting activity led by your local authority?
- Have there been any specific projects started which have helped your patients or the local community?
- Is anything new being done to help individuals who have special needs, for example the mentally ill, the learning disabled, the unemployed, older adults and those with long-term conditions?

Reflections

At the beginning of this discussion an argument was made around the current need for UK governments to pursue a more broadly based public health agenda than has traditionally been the case, both to promote health and to reduce health inequalities. Well over a decade on, we can reflect on how far the various governments' health policy agendas have moved us along the path proposed and what degree of success has been achieved.

Sadly, Harteveldt's (2005) scepticism about the ability of White Papers or political speeches to reduce health inequalities seems to have been justified. More efforts continue to be needed in the pursuit of achievable and affordable policy solutions to the seemingly intractable problems of persisting health inequalities and poor public health (Oliver, 2009; DOH, 2010d; *BMJ*, 2010). Reasons for this are clearly complex, with policy responses needed that will involve a massive collaborative will and effort across many fields of life. Marmot (2010) and others (*BMJ*, 2010) refer to the continuing need for a totally coherent and coordinated health policy programme that links income, employment and housing inequality with all the other broader health outcome inequalities.

Our overview of health policy activity in the second half of the last century, and specifically during the past two decades, has witnessed significant changes around the NHS, ostensibly underpinned by a serious commitment to health promotion (Bennett et al., 2009) In spite of all this effort, however, analysis of the wide variety of policy activities and research findings have cast doubts on their effectiveness and coherence. While there have been many important health improvements for the public in general, the health inequalities gap remains wide for a significant minority (Wintour, 2009; *BMJ* 2010).

Very worryingly, the well-reported and continuing economic recession remains a major threat to all new attempts to revisit and to reinvigorate the public health and inequality project. As Campbell (2009c) reminded us, public health remains an expendable project when financial times and budgets are tight. While the focus on health promotion, high-quality care, safe practice and innovation is immutable in whatever we do as professional nurses, the current economic environment may well make these aims a great deal harder to achieve in practice – not least for those who need the greatest help. It clearly remains to be seen whether Public Health England is able to transform public health and to create at last an effective and much-needed 'wellness' service across the whole of the UK.

Learning outcomes

- a picture of the links between policy, the promotion of health and the reduction of health inequalities;
- an understanding of the developing policy agendas over time, both to promote the nation's health and also to reduce health inequalities;
- an overview of the current policy opportunities and challenges;
- the importance of nurse involvement in the public health and inequality agenda.

Further reading

Benzeval, M., Judge, K. and Whitehead, M. (eds)(1995) *Tackling Inequalities in Health: An Agenda for Action.* King's Fund.

Giddens, A. (1998) *The Third Way.* Polity.

Graham, H. (2007) *Unequal Lives: Health and Socioeconomic Inequalities.* Open University Press.

Scriven, A. (2010) *Promoting Health: A Practical Guide.* Baillière Tindall.

9 Working with Diversity and the Policy Agenda

> **Aims**
>
> - to discuss the concept of diversity and its application in practice, both for patients and for colleagues;
> - to reflect on the positive effects of having a diverse workforce that mirrors the increasing diversity of UK communities and individuals;
> - to consider the implications of a fragmenting and changing NHS for the future delivery of a diversity-sensitive national health service.

'Diversity: a state of being diverse; difference; dissimilarity; variety.'
(*Chambers Dictionary*, 2008)

'Every member of society, at some point, is likely to be a recipient of health and social care. The Department of Health can only achieve its aim of better health, better care and well-being for all by building an explicit commitment to equality, diversity and human rights throughout the system. All public organisations including the Department of Health, public providers and commissioners of health and social care services have a duty to promote equality. To do this, the diversity of the population has to be recognised, from policy development through to service delivery and patient care, acknowledging the diverse experiences, aspirations and needs of staff, patients and the service.'

(DOH, 2008b; 2010b)

Among the many challenges facing all nurses working in the NHS today is that of being able to respond appropriately and effectively to the health needs of the now very diverse UK population (www.statistics.gov.uk). This diversity reflects the global shift over past decades where people have increasingly chosen to live in relation to their families and work opportunities, or because of war, political unrest, conflict, persecution, hunger, adverse economic conditions or social upheavals (Hearnden, 2008; Holland and Hogg, 2010). The implications of such issues are significant for all UK healthcare professionals working in both hospital and community settings, and who seek to ensure both quality and equality of healthcare provision and access across all ages and cultures (Holland and Hogg, 2010).

At the same time, there is a parallel agenda which is equally important. The NHS workforce itself is diverse and also requires special attention. As John Reid, Secretary of State for Health in 2004, put it, the NHS is based and run on diversity (Kendrall-Raynor, 2007), and it continues to be so today (McCargow, 2010). This reflects in great part the international recruitment of nurses from the late 1990s onwards to address the problem of nurse shortages and to maintain staffing levels in the NHS (Hearnden, 2008). Many came from outside the European Union (EU), from India, the Philippines, South Africa and Australia (Buchan et al., 2005). In 2005 the RCN noted that such nurses accounted for more than 60 per cent of the nursing workforce in some healthcare organizations.

However, tighter restrictions on entry to the UK and work permits for non-EU nurses since February 2007 have slowed down the level of recruitment from overseas. A lighter touch in terms of language ability and immigration restrictions has continued to be applied to nurses from the EU. Broadly, as McCargow (2010) notes, NHS employees currently comprise a diverse body of healthcarers, who need to work together well in order to provide congruent care for their similarly diverse populations.

For nurses, the achievement of a diversity-sensitive approach, whether to patient or colleague, is both assumed and required by professional code, government policy and the law (Griffith and Tengnah, 2010). Importantly, this agenda encourages us all both to recognize and to show respect for the diverse communities and individuals with whom we live and work. It is about valuing people, whether patient or colleague, and ensuring their representation and inclusion, whether in a caring situation or elsewhere; it is also about good communication and about working effectively in partnership and being open and accountable for the services we provide, making improvements that are sensitive, appropriate, responsive and supportive. Our mantra as professional nurses and citizens should surely be to treat everyone as we would wish to be treated ourselves. Our patients, colleagues and the public deserve nothing less.

📋 Activity: discuss with your fellow students or colleagues

- How diverse are your patients?
- How diverse is your team and the broader workforce?
- Do these reflect your patient group or your community?
- Are people respectful towards each other?

Diversity and the professional code

The Code (NMC, 2008) clearly sets out the professional responsibilities of nurses to both patient and colleague alike. We all have to act with integrity, demonstrating a personal and professional commitment to equality and diversity, and adhering to the laws of the country in which we live and practice. Nursing is based on ethical values, which repre-

Table 9.1 *The Code*: professional responsibilities

Expected behaviour towards patients	Expected behaviour towards colleagues
You must treat people as individuals and respect their dignity	You must work cooperatively within teams and respect the skills, expertise and contributions of your colleagues.
You must not discriminate in any way against those in your care	You must treat your colleagues fairly and without discrimination
You must treat people kindly and considerately	
You must act as an advocate for those in your care, helping them to access relevant healthcare and social care, information and support	
You must make arrangements to meet the language and communication needs of your patients	
You must be aware of the legislation regarding mental capacity, ensuring that people who lack capacity remain at the centre of decision-making and are fully safeguarded	

Source: NMC, 2008

sent the dignity, autonomy and uniqueness of all human beings, and *The Code* is very specific about our behaviour to and with others in our professional lives (see Table 9.1).

Government policy statements also guide our actions in this respect. The Darzi Review (2008) called for care to be fair and 'equally available to all, taking full account of personal circumstances and diversity – to be personalised and tailored to the needs and wants of each individual'. Lansley (2010) strongly reaffirmed this commitment on becoming Secretary of State for Health for the Coalition government (DOH, 2010b). He wanted everyone involved to remain true to the values and principles of the NHS as set out in the NHS Constitution. This clearly sets out the duty for us all not to discriminate against patients or staff and to adhere to equal opportunities and to equality and human rights legislation.

Professional code and policy imperative are, therefore, clearly reinforced by the legal requirement for public sector bodies to treat their staff and patients fairly. According to law, diversity as a concept is not just about race and ethnicity. Rules that came into force under the 2006

Equality Act required all public sector providers in England to produce a gender-equality scheme which would come into force in April 2007. All public authorities throughout the UK had to demonstrate that they were promoting equality for men and women and eliminating sexual discrimination and harassment. In addition, all NHS trusts had to ensure that transgender staff and patients were treated equally.

These issues were subsequently pulled together within the 2010 Equality Act, which brought together and harmonized the previous equality and anti-discrimination laws. The Act aimed to make the law simpler, more consistent, clearer and easier to follow. Broadly, it strengthened the law in important ways to help tackle health inequality and opportunity – a theme discussed earlier in relation to the promotion of health.

The Act was to be applied to all organizations that provided a service to the public or to a section of the public. It included anyone who sold or provided goods, facilities or services, whether or not a charge was made for them. In effect, it applied to everyone in any way involved in healthcare delivery. This is an important point to remember as we reflect on all the changes taking place within the NHS today and, in particular, as we work increasingly within a very mixed economy of care providers and commissioners right across the UK and beyond.

When proposals are developed or policies made, including those around finance and service provision, the organization must ensure that decisions are made in such a way as to minimize unfairness and not have a disproportionately negative effect on people from different religious, ethnic or gender groups, or those with disabilities (Equality and Human Rights Commission, 2009).

📋 Activity: discuss with your fellow students or colleagues

What if some people believe they are above or beyond the law or professional code and NHS policy directive, or feel that they are unseen and can behave as they wish? The development of a very fragmented, multi-sectoral service is surely much more difficult to police and check than a very cohesive organization like the NHS. However, even that can hide bad practice, as we all know (see Kennedy, 2001; Shipman, 2005; Francis, 2009).

- What can you do in practice to ensure high standards of care and to challenge bad practice in respect of being diversity-sensitive in the very broadest sense?
- Have you had any experience in practice in which a diversity-sensitive approach has not been applied and you have felt upset or angry?
- What happened?
- What have you done about it?
- Have things changed for the better?

Who is protected in our diverse community?

The 2010 Equality Act legally protects people from discrimination on the basis of 'protected characteristics'. For services and public functions, these include:

- disability – a person who has a physical or mental impairment that has a substantial and long-term adverse effect on their ability to carry out normal day-to-day activities;
- gender reassignment – the 'protected characteristic' will apply to a person who is proposing to undergo, is undergoing or has undergone a process to change their sex;
- pregnancy and maternity: the Act specifically clarified that it is unlawful to discriminate against a woman because she is breastfeeding – there is a requirement to allow women to breastfeed in situations where goods, facilities or services are being provided;
- race – includes ethnic or national origins, colour and nationality;
- religion or belief;
- gender;
- sexual orientation.

Direct discrimination

The law prohibits direct discrimination in services and functions. This might happen when someone is treated less favourably than another person because of a 'protected characteristic'. (The examples that follow are all taken from the Equalities Office, 2010.)

> *For example: a local authority advice centre refuses to provide advice to Denise, a person with a learning disability, as staff assume that she will not be able to understand the advice because of her disability.*

Direct discrimination can also happen when a person is treated less favourably because of a 'protected characteristic', even though that person does not have that characteristic (discrimination by association). It might involve a person being treated less favourably because he or she is linked or associated with someone who has a protected characteristic.

> *For example: Jonathan is the partner of Kate, a resident in a local authority care home. Jonathan decides to undergo gender reassignment, and staff at Kate's care home discover this. As a result, Kate is now treated less favourably by staff compared with other residents. This is discrimination because of association with a transsexual.*

If a person is wrongly thought to have a particular 'protected characteristic', or is treated as if they do, this is also direct discrimination (discrimination by perception).

> *For example: Sam is a local authority tenant who calls the local authority to query an electrical repair. Sam has a high voice and Bob, the engineer dealing with the query, thinks that Sam is a woman. Bob is*

very dismissive of Sam's query and refuses to explain the issue properly because he believes that a woman would not be able to understand it. This is sex discrimination against Sam because he has been wrongly perceived to be a woman.

Harassment

Harassment is linked to direct discrimination. If a person is harassed because of religion, beliefs or sexual orientation, and is consequently treated less favourably than someone else, he or she can claim direct discrimination.

For example: Janice, a black woman, is queuing at the Passport Office when she overhears two members of staff making racially abusive comments. As this conduct was unwanted by Janice and it made her feel humiliated and degraded, she can bring a claim of harassment.

Victimization

Victimization is another example of direct discrimination. It occurs when someone is treated badly because he or she has done something in relation to the Equality Act, such as making or supporting a complaint or raising a grievance about discrimination, or because it is suspected that the person has done or may do these things. People are not protected from victimization if they have maliciously made or supported an untrue complaint.

For example: Fabio makes a formal complaint against his Primary Care Trust, as he feels that the Trust has discriminated against him because he is gay. The complaint is resolved through the organization's grievance procedures. However, as a result of making the complaint Fabio is subsequently removed from his GP's list. This is victimization.

Indirect discrimination

Indirect discrimination happens when there is a rule, a policy or even a practice that applies to everyone, but which particularly disadvantages those who share a particular protected characteristic.

For example: A local authority housing department has a policy of reminding tenancy applicants of forthcoming appointments by telephone. This puts deaf people who cannot use the telephone at a disadvantage, as they do not receive a reminder of their appointment. Unless the department can justify its policy of making contact only by telephone as being a proportionate means of achieving a legitimate aim, this is likely to amount to indirect discrimination.

Discrimination

Discrimination arising from disability occurs when a person with a disability is treated unfavourably because of something connected with the disability and this unfavourable treatment cannot be justified. This form of discrimination can occur only if the service provider knows or can reasonably be expected to know that the person has a disability.

> *For example: Vickram, who has an assistance dog, is not allowed to enter his local mobile library because staff say there is not enough room for his dog. This may be discrimination arising from disability, unless it can be justified (e.g. the dog poses a genuine health and safety risk as opposed to merely being inconvenient for staff).*

Positive action provisions

Some people with 'protected characteristics' are disadvantaged or under-represented in certain areas of life, or have particular needs linked to their 'characteristic'. They may need extra help or encouragement if they are to have the same chances as everyone else. Positive action provisions enable public sector organizations to take appropriate steps to help people overcome their disadvantages or to meet their needs.

This issue takes us back to the earlier discussion on promoting health and reducing health inequalities. There are many people who need to be 'helped to health', perhaps more so than others, especially in the new and developing environment of austerity and tightening focus on who gets what and when from the NHS – for example, someone with a long-term condition or someone living in the less affluent, less well-resourced parts of the country (Hurst, 2011b). It is important to note, however, that there is no requirement to take positive action. Also, there is no restriction on treating people with disabilities more favourably than non-disabled people. So although there is potential for responding positively to concerns raised, there is no duty to do so.

> *For example: A police force becomes aware of serious homophobic incidents taking place locally, most of which seem to be going unreported. Following consultation with the local lesbian, gay and bisexual (LGB) community, which reveals little confidence that any complaints raised will be investigated fully, the police force appoints a specific liaison officer to act as the first point of contact between the service and local LGB residents.*

🗒 Activity: discuss with your fellow students or colleagues

- Reflect on some of the examples given above, which come from the Equalities Office.
- Are any of the issues relevant to your patients or groups in your communities?
- What actions have been taken?
- Did you feel able to act on behalf of your patient(s)?

The dual responsibilities of working well and in a non-discriminatory way with a diverse population of patients, together with colleagues in the NHS workforce, remain a continuing challenge for all nurses across the UK. There is a great deal of progress still to be made, not least set against the rapidly diversifying current health service provider back-cloth. Potentially, the overarching requirement already noted to obey the laws and to abide by the spirit of professional codes and policy requirements could become a questionable focus for achievement in a very fragmented and commercially oriented organization, where value for money is central and the provider and commissioner bodies are disparate and, subsequently, potentially more difficult 'to police'.

Conference attendees at a 2011 'Equality, Diversity and Human Rights' conference in London expressed much concern at the detrimental impact of the NHS reforms already being felt by black and minority ethnic (BME) staff. Anxiety was rife about GP consortia not being interested in the equality and diversity agenda when they take over from PCTs and strategic health authorities (Dean, 2011b). In response, Clare Chapman (NHS Director General of Workforce) said that she had no evidence that BME staff and other marginalized groups were being treated unfairly, but would make efforts to guard against this happening by issuing official guidance. Although this appeared to be a helpful response, guidance, like mission statements and policy edicts, can only be as good as those who deliver the approach in practice. Indeed, the proposed government plan to stop publishing annual reports on the experiences of BME patients, for example, rather compounds the feeling that this agenda is not to the fore – a major concern when there are currently 'severe, persistent and systemic health inequalities' experienced by BME and other minority communities across the country (Francis, 2011; RCN, 2011). If improvements are to be made, then surely it is important to gather evidence on which to base decision-making on the specific changes that are needed to ensure fair treatment for everyone.

McCargow (2010) described the NHS as being in one of the most challenging phases of its history, not least because of the complex set of changes under way, with the focus on quality, innovation, productivity and prevention (QUIPP), and with all healthcare employees being asked to do more with less. He cautioned strongly against employers who might be tempted to overlook the need to focus on diversity-sensitive approaches for both staff and patients, in the midst of managing the required major efficiency drive to balance the books across the whole of the public sector.

As RCN diversity and equality coordinator Wendy Irwin noted, while recognizing, for example, support given to LGBT staff, she also feared efforts could diminish as a result of the financial pressures on the NHS. King (2010) agreed, arguing however that 'the economic situation should not to be seen as an excuse to push diversity onto the back burner' by any organization working with or for the NHS.

The bottom line for nurses is surely that the diversity agenda is not just about our professional code, government policy or legislation. It is fundamental to all good patient care and well-being and is a major concern. It is to be hoped that it is an innate given for all professional nurses to want to harness, value and work with different approaches, ideas and philosophies. It is all about listening to and making patients – especially the most vulnerable of them – central to decision-making and care delivery. As McCargow (2010) reminds us, the key challenge for everyone working in the NHS at this time is how to increase productivity and, at the same time, ensure that frontline services are protected and improved for the people who need them most. He believes in the importance of working within a diverse workforce which reflects the population it serves, and describes diversity as 'the power of collective difference', a way of finding new solutions, new ways of working and new innovations through groups of people challenging and stretching each other. It is perhaps through this route that we as nurses can really start to make good progress in delivering a fairer NHS, not just for our many colleagues, but for the diversity of patients and public who, we know, continue to value and want professional nursing care (Maben and Griffiths, 2008).

McCargow (2010) suggested that there was a desperate need to bring diversity up the value chain within the NHS hierarchy. Although he believed the employee base was already very diverse, the problem was that this typically ended just above middle management – a view endorsed by Serrant-Green (2010). This means that NHS leadership for the most part is missing out on the value of 'collective difference' at strategic levels. There remains much work to be done in pushing a diversity-sensitive approach higher up the policy agenda pecking order within today's rapidly morphing NHS.

📋 Activity: discuss with your fellow students or colleagues

- Reflect on McCargow's idea of 'the power of collective difference' helping the development of new ways of doing things for some individuals or groups who do not like what you do or maybe want you to do things in a different way for them.
- Can you think of any experience where you or your team have worked together with a particular group and together made changes to your service or approach which you had never considered before, probably because you had no idea that a different approach would be more relevant or appropriate to the needs of that group or individual?

Issues for patients

The duty to promote the interests and dignity of all patients and service users, irrespective of gender, age, race, ability, sexuality, economic status, lifestyle, culture and religious or political beliefs, continues to need a great deal of attention. A look at the experiences of NHS patients today presents a very mixed bag of findings, some of which are very worrying indeed (Sprinks, 2010a; Parliamentary and Health Service Ombudsman, 2011). While no doubt many good efforts have been made to respond positively to diverse health needs and situations, there is still much work to be done.

Black and minority ethnic (BME) patients

In June 2009, the DOH national patient survey revealed that patients from BME backgrounds are less likely to report a positive experience than their white counterparts across all healthcare settings (King's Fund, 2010a), a finding which continues to date (CNO Directorate, 2011). It is therefore difficult to understand the government's rationale for not continuing to publish annual reports of the specific experiences of BME patients (RCN, 2011).

It has been argued by the DOH that it needs to consider the cost-effectiveness of producing yearly reports giving similar results. It has promised that there would be a continued examination of any identified BME issue of concern, which would then be subject to a thorough analysis and action. However, this is surely predicated on its selection at DOH level and appears to be a less transparent and rigorous process than hitherto. We might consider this to be one way of hiding or subsuming the differences between different groups – potentially diluting the evidence and impetus to respond to the diverse needs clearly evident within BME communities and individuals.

Older adults

In August 2009, a report from the Royal College of Psychiatrists about psychiatric services for older people found there had been little improvement in services since their last report in 2001 (Myers, 2009). Redding (2009) similarly reported that more improvements in care and support are needed for many vulnerable and elderly patients in the community who have continuing care needs. Age discrimination and treating older adults in patronizing and inappropriate ways unfortunately remain prevalent within today's NHS (Goodman and Clemow, 2008, 2010; Keenan and Atkins, 2011). Such concerns have been reiterated and reinforced in the very shocking and distressing Ombudsman's report on the appalling lack of good nursing care given to a number of older adults in NHS care across the UK (Parliamentary and Health Service Ombudsman, 2011).

First responses to the report included many mentions of unregulated support staff activity, and less about professional nurses (Waters, 2011). However, such divide-and-rule focus for blame is surely inappropriate. Fradd (2011) helpfully notes, from her experience in reviewing services where things have gone wrong, the importance of considering whole system failures, where there has been too great an emphasis on operational and financial performance, rather than on quality and safety – remember the relatively recent mid-Staffordshire experience (Francis, 2009).

The responsibility of all staff working at whatever level and wherever in the NHS is to provide compassionate and safe care. While nurses and support workers appear to be the frontline scapegoats, there is a raft of others behind them in the organization who are just as culpable. It is up to the whole organization to think about how to care compassionately – board members, clinical leaders, doctors and nurses, support staff: no one is immune from the responsibility of caring or responding if they see bad practice and unkind care. As Allen (2011) reminds us, the harrowing accounts of neglect and abuse in NHS hospitals makes headline news, but the findings are just the latest in a long list of damning reports. Surely we have enough evidence to accept there is something radically wrong with our treatment of older people.

Lesbian, gay, bisexual and transgender (LGBT) patients

A 2009 Department of Health guide on sexual orientation aimed to ensure that lesbian, gay, bisexual and transgender people received appropriate care within the NHS. Importantly, guidance was given on how to reduce health inequalities among these groups. It acknowledged that they have specific concerns that are not necessarily met by service providers, and that they can experience many social and health inequalities. Men are twice as likely to attempt suicide as women, with gay and bisexual men most at risk. The charity Stonewall's research into lesbian health found that one in five had self-harmed and a similar proportion had an eating disorder (Moore, 2011).

Interestingly, in spite of DOH policy guidance, the specific health needs of LGBT people according to PACE (a health and well-being charity) are poorly met. A conference held in Cornwall, supported by the NHS, the police and local authorities, found that many LGBT people feel that public services are not always welcoming or non-discriminatory (Moore, 2011). Karen Wells, a RCN council member, describes her experience of nurses interacting with transgender people as 'not good', noting that many found it hard to work alongside transgender people or to care for them as patients (see Waters, 2011).

Like Wells, Cavender (2011) believes that sexuality is a taboo subject for many nurses. This reflects a lack in training in talking to patients about diverse gender and sexuality issues or to advocate for their rights. She refers to the skills required to talk about trans-health screening, new legal rights of LGBT people, gay parenting or same-sex violence. This low awareness of issues is not only bad for the patients, but also leaves nurses vulnerable to legal challenges, as the LGBT communities are likely to complain about services that fail to live up to the new equality expectations (DOH, 2010d).

Potential changes to NHS provision in the current climate of retrenchment are just as threatening to LGBT patients as they are to the general population. Concerns are felt, for example, on the current imposition of restrictions on non-urgent treatments which could see an increase in discrimination against LBGT people. Gender-reassignment surgery, along with fertility treatments accessed by lesbians, may well be reduced or stopped as part of cost-cutting measures across the NHS. According to Stonewall, the clear lack of understanding of, and efforts by, the NHS to work well with LGBT individuals and groups is seen as worrying and unfair. As Angela Saxby, equalities and diversity manager at NHS Plymouth, noted, this apparent lack of interest in the sexual orientation and transgender agenda may prevent the development of relevant care services for a number of often marginalized individuals and groups. It required a much greater community-based effort to work with the local LGBT community, to reduce the prevalence of health inequality for such groups and to improve health outcomes for all (Gooding, 2009). The bottom line for nurses, however, is that every patient, whatever their sexuality, should be treated with respect and dignity. In turn, our own colleagues, with whom we work, also deserve no less.

The workforce experience

If we wish to create a culture of inclusivity for all the communities and patients with whom we work, there is surely a need to create a diverse, reflective and responsive workforce – an essential precursor to the development of effective and inclusive services (Hearnden, 2008). If the staff reflect the make-up of the local community, they are potentially better able to engage with individuals, providing the right treatment or support, at the right time, in the right way (Bradford University, 2011). Carol Baxter, Head of Equality, Diversity and Human Rights at NHS Employers, looks to employing organizations to create an open, safe and positive workplace, one in which all staff are supported and treated fairly and are able to flourish and deliver high-quality nursing care (Gooding, 2011).

Black and minority ethnic staff

As with BME patient experiences, there is still some way to go in the creation, development and support of an effective and diverse workforce. Policies aimed at ensuring that staff from BME backgrounds do not suffer discrimination are not working, according to a leading black nurse (Lewis, 2009), a situation that is, sadly, of long standing. A survey on diversity and the NHS by *Nursing Standard* in 2004 found examples of both direct and indirect discrimination experienced by BME nurses.

Box 9.1 Examples for reflection

- An Asian grade F nurse is convinced her race means she is treated unfairly at work. 'I was left to take all the patients to the toilet and clean commodes all the time for 11 years because of my colour and ethnicity.'
- A white grade E nurse, said: 'I hear racist comments on a daily basis from unqualified staff, such as healthcare assistants, boasting about joining or voting for the British National Party, and ignorant comments are made on a frequent basis.'
- A grade D black nurse said she had been called names such as 'bitch or bastard', especially by patients.
- A white grade D nurse referred to snide comments made by some people – e.g., 'one type of ethnic group of women always make a fuss after surgery'.

(*Nursing Standard*, 2004)

Children's nurse and equality campaigner Rosie Purves, who died in 2011, was awarded £20,000 compensation in 2004 after taking action against Southampton University Hospitals NHS Trust. She argued that managers failed to support her when a white woman demanded that white staff should care for her child (*Nursing Standard*, 2010c).

A Royal College of Nursing workforce survey found that 65 per cent of BME respondents felt that their pay band did not reflect their role and responsibilities. While there are many supportive diversity policies, BME nurses believe that it is harder for them than it is for their white counterparts to access training and win promotion (Serrant-Green, 2010). Myers (2009) agreed, arguing that the lack of BME staff in NHS leadership positions provided stark evidence of widespread inequality within the overall workforce, a situation further reinforced by Dean (2011b), who also expressed concern about BME staff suffering disproportionately from the cuts in employment currently taking place across the UK.

Efforts have been made, of course, to redress this balance and some success has been achieved, not least in memory of the Jamaican-Scottish nurse Mary Seacole (Chifulya, 2010; Jennings, 2010). The Mary Seacole Development and Leadership Awards were established by the DOH in 1994 in response to the poor representation of BME nurses in senior NHS positions. As Joan Myers explains, the main aim of the scheme was to recognize Mrs Seacole's contribution to nurse leadership by celebrating and encouraging diversity in the NHS workforce. The awards are intended to support nurses from BME backgrounds in achieving promotion to senior positions, where traditionally they have been under-represented. Established in 1994 by the DOH, the awards were also an attempt to eliminate health inequalities in BME populations

Winners of the awards have improved nursing care practice for the

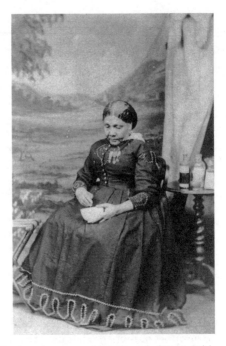

9.1 The work of the Jamaican nurse Mary Seacole (1805–81) has inspired an annual prize which celebrates diversity in the NHS workforce.

BME population covering many relevant themes – for example, the recruitment and retention of BME nursing students, the care of those with sickle cell disease, antenatal classes in the homes of south Asian women to encourage breastfeeding, special training for midwives working with asylum seekers, and outreach work with the south-east Asian community to increase testing for hepatitis C (Snow, 2010e). Many award-holders have developed their leadership skills and some have subsequently gained promotion and helped to improve BME patient outcomes. It is to be hoped that current economic circumstances do not jeopardize the future work of this important development.

Older workforce members

In a similar vein, although older members of the NHS workforce have accumulated rights over the past decade to be treated fairly, there is still some distance to go in making this situation a reality across the NHS as a whole. Wright (2008) referred to the rising ages for retirement and the collapse in occupational barriers, with many nurses wishing to continue in work way beyond the long-established retirement age of 65. (The employment of people over the current retirement age is seemingly becoming increasingly popular with government, not only to retain staff with experience, but also in an attempt to reduce the cost of pensions and other benefits. New legislation announced on 29 July

2010 enacts that no employer can force people to retire from work at 65 as from 1 October 2011.) Older nurses can now demand and expect the same opportunities for training as younger staff. In addition, any kind of work harassment on the grounds of age that creates an intimidating, hostile or degrading environment is out of bounds – as are age-related jokes.

Support is patchy across the NHS for the employment of older people, but there have been some good examples. The Royal Liverpool and Broadgreen University Hospitals NHS Trust aimed to eliminate age discrimination by employing people across a wide age range and with a broad range of knowledge and skills. Wake reported that being age-positive contributed to the performance of the workforce; what was needed was a workforce that was flexible, diverse and competent (see Davis, 2008). According to the Trust's Director of Human Resources, many staff have been employed in their 60s, including a healthcare assistant aged 68 and an A&E bank nurse of 62 (Davis, 2008). It was seen as good both for delivering the aims of the trust and, more importantly, for providing experienced, effective and appropriate patient-responsive care. Tola Rowe, for example, paediatric nurse at Barnet and Chase Farm Hospitals Trust, retired from her post days before her 78th birthday in July 2010 (*News*, 2010).

Lesbian, gay, bisexual and transgender staff

Discrimination in terms of sexual orientation remains an issue that continues to need more attention (Scott, 2011a). The LGBT lobby

---

Box 9.2 Efforts made by non-NHS organizations to support the diversity agenda

The Chartered Institute of Housing (CIH) set up a two-year traineeship for people with disabilities to increase the number working in the housing sector. Starting in the autumn of 2010, it aimed to help 120 people with disabilities to get jobs with housing associations over the following five years.

- Allan Barr, 33, who has cerebral palsy and is a wheelchair user, is now a trainee housing officer at Glasgow Housing Association.
- Marcus Grazette, aged 24, who is of African and Indian descent, joined the civil service's fast-stream graduate programme in October 2010.

Although the scheme is not exclusively for BME candidates, it has been designed to remove discriminatory bias from the recruitment process. Once in the Foreign Office, his induction involved diversity training. The managers were very conscious of its importance. Any progression to a more senior level is predicated on meeting diversity objectives in appraisals. (Batty, 2009)

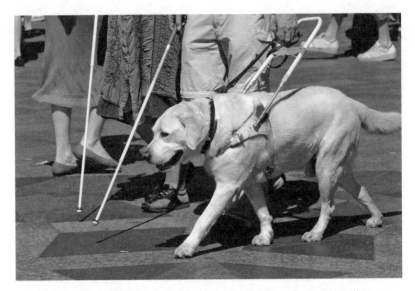

9.2 People with disabilities are a traditionally disadvantaged group in society, and they can face complex difficulties when they attempt to find work in the nursing profession.

group, Stonewall, publishes an annual report of the best places to work – a survey of gay-friendly employers (Gooding, 2009). In 2011 only a handful of NHS organizations made it onto the list of the UK's top 100 employers, with Nottinghamshire Healthcare NHS Trust the highest ranked, in twelfth place. Scott expressed disappointment that other government departments, local authorities and private firms demonstrated a greater commitment to their LGBT and other disadvantaged staff than the NHS.

Attempts to enter the nursing profession – another barrier for those with disabilities?

Sin (2008) highlighted the complexity of difficulties around the rights and responsibilities that people with disabilities face in their quest to study, qualify, register and work in nursing. He noted that they were portrayed as recipients of care and not as potentially valuable contributors to the caring enterprise. The NMC/DOH requirement for registrants to be of 'good health and fitness' has led to accusations of discrimination. As argued by Sin, this has led to a focus on diagnosis rather than on competence and the requirements of the role and work involved, and thus to direct discrimination. He believed that professional regulation, and indeed entry to the profession and employment within the NHS, should be based on assurances of competence and conduct, not on judgements of health and fitness.

It is disheartening to find that the NHS appears to perform badly in relation to the employment and support of some traditionally disadvantaged groups, like those with disabilities and LGBTs. This is despite new legislation and several public service initiatives which should mean that employers in the public sector support and choose their staff on skills and talent alone. Although work was being done on diversity, the issue was being tackled on an ineffective 'one issue at a time' basis and there seemed to be a hierarchy of diversity strands in the way the NHS delivered the policy. Work on gender and race, for example, seemed to receive much greater attention, with disability and sexual orientation issues left off the agenda or dealt with in a perfunctory manner (Gooding, 2009).

Activity: discuss with your fellow students or colleagues

- Reflect on the diversity of people in your team.
- Are you able to involve everyone or are certain individuals left out?
- Are there any difficult issues within your team which relate to differences of belief, culture, age or sexuality?
- Are there any positive issues?
- Look at the picture on the previous page. Consider the impact of employing a blind person who has a guide dog.

Moving forward: embedding the diversity agenda in the NHS

In a 2010 bulletin, the Chief Nursing Officer expressed awareness of the many failings and also of much progress made within the NHS. As she acknowledged, however, 'embedding the broad equality and diversity agenda requires consistent engagement and communication with healthcare stakeholders to ensure the necessary changes are embraced, supported and taken forward'. From a personal and professional perspective, we are all required to work towards creating a positive team environment, one in which diversity is a welcome and necessary attribute for delivering high-quality care. We are encouraged to:

- challenge attitudes which impede approach;
- welcome and encourage diversity and difference – in teams, amongst patients and the wider public;
- think and act broadly – include everyone;
- challenge those who do not respect others.

Conclusion

In this current climate of financial retrenchment, there is a danger that diversity issues will become less of a priority for managers. Financial constraints have resulted in organizations making important decisions about their operations, the services they provide and the numbers of people they can employ. These decisions have included efficiency drives, budget cuts, reorganizations, relocations, redundancies and service reductions.

Concerns have been expressed that these moves have had a disproportionate effect on certain groups of people. For example, according to the Equality and Human Rights Commission (2009), women are more likely to be affected by redundancies than men, with organizations revising their maternity and flexible working policies in an attempt to save money. The Commission was thus emphasizing the importance of all organizations, including the NHS, being mindful of how they implement required policy changes, not least when reducing the size of the workforce to reduce costs.

However, the idea that 'diversity' issues will become a lesser priority for managers and nurses is rejected by some as scaremongering. According to Wake, there is a business argument for promoting diversity in the workforce, as this provides flexibility and an appropriate mix of experience and competencies, which are good for delivering high-quality nursing and management and for improving the working lives of the staff (see Davis, 2008). White (2009) believes that engaging with the range of communities will help the NHS address health inequalities and meet its statutory requirements. In turn, it also helps to ensure that care is sensitive and, it is to be hoped, more relevant to the diverse needs of the patients.

Baxter argued that success starts with employing a diverse workforce that reflects the make-up of the local community, listening to the views of the service users and colleagues, and acting on these perspectives (see Gooding, 2009). As Oona King, Head of Diversity at Channel 4, noted, 'it seems obvious that the closer the workforce reflects the community it serves, the better patient care will be' (King, 2010).

Concerns as to the primacy of the diversity agenda during a period of austerity is, however, a worrying reality. Economic necessities may force NHS providers to apply a very stringent approach to care delivery in order to contain costs and remain within budget. While specific and individualized services for all patients are clearly desirable and, one hopes, 'diversity-sensitive', it remains important to keep the service going more generally for the whole population and to consider priorities very carefully. This business-like approach is de rigueur in today's NHS.

Pamela Chandler, however, Head of Equality and Diversity in the Heart of England NHS Foundation Trust, is adamant that this sharper commercialized approach to healthcare will not stop continuing efforts to develop a diversity-sensitive service in the NHS (see Weekes, 2009). She said that equality and diversity were now inextricably linked to the commitment to quality care and good health outcomes for patients. She acknowledged that spending more generally had to be curtailed. Overseas recruitment was no longer a priority, not because of discrimination, but because of economic necessity. Joan Myers (2009), a professional officer for diversity for the DOH, concurred with this view, noting that while the NHS would have to change during the recession, the diversity agenda would remain one of its major priorities.

Currently then, we have the law and government policy behind us in supporting and delivering a positively diverse service within the NHS. There are clearly barriers to its success which need to be overcome. However, as professional nurses and citizens, we all have a responsibility to work to ensure a viable, sustainable and diversity-responsive health service. There is a need to be patient and colleague-centred in the development and organization of our services, to listen to others' views and act on these perspectives. By these means we can hope to provide the opportunity for everyone to be treated fairly, promote equality of opportunity for effective care for all, and indeed achieve the much-desired ambition of achieving a diversity-friendly NHS.

Learning outcomes

- an understanding of the concept of diversity and its application in practice both for patients and for colleagues;
- an understanding of the positive effects of having a diverse workforce that mirrors the increasing diversity of UK communities and individuals;
- an understanding of the implications of a fragmenting and changing NHS for the future delivery of diversity-sensitive national health services.

Further reading

Barr, J. and Dowding, L. (2008) *Leadership in Health Care.* Sage, ch. 3.

Hafford-Letchfield, T., Leonard, K., Begum, N. and Chick, N. F. (2008) *Leadership and Management in Social Care.* Sage, ch. 5.

Holland, K. and Hogg, C. (2010) *Cultural Awareness in Nursing and Health Care*, 2nd edn. Hodder-Arnold.

Llewellyn, A., Agu, L. and Mercer, D. (2008) *Sociology for Social Workers.* Polity.

Parliamentary and Health Service Ombudsman (2011) *Care and Compassion?* Report of the Health Service Ombudsman on ten investigations into NHS care of older people (www.ombudsman.org.uk/care-and-compassion).

10 Supporting People with Long-Term Conditions: A Policy Perspective

> **Aims**
> - to discuss the implications of the developing care needs of those people with long-term conditions (LTCs);
> - to consider the impact of the Coalition's policies for health and for cutting public expenditure;
> - to promote a positive professional response to the challenges being faced across the NHS in working with people with LTCs.

> 'Delivering improvements for people with long-term conditions isn't just about treating illness. It's about delivering personalised, responsive holistic care in the full context of how people live their lives. Our journey to achieve this has started, our challenge is to continue to take it forward.'
>
> (Colin-Thome, 2008)

> 'Long-term conditions are those conditions that cannot, at present, be cured, but can be controlled by medication and other therapies. The life of a person with a LTC is forever altered – there is no return to "normal".'
>
> (DOH, 2008c)

Demographic and societal changes have led over time to an increasing incidence of chronic illness and life-limiting conditions. As such, the NHS continues to face the challenge of responding to the varied needs and expectations of a growing number of people with long-term conditions (LTCs) (Wanless, 2006; DOH, 2010d). There are some 15.4 million people in England, almost one in three of the population, who live with some form of LTC (Gould, 2010). Managing these conditions accounts for almost 70 per cent of the NHS hospital and primary care budgets. This percentage is set to rise still further, not least because of a reduction in the birth rate, greater life expectancy, an ageing population and the increasingly inactive lifestyles of the general population (Gould, 2010). The Department of Health estimates the number of people in England with LTCs is likely to grow by 23 per cent by 2035.

There are a number of important variables which impact to a greater or lesser degree on the whole policy challenge of providing care for people with LTCs. People with one or more longer-term conditions are heavy users of health and social care services, including community, primary, urgent and emergency care, and secondary and tertiary

Box 10.1 Conditions defined as LTCs

- coronary heart disease
- heart failure
- stroke and transient ischaemic attack
- hypertension
- diabetes
- chronic obstructive pulmonary disease
- epilepsy
- cancer
- severe mental-health conditions (schizophrenia, bipolar affective disorder and other psychoses)
- asthma
- chronic kidney disease
- dementia
- depression
- multiple sclerosis
- Parkinson's disease

(DOH, 2008c)

services. Individuals with multiple needs often receive unplanned and uncoordinated care and are frequently admitted to hospital. This places a significant burden on health and social care providers, not least from a cost perspective.

The incidence of LTCs is highest among the most disadvantaged groups, older adults, the unemployed, those living on low incomes, the learning disabled and those with mental health conditions. These groups are a major policy concern for a government that is aiming to reduce health inequalities, promote the good health of the population and, at the same time, reduce public expenditure – a difficult proposition. The ageing population means that chronic diseases will continue to rise and so will the costs of providing care. It has been estimated that treatment and care for those with LTCs takes up 70 per cent of the total health and social care spend in England – a cost issue receiving a great deal of attention from the Coalition government.

While the majority of those with LTCs are older adults (Perry et al., 2010), there are also many young children who need long-term care at home and in school (Hewitt-Taylor, 2010; Puntis, 1995). Worryingly, trends also suggest that a growing number of younger adults are now developing LTCs – as a result, for example, of alcohol-related illness, inactivity and the growing levels of obesity within the UK (King's Fund, 2010a). Ill health among the growing number of younger adults places a very significant burden on health and social care. People within this age group with an LTC are twice as likely to be out of work than those of similar ages without such conditions. Furthermore, being unemployed at this stage of life is not only detrimental to both physical and mental health, it is also likely to limit the possibility of any future employment,

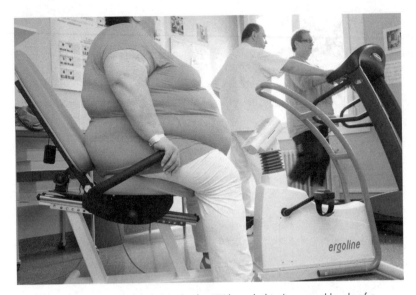

10.1 The growing levels of obesity in the UK have led to increased levels of a variety of long-term health conditions.

and will have a significant impact on health and social care costs. In reality, the needs of this group will develop and grow over a longer period of time, with all that this implies for future public sector spending.

Research into what people with LTCs want in terms of care and support provides us with some answers as to what matters most to them. It has been found that they want services that will provide support to enable them to remain independent and healthy and have increased choice. They want far more services to be delivered safely and effectively in the community or at home; and they want seamless, proactive and integrated services tailored to their needs (DOH, 2005d, 2006e). The consequence of this challenge then – looking beyond the obvious ones of individual ill health and the need for often-complex long-term support – is the growing cost of meeting this agenda against a backcloth of the severe current financial restraints, and a very determined government's search for cost-effective as well as cost-efficient health and social care services (Lansley, 2010) What needs to be done against what can be afforded remains a worrying dilemma for politicians, for us and for the patients concerned. As in previous chapters, we will first look back at earlier policy developments and then consider how we would like to move forwards in meeting this increasingly complex health challenge.

What has happened so far?

Worry about this developing situation is not a new aberration suddenly facing the current government. For decades, politicians, health planners, nurses and doctors have raised concerns that conditions of lifestyle, affluence and indolence, coupled with a growing elderly population, could become an unaffordable problem for the NHS. Predecessor governments of recent times have responded in many different ways to the financial and practical policy challenges of meeting the health and social care needs of this expanding group of people living within communities across the UK.

Efforts made to provide appropriate and acceptable care have focused on people's own homes, nursing and residential homes and other intermediate care settings (SCIE, 2006). Where possible, many have been supported at home to help themselves, with an emphasis on independent living (DOH, 2001b). Much policy attention has also been given to providing better and more dignified palliative care and supportive end-of-life services (DOH, 2006e; National Council for Palliative Care, 2006) It has been argued that high-quality health and social care should be delivered in a person-centred way, one that respects the rights of people and patients to privacy and dignity, is responsive to what people want and request, and is provided in an appropriate home environment in their own community. Our earlier look at the reforming health service, for example, has shown a relentless policy shift over time from long-held favouritism towards the hospital sector and secondary care towards primary and tertiary care in the community, and the promotion of greater individual responsibility for health and well-being for people in their own homes – in particular for those with an LTC (DOH, 2008a).

The publication of National Service Frameworks (DOH, 2005b), combined with published national targets (DOH, 2004e) for improving long-term care, helped to focus community matron, nurse, general practice and social care activity. As Sir Derek Wanless put it, it was all about the importance of collaborative working between organizations, planning for the future and putting in place systems which would truly meet the changing and challenging needs of this population.

At the same time, the new general medical services contract of 1 April 2004 offered rewards to general practices for evidencing the quality of their management and delivery of care to patients with LTCs. Many nurses in general practice contributed to this work, helping to care for people with heart disease, diabetes, cancer, stroke, hypertension, lung disease, epilepsy, hypothyroidism, mental illness and asthma. The Chief Nurse made clear her support for these policy and practice developments, noting that improving care for people with long-term conditions was an important and continuing priority for the government (DOH, 2005b, 2005d).

Self-care and self-management

Many different services have been set up across the UK to help people self-care, providing them and their families with relevant and accessible support, and also acknowledging the central role and responsibility of each individual in managing their own care and health. In Birmingham, a partnership between Birmingham East and North Primary Care Trust, Pfizer Health Solutions and NHS Direct delivered proactive telephone-based healthcare support 'care management' to individuals in the region with LTCs. This service supported people with cardiovascular disease, heart failure and diabetes to take a more active role in managing their own health. It reminds us of our earlier discussion on the benefits of new technologies in improving and modernizing care provision.

Innovative self-care

An award-winning project was run from 2004 to 2006 at Chilcote Surgery in Torquay. It was supported by the Met Office, Torbay Care Trust and the Improvement Foundation. The project involved the forecasting of weather conditions that might exacerbate symptoms of respiratory disease, and resulted in a reduction of hospital admissions of those with chronic obstructive pulmonary disease (COPD) by 82 per cent. The patients were given special information packs, including room thermometers and a guide to the actions they could take to prevent their symptoms from worsening and requiring professional intervention. The Chilcote Practice developed a COPD register and appointed a specialist nurse coordinator to make it easier and faster to communicate with patients. This project reflects the promotion of innovative ideas, cross-sectoral partnership working to improve health, and the empowerment of individuals and the encouragement of responsibility for their own health and well-being.

Self-directed care

Directed self-care was another approach that was introduced in Barnsley, whereby individuals were given relevant support to assess their own needs and to manage their own care and individual budgets to purchase what they needed from the local health and social care services. This was set against a very strong integrated whole systems approach, in which education, employment, housing, community care and public health worked closely together in partnership with the patients, their families and carers. This is a good example of the patient centredness and partnership approach required by previous government policy which we have considered in earlier chapters.

Proactive disease management and well-informed patients

This process was seen as making a real difference to people with single conditions or a range of problems. As prompted by the National Service

Frameworks, effective interventions involved early identification of problems, a prompt response, the right care package and the right support; personalized care planning was of key importance. In North Tyneside, Northumberland, this approach was used to change the way in which diabetes care was delivered, enabling people with diabetes to become fully involved in their own care.

Clinics were reorganized so that patients had their tests performed and were then informed about their results before the care-planning consultation. This gave the patients the chance to think about the results, and to make a note of questions or anything else they wished to discuss. The consultations focused not only on diabetes, but also on other wider issues. Healthcare professionals involved were trained to elicit the patient's agenda, agree priorities and set goals and actions in collaboration with the patient – a user-centred approach that is both informative in nature and encouraging of responsibility for self-care and a knowledgeable interest in their own condition (DOH, 2008c).

Disease management and end-of-life

In 2002, Bradford City, Bradford South West and Bradford North PCTs all appointed heart failure nurse specialists (HFNS), who formed a team to support people at home following a hospital admission for heart failure. None of the nurses, however, had specialist palliative care expertise, and they needed help. They contacted and formed a team with local specialist palliative care services. It became clear from positive patient and family feedback that the HFNS team was then able to provide excellent end-of-life care, not least with additional support or telephone advice from a palliative care consultant or Macmillan nurse. This example emphasizes the value and positive nature of partnership working for the benefit of both patients and their families, and from learning and sharing skills and knowledge with other care-providing colleagues.

Multidisciplinary teams

People with LTCs have a range of complex needs and can often require care and support from a wide range of services and professionals. The importance of good team working is of paramount importance, as it underpins a coordinated seamless approach to delivery of care and support, avoiding fragmentation, confusion and duplication of effort. The Tremeduna Team in Sedgefield, County Durham, worked as an integrated, multidisciplinary locality team. Staff involved were in a single location, used a single assessment process and a single client-recording system, took referrals via a single point of contact and were assessed by a single set of performance measures (DOH, 2008c).

Community matrons

Policy responses to the growing problem of LTC care, ostensibly in an effort to manage costs and services better, resulted in many positive developments for professional nurses, particularly within the community nursing field. The reintroduction of the role of matron, as set out in the 2000 NHS Plan, was part of the Labour government's modernizing agenda, and also an opportunity for professional enrichment for experienced nurse practitioners. The public's long-held perception of the power and gravitas of the traditional matron figure was an important and very enduring force (DOH, 2003a) – seen as someone likely to sort out the issues raised in press complaints of dirty, ineffective hospitals and poorly disciplined staff.

Old-style matrons – what were they like?

The traditional matron of 40 years ago was the most senior nurse in a hospital. She was responsible for all the nurses and the domestic staff, overseeing all patient care and the efficient running of the hospital, although she almost never had real power over the strategic running of the hospital – that was left, in the main, to the doctors. Matrons were described as 'fearsome individuals' (as indeed they were!), 'scary' and 'able to strike the fear of God into hospital staff', 'looked up to as an individual of great authority' and as 'a mother figure' for their hospital (Satchell, 2008). The matrons of the past had a very distinctive uniform, usually a dark-blue dress, in a slightly darker hue than that of her direct subordinates (the sisters). She also wore an elaborate, white starched hat.

The modern matron

The re-creation of this role, albeit very different from that of the now stereotypical 'Hattie Jacques' matron of the 1950s and 1960s (see Box 10.2), was presented by the government as being a user-responsive gesture. It was said that the public wanted changes to be made by someone with the power to do so – someone to get the basic things done right. The need for effective case management of individuals with chronic

Box 10.2 Josephine Edwina Jacques, 1922–1980

Josephine Jacques was a British comedy actress, known as Hattie Jacques. From 1958 to 1974 she appeared in 14 *Carry On* films, playing roles such as a stereotypical, frightening, no-nonsense hospital matron. She was powerful, domineering and, above all, large. She can be seen in the following films: *Carry On Matron*, *Carry On Nurse*, *Carry On Doctor* and *Carry On Again Doctor*.

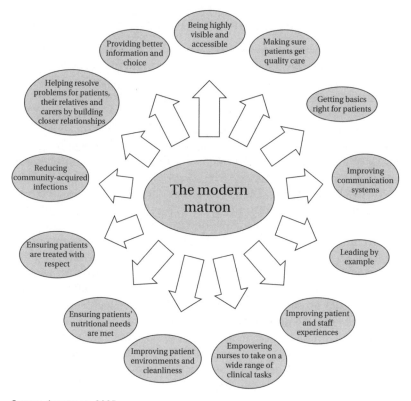

Source: Armstrong, 2005

Figure 10.1 Key responsibilities of the modern matron

disease was emphasized, not least by putting the patients and their service at the centre of everything that was done. The proposed intro-duction of a new-style community matron was to be the way to achieve this aim. Unlike the formidable, traditional matrons of the past, the modern matrons were clearly a new and very different breed of nurse, who were to provide a high-level lexicon of skills and knowledge, com-bined with both management and leadership ability (see Figure 10.1).

The White Papers *Choosing Health* (DOH, 2004a) and the *NHS Improvement Plan* (2004f) both focused on community matrons, and said they were ideally placed to promote the health needs of people with long-term conditions. With their hands-on case-management expertise, they could identify those whose health was at greatest risk, and could work with patients and carers to reduce the effects of disease and prevent accidents, dehydration, infections or other conditions that could result in admission to hospital. Community matrons would be able to put their patients in contact with NHS-accredited health trainers, who could provide additional practical support to the patients and carers for changing their behaviour to prevent ill health.

A broader health-promotion role

The matron's population-wide responsibility and breadth of vision in assessing community health needs was important to the government's objective of reducing health inequalities. This proposed whole population approach looked beyond patients already on nurses' caseloads, or those who presented or were referred for care. It encouraged the identification of those who could benefit, but who, for all sorts of reasons, whether by choice or through ignorance, did not appear normally or easily on the radar screens of primary and community care services.

By the time of the change of government in 2010, a range of initiatives had been introduced to support people with chronic, long-term conditions. These included training for patients to manage their conditions themselves (DOH, 2001b), more intensive support packages from nurses and other primary care professionals for those with complex needs (DOH, 2004g) and financial incentives for general practices to manage patients with LTCs effectively. Many solutions were devised around the country, including high-tech care at home with arm's-length monitoring, all in an effort to reduce hospital admissions. Broadly, the many different services had worked well and had been popular with patients and their carers. In spite of this, however, there had not been significant improvements in terms of avoidable and expensive admissions to hospital (King's Fund, 2010a).

Box 10.3 Case study: A positive Expert Patient Programme (EPP) experience

'Self-management support can help to increase confidence, particularly in people with long-term conditions, to manage their health and well-being, and improve their quality of life' (EPP, 2011).

Between April 2009 and March 2010 an examination of the effects of an EPP in the Wirral focused on people recovering from drug and alcohol misuse. The programme had helped participants to meet new people, and gain better control of their emotions and increased self-awareness and self-worth; it encouraged a more appropriate use of services, leading to decreased anxiety, better sleep patterns and diet, an ability to try new things, increased motivation, improved self-presentation, new skills, confidence, self-esteem, better communication skills and improved relationships with family and friends. Some took up volunteering initiatives or further education courses or had positive job-related outcomes, such as increased work hours. Some were offered opportunities to learn new skills to help them integrate back into their local community.

(www.selfmanagement.co.uk)

Where to now?

The financial and professional challenges of caring for people with LTCs in their own communities are clear. No frontline services, including that of community nursing, have escaped the attention of successive governments in this respect. Incremental policy developments have slowly changed the focus of NHS care and, in turn, attempted to ally economic stringency with high-quality responsive 'personalized care' – an equation which may well become very hard to deliver in the currently developing primary and community care environment (DOH, 2010c). The difficulty of responding effectively and appropriately, and within very tightly defined financial parameters, to the varied needs of people with LTCs remains a major concern, not least for the patients concerned, but also for the many nurses and other primary care professionals who have been, and still are, centrally involved in this complex and costly work.

Gould (2010) noted that good developments had been patchy and not well diffused across the service. He commented on the inability of the NHS to 'efficiently identify and implement effective solutions', because the process of analysing information about them and then sharing it with the whole organization was a 'long, grinding process', which stultified progress and militated against rapid change. Local innovative work about LTCs had not always been picked up and then replicated across the service. All of this perhaps reflects the lack of political sexiness around LTCs, as compared with new cancer treatments, innovative surgery and cutting waiting times for admissions to hospital. Managing arthritis, chronic depression and diabetes, while important for the individuals concerned, are less attractive to the general population at large and seemingly less newsworthy for the politicians.

Current suggestions on making strategic improvements include a greater use of the private sector and not-for-profit social enterprise companies, with their ability to create a single model of care delivery which could then be adapted locally, rather than trying to support a hybrid network of responses across the NHS – some good, some not. However, these moves could interfere with the already working integrated pathways and initiatives between hospitals, general practices, community and third sectors and might well result in people falling through the net and losing out.

Other aspects of importance which need to be nurtured are the 'expert patients', who have a great deal of knowledge about their conditions, which needs to be exploited and shared. Their insight into care and services needs to be collected and applied. Greater efforts should be made to ensure that enough information is given so that patients can make well-informed choices about their own lifestyles, care and treatment. Healthcare records should be much more freely available, so that there is communication between participants in the healthcare relationship and decisions made are available to all. In a sense, a right to healthcare is balanced with the responsibility of taking the advice given, discussed and agreed together in a contract.

This sort of approach, which appears to shift power in favour of the user with a LTC, is, however, predicated on individuals who wish to be in greater control of their healthcare. According to Gould (2010), this may not always be the case. The Picker Institute estimated that '25% of patients want to be told what to do, 50% want to be involved, and only 25% want to be in the driving seat'. A new way forwards would clearly involve a large cultural change, on the parts of professionals and patients alike, and of course the politicians. This particular issue is going to require much more action and investment by the Coalition government.

New solutions?

> The best care and support is delivered by professionals and others working together as parts of teams to meet the needs of communities, groups and individuals. There are huge benefits for everyone – NHS, local authorities, the third sector, but most of all for those people whose lives can be transformed by being given the support that is right for them. (Behan, 2008)

The Coalition government's initial Health White Paper, *Equity and Excellence* (DOH, 2010c), looked to general practice as the new focus for the NHS and to GPs as the future commissioners for care. PCTs were to be abolished and public health was to sit within local authorities. All areas of public expenditure were immediately put under sharp scrutiny, with no sector being immune from daily announced cuts and changes. The future of primary care and community nursing faced many serious challenges at this time and, implicit within these, questions as to the new and potential contexts for their work.

Who would employ community nurses? Would the private sector take over their work? How would GPs manage in becoming commissioners for care? Would there be a return to the past failures of the GP budget-holding experience of the 1980s? Most importantly, what did this unsure future hold for all the people with long-term conditions in our communities who rely upon strong and coordinated services? Would their rights to services be reduced, and would they now have to start paying for certain support services and medications previously provided without an additional charge? These were all worrying questions for both patient and professional alike.

🗒 Activity: discuss with your fellow students or colleagues

- What sorts of issues have come into play for those with long-term conditions with whom you work?

- Have worries been expressed by patients or their informal carers?
- Has your ability to care or provide certain services been curtailed or changed?
- What positive changes, if any, have happened?

Professional issues

Positive commentators referred to the potential for many new and exciting opportunities being opened up, not least for community nurses who were described as multi-skilled, resourceful professionals, willing to expand their expertise and to try out new ideas for the benefit of their patients and their profession. The developments already noted around the LTC agendas of previous years exemplified and confirmed that belief. In turn, *Equity and Excellence* looked to the well-developed skills and knowledge of NHS primary care: 'We will hand back power to the patients and the NHS professionals who treat them . . . we want to set frontline professionals free to innovate and make decisions based on their clinical judgement and the needs of their patients . . . for example with groups of GPs and nurses commissioning services for their local communities.'

Taking up this agenda involved building on skills already gained and entering into new relationships, particularly as the private sector and social enterprises were already bustling into position, ready to compete and to offer the required skills in cost-effective and competitive packages (Booth et al., 2010a). This was not, however, a recipe for expansion. The government was intent from day one on removing any perceived layers of duplication in public services, to untangle the mass of bureaucracy seen as unnecessary within the NHS, and to put the money saved back into patient care, while also expecting financial savings. Community nurses were going to have to show their professional and political muscle and become serious players in the new competitive environment if they were to continue to provide care for those with long-term conditions as they had in previous years – or even to stay in employment (RCN, 2010).

Advice on implementing the new government's policies for health were not short on detail – both encouraging and, by turn, concerning. Those nurses who were willing to embrace change needed to become entrepreneurial and to attract the attention of the developing commissioning consortia. According to the White Paper (DOH, 2010e), these would be made up of GPs or perhaps former PCT commissioners or, indeed, a private sector group employed on behalf of a feeder body of GPs (*Daily Telegraph*, 2010). Former nurse Anne Milton, a minister at the Department of Health, suggested that nurses could also become consortia members, noting that the government had 'created the field and that it was up to nurses to step up to the mark' (Milton, 2010d). Unfortunately, this was not stated in the White Paper and, indeed, a role for nurses had not been mentioned in any document. According to the Chief Nurse, 'nurses will have to work hard with consortia to make sure they play a part because that is best for patients' (Beasley, 2010).

It would continue to be important to enhance knowledge and skills and to adopt with some seriousness the approach that 'learning was for life'. This relates especially to updating and applying the skills of assessment in the identification of the needs of individuals and communities, and collecting and using that evidence to ensure appropriate, adequate and effective service provision. This ground-level professional knowledge, combined with rich practice experience, could help to steal a march on others, who might only rely on desktop knowledge and an ability to define budgets. The desire to continue to act as advocates for patients with LTCs – matron or not – requires the skills of professional self-promotion, continuing knowledge and skill development and an ability to work in an integrated way with other sectors right across the community, diagonally with mental health trusts and vertically with the acute hospital sector.

Specialist nurses are crucial to the care of patients with LTCs, and community nurses need to continue to develop and maintain strong networks with all sources of expertise, not least that which is found within the hospital setting. Specialist hospital nurses themselves, however, also have to be increasingly aware of the developing NHS primary care environment with its mixed economy of providers. While a proactive, vertical and integrated approach to delivering care has been encouraged in the past (Abel et al., 1995) in order to maintain the continuity of care for patients with LTCs, the future could be very different.

Other sectors have prepared well and are increasingly interested in providing out-of-hospital care for patients, from support for home parenteral feeding for children, to 24-hour care for older adults with mental illness or learning disability. Hospital trusts in the current, financially challenged environment are, in turn, increasingly keen to provide only care for which they are paid and which takes place within the defined confines of their organizations. It is clear that well-worn laurels of the past gained for innovative practice need to be re-won by all nurses concerned with LTCs, whether in the hospital or community setting.

In conclusion, policy efforts made by successive governments over the past decade have promoted many constructive developments in the care of people with long-term conditions in the community. That said, much work clearly remains to be done. The changing organizational environment set in train by the Coalition's White Paper is continuing to provide a very difficult backcloth against which any new developments must be made. Many will be fearful that an acceleration in the privatization and fragmentation of health services, especially in primary care, will make access for the most vulnerable, such as older people, those with long-term conditions and the marginalized, much more difficult. This would clearly have negative implications for any hopes of reducing the problem of widening health inequalities as discussed elsewhere.

Concerns also arise around GP commissioning. Will this be a revisiting of the GP budget-holding experience of the 1980s, with its

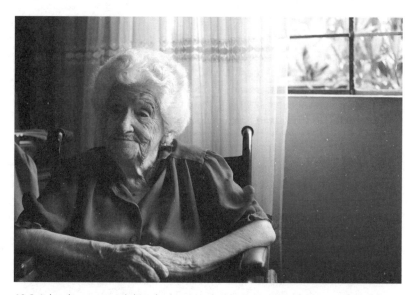

10.2 It has been argued that the increased privatization and fragmentation of health provision will have a particular impact on older patients, who are among the most vulnerable groups.

creation of a 'postcode lottery' of services and inequalities in access to secondary and tertiary care? Will the private sector's known (and well-geared-up) pursuit of consortia-commissioning work on behalf of GPs have an effect on services subsequently provided? Indeed, what level or type of services will remain free at the point of need within the NHS? What sorts of services will NHS nurses be allowed to offer in the future? Will they begin to have a two-tier menu of services on offer, with added extras requiring payment? This is surely a major concern for many people who have a long-term chronic condition and also without a doubt for many caring professional nurses who may see their practice curtailed out of financial necessity.

The Coalition government has promised to aspire to an NHS that can deliver high-quality care to all patients, in all areas, all the time – in ways that are demonstrably fair, efficient and accountable. It is to be hoped that the care of people with long-term conditions remains at the forefront of this agenda and that the nursing profession is able to continue and further develop its effective contributions to date. While it still remains hard to imagine exactly what the new NHS will look like in the next few years, there is no doubt that professional nurses will be crucial to its success.

Learning outcomes

- the implications of the developing care needs of those people with LTCs;
- the potential impact of the Coalition's policy for health and the need to cut public expenditure;
- positive professional responses to the potential challenges being faced across the NHS in working with people with LTCs.

Further reading

Cuthbert, S. and Quallington, J. (2008) *Values for Care Practice: Health and Social Care Theory and Practice.* Reflect Press.

Llewellyn, A. and Hayes, S. (2008) *Fundamentals of Nursing Care.* Reflect Press, ch. 7.

Mason-Whitehead, E., McIntosh, A., Bryan, A. and Mason, T. (2008) *Key Concepts in Nursing.* Sage.

Williamson, G. R., Jenkinson, T. and Proctor-Childs, T. (2008) *Nursing in Contemporary Healthcare Practice.* Learning Matters, ch. 7.

11 Policy and Nurse Professionalism Today: A Threat or a Promise?

Aims

- to define what is meant to be a professional;
- to consider the implications of current policy developments for the nursing profession and its future;
- to reflect on the need for all professional nurses continually to refresh and to develop their professional skills and knowledge.

'Nurses in Europe are not a homogeneous group: large differences are found in the roles they play, the tasks they perform, the training they receive, the status they have in society and the remuneration they get for their work. They comprise a formidable workforce that provides some of the most essential services to keep people healthy, to take care of the ill and injured, and to nurse the frail and elderly throughout the region.'

(Dr J. E. Asvall, former WHO Regional Director for Europe, cited in Salvage and Heijnen, 1997)

Asvall's statement of over a decade ago very much reflects the focus for the discussions that follow. While the policy agendas for health and healthcare delivery within the UK (as elsewhere across Europe and beyond) grow, develop and change, the necessary role of the professional nurse carer has an unremitting allure and presence. The potential of the role continues to be explored today, against the backcloth of the ever-developing health policy agendas of the current government (DOH, 2010b, 2010c, 2010d).

It is by taking up and preparing for the future opportunities proposed or implicit within the government's policy statements that professional nurses can hold onto and maintain the interesting and worthwhile career so needed and supported by the public at large. That said, while public esteem for professional nursing is generally high and perceived as an important role in society, it does not necessarily ensure a comfortable ride against the buffeting of current health policy imperatives or the impact of economic pressures. As noted already, no health professionals within the NHS have been immune, or are likely to remain immune, from the developing impact of a more managerial and business-like approach to healthcare delivery, so evident over the past two decades.

An understanding of the continuing fallout from these policy

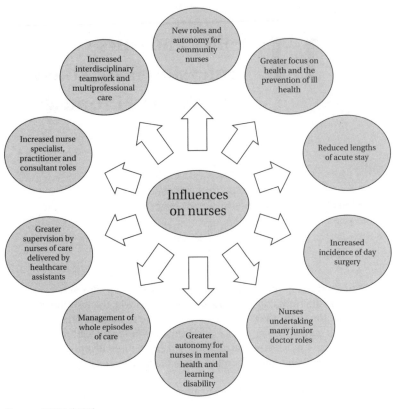

Source: NNRU, 2009b

Figure 11.1 Influences on the changing role of nurses

changes, and of course potential professional routes for the future, make for a worthwhile discussion for any nurse of whatever discipline. As Rafferty (2009) aptly reminded us, 'it is a question of understanding the demands that modern healthcare make on nurses. Nurses need to be well educated to support patients in the fast-moving world . . . Caring, compassionate *and* clever are what the public and healthcare system demand and deserve from modern nursing' – in addition, I would add political nous and resilience.

NHS reforms: the challenges and opportunities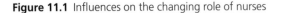

The role of professional nurses, together with their associated values and achievements, have been both challenged and developed during the past decades. A number of influences have changed and redirected nursing care across the UK (NNRU, 2009a, 2009b; see also Figure 11.1). While some nurses have found it impossible to survive the demands made upon them, others have thrived and created positive niches for themselves and, as of now, are still looking forwards to an interesting career in the future (Belfast Health and Social Care Trust et al., 2011; DOH, 2010c; Scottish Government, 2010; WAG, 2010).

Much work still to do

In spite of the development of the many new approaches in practice, there clearly remains much work for all nurses. The policy reforms of recent times have not always delivered the outcomes promised. Health inequalities have widened in spite of continuing efforts to close the gap (Marmot, 2010). Healthcare consumers have not necessarily been further empowered; rather, they have been offered a 'window dressing' type of choice (Mahon, 1992; Patients Association, 2009). The avowed intention of making the NHS more concerned with the promotion of health is still questioned, because of its long-held emphasis on the more easily measurable and 'costable'.

In turn the right to NHS care is now increasingly linked to individual responsibility for the maintenance of good health – potentially a problem for the most vulnerable in our communities. In addition, the emphasis on diversity sensitivity, for patients and for healthcare colleagues alike, remains an elusive goal, in spite of legislation, government desire and professional codes. Finally, the often stated support for effective multidisciplinary collaboration in care appears to have been made ever more difficult by the creation of competitive and fragmented structures within and without the currently changing NHS. All this policy activity has been underpinned by a number of important themes:

- the growth in a much sharper, commercialized approach to health services in the search for cost containment and value for money;
- a diversification in healthcare providers, creating a mixed economy of carers and providers;
- the continuing search for more affordable, effective and efficient health services;
- attempts to rein in, manage and define professional activity;
- the shifting of responsibility for health status and some health services back onto individuals and families and away from public provision.

Against this challenging backcloth, professional nurses have to work hard to keep up with the demands of policy change, and to deliver high-quality care in the rapidly moving and often difficult environment of care which is the NHS business of today.

📋 Activity: discuss with your fellow students or colleagues

- Are you, and those with whom you work, worried or excited about their future role as nurses in the NHS?

- What sorts of issues have been discussed around nursing and role opportunities?
- Do the patients seem pleased with their healthcare services or are there concerns?

Challenges to professional nurses: a continuing agenda

Many nurses, perhaps understandably, express differing degrees of exasperation as one policy development is followed by another. This conveyor-belt like experience, in all fairness to the government (and indeed any others before), is not just a recent phenomenon. Changes in policy direction and detail have taken place in the NHS in quick succession ever since its inception in 1948. Generations of nurses have had to ride many uncomfortable waves of policy, not least when the economy has demanded restraints and cutbacks in public expenditure. The efficiency reforms of the 1980s and 1990s were prime examples. Gough (1997) described them as, 'a stunning case study of the marginalization of the nursing contribution'. Many nurses felt compromised during that time, because of their inability to respond to patient need as fully as they may have wished.

Others (Mangan, 1983; Allsop, 1995) saw the impact of the more market-like approach to healthcare delivery as bad news for nurses, with its primary focus on the measurement of costs, contract making and money flows. In turn, a secondary interest appeared to be shown by the government in the seemingly peripheral qualitative concepts around service to the users, health promotion, or indeed, for this discussion, to the professional growth and development of professional nursing. Meehan (1996) described nursing care as being sacrificed on the high altar of finance, as nursing posts were being shed left, right and centre in a desperate attempt by healthcare trusts to balance the books – a theme which certainly reverberates today (Carter, 2010a; Cole, 2010; Scott, 2010c; Dean 2011a).

Many commentators noted the deafening silence about nurses in the Coalition's initial Health White Paper, *Equity and Excellence* (DOH, 2010e). It was strange and perplexing to see that the majority of the health workforce merited only two mentions. The media discussions on television and radio in the early weeks after its publication were similarly lacking, with barely a mention of nursing. As Cole (2010) said, 'it is hard to imagine what the new health services will look like, but one thing is certain, nurses will be crucial to its success. Politicians would be wise to put nurses, alongside doctors, at the centre of such change.'

The eventual announcement of a replacement Chief Nursing Officer (CNO) for Dame Christine Beasley when she retired, for example, only came after months of speculation and anxiety about the continued presence of such a role at the DOH. The failure to announce a successor early on caused many to fear a watering down or even a removal of the role. In a similar way, other more supportive proposals for nurse

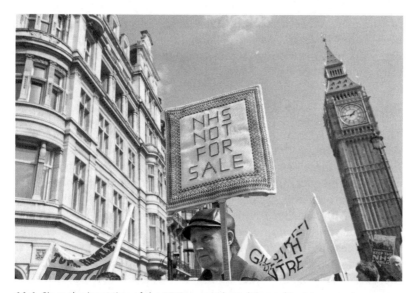

11.1 Since the inception of the NHS, nurses have been subject to several waves of economic challenges and cutbacks, making their position uncertain and volatile.

developments and contributions more generally have slipped out in a somewhat dilatory fashion – as though as an afterthought. Without a doubt, health policy imperatives have created an often difficult and challenging life for all professional nurses. This is, however, an unsurprising observation. Nurses are, and always have been, central players in the NHS. There is no way they could have been above or removed from the various outcomes already noted.

📋 Activity: discuss with your fellow students or colleagues

- Is the current government's health policy agenda a difficult challenge for you and your nursing colleagues? As a back-up to this question, look at the nursing press and find out what nurses are saying
- How are the patients responding to the changes? Do they comment?

Continuing challenges

One major aspect of the introduction of the managerial and market-like culture in the 1980s was the intention to control and shape professional carers of whatever discipline – nurse, doctor or professional allied to medicine. After all, high-status professionals are expensive to employ, and it was easy to see the appeal to cost-conscious managers of a more flexible, less powerful and much cheaper support carer workforce. This threat, and all that it entails, currently remains firmly on the agenda (Dean, 2010). As Charman (2009), the NHS Employers' Head of Employment Services, said: 'There will be more healthcare support workers in five years' time. Professional nurses will become a smaller, elite workforce overseeing the work of an increasing number of Health Care Support Workers (HCSWs).'

Why the concern? What is the evidence?

The training, education and employment of HCSWs across all disciplines is already very well established (Scott, 2010). In addition, the increasingly growing entrance of private health companies being welcomed by the government into NHS life (Booth et al., 2010) rings yet another warning bell. Clearly they are already well prepared to inject the NHS with their well-honed financial acumen and knowledge of residential, nursing home and private hospital care. However, cost effectiveness in those areas is often based on non-professional carer employment, a lean application of legal requirements and tight profit margins (Lister, 2008). If such approaches are applied to the NHS, then it is easy to see how the small, elite force of professionally qualified nurse leaders of care delivery might just become a reality.

While this may be good news for those who aspire to be in this elite professional nurse group, the negative implications could well be a lowering of standards to dangerous levels. Dr Simon Jones, chief statistician at Dr Foster Intelligence and senior research fellow at the National Nursing Research Unit at King's College London, said: 'research demonstrates that it is vital for Trusts to maintain good levels of professionally qualified nursing staff in order to safeguard patient safety' (cited in Ford, 2009).

Community nurses and others told the Queen's Nursing Institute that patient care was suffering because district nurses were being routinely replaced by healthcare assistants, with care 'dumbed down' to dangerous levels because of pressures to take on responsibilities for which healthcare assistants had little or no training (Snow, 2010d). Hurst's (2011a) research similarly supported the notion that the quality of care falls as skills are diluted and staffing pressures bite. We only need to look back to the experience of the Mid-Staffordshire NHS Foundation Trust to realize the potential detrimental effects of such moves for ourselves, for our patients and for the reputation and survival of the NHS (Francis, 2009).

The beginnings of such change in the workforce balance

The expressions of doubt as to the need to employ professional nurses surfaced in the early 1990s (Caines, 1993; Downey, 1993). Different ideas abounded, including the development of the support worker role (Fatchett, 1996), the up-skilling of cleaners to care for the elderly terminally ill (Goodchild, 1995; Leifer, 1996), the use of robots to deliver records and samples (Brown, 1996), questionnaires to replace health visitors (Kenny, 1997a) and health-promotion leaflets to replace school nurses (Kenny, 1997b).

Finally, a proposal was made that serious consideration should be given to replacing the role of the professional nurse with that of a generic carer with a broader based carer role, encompassing the responsibility for coordinating patient care and for delivering most of it in the NHS of the future (Manchester University, 1996). Responses to the last proposal were, unsurprisingly, polarized. Caines (1993) argued that it was time to scrap the boundaries between doctors and nurses and to create a single clinical group. Everyone interested in healthcare could take the same basic training and education, but then progress as far as individual inclinations or intellect permitted.

Conroy, however, argued that tinkering with the then-current health-care roles was not enough (in Leifer, 1996). She believed that patient needs and requirements for nursing care should define the package of skills required. Employment of professional carers, she suggested, should directly relate to the work needing to be carried out. In this way traditional professional role demarcations could be avoided, and only those who offered a relevant package of updated skills and knowledge would be employed.

The solution thus proposed was a flexible workforce, the centre point of which would be a 'generic health practitioner responsible for the continuity of care'. In addition it was proposed that the 28 per cent of support workers who contributed to nursing care should be expanded to 40 per cent by 2010, a percentage figure which has already been over-taken, according to both NHS Employers (2009b) and also the Audit Commission (see Dean, 2011).

Reactions at that time were unsurprisingly explosive, not least from nurse commentators. These ranged from 'nonsense', through 'out of touch with reality and an unsophisticated response to complex and challenging questions' to 'a cover for managers to cut qualified nurs-ing staff' (see Healy, 1996). The ideas were seen in combination as a potential body blow to the credibility of the nursing profession. One journal editor stated firmly that nurses wished to remain within their distinctively named and known care professions, particularly if the government gave them the recognition, authority and tools to do their job properly (*Nursing Times*, 1996). This statement reflected a strong and sincere belief in the special role of the professional nurse – a feel-ing which continues to be expressed today (Pearce, 2011; Scott, 2011c).

📋 Activity: discuss with your fellow students or colleagues

- Consider the proposals above and reflect on how much has come into being.
- Think how the work of support workers has developed and how many new roles they now take on in practice.

- Think how professional nurse roles have wandered into areas that were previously the remit of doctors.
- Were you shocked by some of the suggestions, or have they already happened or perhaps gone even further than proposed?

The concept of professionalism: why is it so important to us?

In very common usage, the term 'professional' is seen as a symbol of high value, implying dedication and commitment. There is a vast expanse of literature on it, and a multitude of definitions and perspectives. The analysis of the concept has been a major preoccupation of sociologists over time. It becomes evident that, like other concepts – health need and care, for example – the debates around the nature of professionalism are complex, often contradictory, and in the end rely upon individual perception, understanding and experience. Let us just consider some of the ideas introduced by seminal writers:

1 Professionalism represents an institutionalization of personal service and community welfare (Durkeim, 1951).
2 Professionals are not motivated by either personal interests or economic reward (Weber, 1966).
3 There is an ethical focus to the work professionals do and it is about providing a service to others based on technical knowledge (Parsons, 1931,1951).
4 It is about providing a guarantee of objectivity and being above sectional interests (Turner, 1991).
5 An occupation possessing skilled intellectual technique, a voluntary association and *a code of conduct*; the code of conduct was seen as 'the guarantee of integrity . . . the main distinguishing mark of the professions' (Kaye, cited in Prandy 1965).

Other views on the nature of professions are also worth noting. Greenwood (1957) and Millerson (1964) listed the characteristics or traits of professional groups as follows:

- skills based on theoretical understanding;
- autonomy in judgements;
- tested competence in achieving high standards;
- possession of a service ethic, so that work is done for the common good rather than for individual self-interest.

As Hugman (1991) explains, each occupation to be considered as a candidate for the label professional could be compared to the list of traits, and the degree to which it matched was then taken as an indication of the extent to which the occupation was a profession. Following from this, Etzioni (1969) applied the approach to nurses, social workers and teachers, and defined them as 'semi-professionals', because he found them to be highly managed and controlled within their working environments. In addition, he suggested, their work lacked specific (to them) theoretical underpinning and emphasized skills rather than knowledge. By comparison, medicine and law had a much greater claim to professional status than nursing.

📋 Activity: discuss this with your fellow students or colleagues

- Discuss some of the issues raised above – do they worry you?
- Did you come into nursing to become a professional or for some other reason?
- Do you think you are a professional or a semi-professional?
- Does it matter what we are called?

In yet another perspective, professionalism is seen as a form of occupational control (Friedson, 1970; Johnson, 1972). In this way, the profession decides who should or should not belong, for instance in nursing through the use of registration. For example, a qualified nurse is seen as a safer and more knowledgeable practitioner than someone who is not qualified. Such self-regulation is very common amongst healthcarers around the world (Lewis et al., 1978; Willis, 2009)

The specialist knowledge and skills acquired by members of a particular occupation like nursing enable them, to a greater or lesser degree, to claim autonomy in judgements about their care, and to be relatively free from management and supervision. In reality, of course, the ability of any healthcare professional to wield total power or control over their work is constrained by others. This may involve members of the same profession, other allied professions, those who are paying for the care, the consumers or users of the services, and wider social institutions, for example acting on behalf of the government – including the NHS Commissioning Board, the Care Quality Commission, Monitor and the National Institute for Clinical Excellence.

By these and other means, the activities of professionals, in whatever sphere, are determined both within and without, and between professions. The power relationships thus created are obviously complex, with all sides seeking to achieve their own ends by both covert and overt means. Suffice to say, no professional groups, including nurses, have been immune to the complexity of specific forces, which have both influenced and shaped the nature of our professional contribution as it is today.

📋 Activity: discuss with your fellow students or colleagues

- What external factors impinge on your practice?
- Is your code of conduct difficult to deliver?

- What part does the implementation of policy have in defining your practice?
- Can you do all that you wish to do or are there constraints on your practice?
- Does your professional future look promising/interesting/worrying?

The role of professionals in the NHS and beyond

The formal care arenas, including the NHS, are crammed with professionals, who would all, to a greater or lesser degree, subscribe to a traditional vision of their role: the notion of having operational autonomy, a concern with giving service immediately to a person in need, and a belief that their specialist knowledge and skills can only be provided by members of their own profession. Indeed, they must by definition see themselves as protecting the public from outsiders – for example, from unscrupulous practitioners who have been expelled from the profession or who claim the status but are not members, or from quacks, amateurs or practitioners of unscientific methods (Goldacre, 2009).

It is no wonder, then, that any group, including nurses, would wish to be acknowledged as a profession, and of course to have the opportunity both to shape their practice and to garner good financial rewards in the process. It is also no surprise then that the nursing profession has been, and still is, very protective of its role in society and defensive in relation to any challenging influences – whether policy development or diminution in permitted activity. That said, Heller (1978) argued that nursing, unlike medicine, has failed to achieve the desired status and power within the NHS.

📋 Activity: discuss with your fellow students or colleagues

- Does Heller's view hold true today?
- Is nursing as a profession weaker than medicine?
- Are both professions equally constrained and managed?
- What examples could you give from your own practice area, either agreeing with Heller or challenging his views?

Whatever your conclusions, whether as semi- or full professionals, nurses are viewed in a special light by the general public, as indeed is the medical profession. The idea that doctors are seen as even more important than nurses is also probably true – but so what? The nursing profession offers a complementary and different caring role and surely any reasonable debate should not be about competition for the high ground, but about how responsive and effective any professional group's contribution is to meeting current health needs. Making the patients' needs central and applying a judgement on the degree to

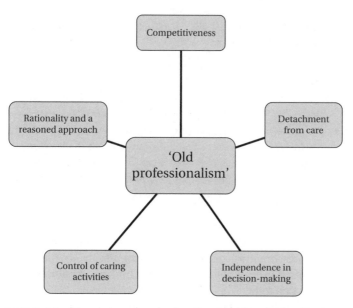

Figure 11.2 A traditional view of professionalism or 'old professionalism'

which any professional group achieves a level of success in meeting those needs surely ought to be the determining factor of their level of professionalism and reward.

By shifting the focus in this way, we can begin to redefine the nature of professionalism into a shape and perspective which is more relevant to meeting the health needs of the twenty-first century. We can potentially see the emergence of a way of working which is modern and a more achievable way of combining and integrating professional skills, something which the historical and traditional professional hierarchies and role boundaries have often made very difficult.

Davies (1996), for example, referred to the 'inhospitable terrain' on which nurses have worked and struggled to develop and consolidate their rights to professional status, and their care contribution to be treated with the same respect as that of the medical profession. She believed that nurses' attempts over time to prove their worth as professionals had fallen regularly on deaf ears, and that the traditional concept or interpretation of professionalism ('old professionalism') was a mirage and impossible to achieve because of the implicit nature of nursing care and its historical subservience to medicine. As Lindberg et al. (1990: 29) described it: 'The early science of nursing was not a separate and recognized discipline, like chemistry or psychology. Instead, it was a loosely defined body of scientific facts and principles underlying *physician prescribed* nursing.'

As Davies (1996) and others (Denny and Earle, 2008; Rafferty, 1996; Wicks, 1998) have noted, the 'old professionalism' traits, as listed in Figure 11.2, relate well to the stereotypical, traditional and masculine

Box 11.1 The Nightingale Pledge: attributed to Lystra Gretta, 1893

'I solemnly pledge myself to God and in the presence of this assembly to pass my life in purity and to practice my profession faithfully. I will abstain from what is deleterious and mischievous and will not take or knowingly administer any harmful drug. I will do all in my power to elevate the standard of my profession, and will hold in confidence all personal matters committed to my keeping, and all family affairs coming to my knowledge in the practice of my calling. With loyalty will I endeavour to aid the physician in his work, and devote myself to the welfare of those committed to my care.'

image of the medical profession. They do not, however, fit with the predominantly female nursing workforce (and many in the current medical profession too), as they are antipathetic to the reflective, attached, caring, interdependent nature of both professional nurse and medical practice today.

The development of specialist and other high-level nurse roles is a good example of these new interprofessional working relationships (Abel et al., 1995; Puntis, 1995; Barklem, 2010; Davis, 2010; Handley, 2011) – something unimaginable in the 1950s, 1960s and 1970s, as noted by writer, broadcaster, social campaigner and former nurse Claire Raynor in her autobiography (2010). *Deference to* doctors, but not *partnerships* in care, were clearly the norm for nurses during those earlier decades. Nurse training was very much about assisting doctors without usurping their position or authority. The art of nursing was focused on care and the softer domestic elements, with the science of medicine strongly focused on diagnosis, prescription and cure – a legacy of the Nightingale era and its core values and principles.

📋 Activity: discuss with your fellow students or colleagues

- Study the Nightingale Pledge in Box 11.1.
- How relevant is this pledge today?
- Compare it to today's NMC code of conduct (2008).

A new concept: 'new professionalism'

Davies proposed the creation of a new, more inclusive conceptual model of professionalism, one which values the collection of a more appropriate group of professional carer traits, which better reflects the changing nature of patient health needs for the early twenty-first century, and which is more relevant to the currently developing NHS care delivery systems and allied organizations. As she put it: 'Nursing should construct a new model of professionalism that reflects the

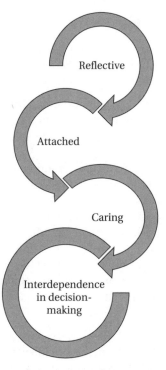

Figure 11.3 'New professionalism': a more relevant concept for nurses?

changing relationships between providers and patients, doctors and nurses. This revitalized understanding of ourselves is essential if we are to respond creatively to health challenges' (Davies, 1996). This aspiration is just as relevant today, because of the changing nature and diversity of healthcare provision, and the complexity of providers from many different sectors. All professionals of whatever discipline have to be able to work in this new and developing environment and be able to work interdependently (see Figure 11.3). The old ways of working in professionally led silos (in ward, unit, discipline or organization) have already changed and developed in complexity and, as such, the new professional practitioners of today have to adopt very different approaches, to be able to work with and to rely upon others – not least, and above all, with the users of their services.

While nursing is thus offered a constructive and exciting objective to pursue, the reality is that any fundamental change of understanding around the concept of professionalism is unlikely to be easily achieved. Indeed, some may well argue that trying to 'change the goalposts' is no way for nurses to achieve the highly prized professional status either. In any event, this particular debate will need to be carried forward by all nurses for some time to come if they are ever to achieve without argument the coveted traditional role of 'full', highly prized professionals.

Survival as a profession

Whatever definitions are in the ascendancy, however, and whatever their appropriateness or otherwise, nursing as a whole needs to give closer attention to a number of important aspects, including:

1 The development of a good understanding of the generality of external political and other forces which currently shape society's attitudes to healthcare on the national stage, and to professional nursing care within it.
2 The development of a clear understanding of current health policy directions and developments, and the potential future pathways for professional nurse careers.
3 An ability to demonstrate and to promote a picture of what professional nursing care has to offer as opposed to non-professional care. This of course requires continuing professional development throughout each nurse's working life, so that what is offered is current, updated and of a very high standard – aspects which can only be offered by those with specific high-level skills and knowledge.

Admittedly, the defence of professional nursing will involve a high level of commitment and motivation. It is not likely to be an easy task, judging by past history. It will be made more difficult by the current period of financial retrenchment and the search for cost-cutting potential both in health services and among health personnel. No professional group, including nurses, is immune. The continuing support and massive development over time of the cheaper and more flexible support worker role across healthcare only serves to rebut claims as to the special professional nature of much nursing care.

Tasks passed to others may have released time for other higher-level activity, but may at the same time have served to diminish the professional nature of the nursing role and nursing activity in the eyes of cost-conscious managers. Why employ one costly person when you can afford two who, on the face of it, achieve the same in practice? This is a belief which has been countered in recent research evidence (NNRU, 2009b), but which is currently being ignored across an NHS scrambling to cut costs and being taken over by private sector bodies in order to survive. As Booth et al. (2010a) commented: 'The private sector boom comes amid the toughest financial climate for public services in a generation, and despite continued assurances from ministers that reforms to public services are aimed at achieving greater value for money and improving efficiency.' According to Andy Burnham, MP, 'some private operators are going to have a field day, making a fortune from a system which will offer less public accountability' (in Booth et al. 2010a).

In the current economic environment there is clearly a very real threat to the continued broad employment of professionally qualified nurses within the NHS, not least when the non-qualified are perceived as offering the same sort of care in practice. So how have we arrived at this current situation? Let's look back at the past decades and see if there are any lessons to be learned.

Professionalism under threat?

From the beginning of the NHS, nurses, together with doctors and the professions allied to medicine, have all developed their roles and contributions to healthcare delivery. Without a doubt, the obvious centrality of their work to the health service ensured both power and a degree of autonomy. This was very evident to the Conservative government in the early 1980s, with the professionals seemingly having greater power than the managers and administrators.

In addition, the multidisciplinary federation of healthcare players, inevitable in an organization as dependent upon professionals as the NHS, meant there was no single focal point of power or decision-making. It was because of this lack of clarity in the management process that the then government decided to introduce a series of changes designed to strengthen NHS management and, as we know already, to begin to control activity and expenditure – not least that of the professionals.

No group in the health service, whether professional or manual, was left untouched, least of all nurses, in what was to be a systematic overhaul of the whole service. Whereas all previous governments in the 1950s, 1960s and 1970s failed to hold on to the professional reins, the four Conservative governments from 1979 onwards put themselves firmly into the driving seat in an attempt to make the healthcare agendas of professionals and non-professionals alike fall into line with their policy direction and focus.

The impact of general management

For some, the introduction of general management in the early 1980s was regarded as an attack on both professional autonomy and clinical freedoms. It attracted a predictably hostile reception from both doctors and nurses. The Griffiths inquiry team (1983) must have expected nothing less. Their specific remit had been to make an assessment of NHS management, and their conclusions came as no surprise. They said the power of professional groups overrode management decision-making. The multiplicity of professional role players all demanding that their voices be heard in management circles led to consensus decision-making. This dulled the effectiveness of management and ensured that NHS change was slow and incremental. General business management, as in industrial and retail settings, was proposed as a more successful route to take.

A knowledge of levels and quality of service, of employee motivation and of evaluation of activities and a commitment to the consumers were all perceived as needed within the NHS at large. It was argued that such a move was the only way of taking it forward, to ensure value for money for the taxpayer, together with the provision of a much more effective and responsive health service which would benefit the whole community.

The new management

In the wake of the management inquiry, all NHS organizations were ordered to appoint general managers by the end of 1985. The new managers were to take responsibility for the overall direction and strategic management of the NHS and for applying clear business principles throughout. They were mostly in place by 1986 (Holliday, 1995), with only 36 of these new-style managers being nurses. In the main, the managers came from industrial and commercial backgrounds and were brought into the NHS to drive through the necessary changes.

Short-term contracts, performance-related pay and regular reviews were introduced, all of which were intended to sharpen each general manager's personal commitment to delivering the required managerial approach. While manual workers had already felt the sharp edge of compulsory competitive tendering of their services, professional nurses and doctors were now about to feel the impact of this new managerial philosophy. It required everyone to come under sharp commercial scrutiny and to prove their value and effectiveness, if they were to stay in business in the NHS.

Nursing's response – a concerned profession?

Elements of the traditional nursing hierarchies were dismantled to make way for the new managers, including the demise of the traditional matron figures. This, in particular, represented a rejection of the former system of nurses being rewarded simply for the length of time served in the NHS. In its place came new ideas linking reward and career opportunities to evidence of developed skills, experience and managerial ability. We can see the legacy of this approach in the expectation of the demonstrably higher levels of continuing professional development and ability needed to be a 'modern matron' in the twenty-first century NHS (DOH, 2003a) and, even more so now, for those professional nurses who aspire to advanced nursing practice status within today's rapidly changing NHS (DOH, 2010c; Harrison and Snow, 2011).

Doctors also concerned?

Many doctors also found the introduction of the new managerial culture worrying. That said, appeals to the doctors' sense of responsibility to the public, particularly in a period of economic stringency, provided the essential backcloth to the reality of other managerial strategies. They were encouraged at that time to become responsible for clinical budgeting, performance reviews and performance indicators – aspects which have now become accepted custom and practice. In addition to this, improved distinction awards were offered to consultants to oil the wheels of change – a move harking back to Aneurin Bevan's days of 'stuffing the consultants' mouths with gold' in his efforts to bring in a national health service (Foot, 1973).

Some doctors, like nurses, became general managers. Others who remained unconvinced held out for a long time, but slowly conceded points in order to survive. It became obvious to the government that further reform was needed to develop and enhance the required cultural change, and to force all the professions into a context in which they had to become a working part of the new NHS tanker or leave.

The pressure on professionals continues

The traditional ways of running a service in which professionals held absolute power were poised at this stage to be pushed into the sidings by the introduction of the internal healthcare market reforms. It was argued that the managed competition between the purchasers and providers of the service would both open up and sharpen the delivery of professional services. Those who delivered 'the business' would benefit financially and professionally, as would their employer institution; those who did not would lose out. As Mangan (1993) said at the time, nurses needed to demonstrate their worth if they wanted to remain as (professional) clinicians, teachers and managers in the new NHS – a call which must sound very familiar to all nurses today.

📋 Activity: discuss with your fellow students or colleagues

- What are your thoughts on general management?
- Are there circumstances or issues in organizations that can only be led by professional managers?
- What are the upsides/downsides of having a business-like approach in the NHS?
- What efforts have you made to refresh and update your practice?

The NHS internal market reforms: impacts on professionals

By January 1989 the change to general management in the NHS was seen as an effective tool for making inroads into rectifying the many faults found in 1983 by Griffiths and his colleagues in the inquiry team. New management information systems had shown variations in performance up and down the country, different waiting times

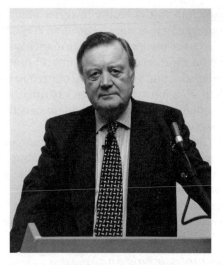

11.2 After his appointment as Health Secretary in 1988, Kenneth Clarke was responsible for introducing the controversial idea of an 'internal market' within the NHS.

for treatment depending on where one lived and variations in referral rates and prescribing habits. The then Conservative Secretary of State for Health, Kenneth Clarke, said that 'all professionals could do much better in putting the patients first'. This of course provoked a considerable reaction, not least from other politicians.

Robin Cook, then Labour Party Shadow Health Secretary, clearly aware of all the managerial activity discussed above, wondered: 'How many more bureaucrats will the NHS need to make this package work? Will he [Kenneth Clarke] tell us how much more time doctors and nurses will have to take off patient care to file their financial returns? Will he tell us how much more the monitoring, the pricing and the bargaining over every treatment will add to the cost of administration?' (Hansard, 1989). He also queried the apparent lack of discussion with, and lack of advice taken from, the caring professions in the health service. Clarke responded: 'There is no reason why the public service should not be run with the same efficiency and consumer consciousness as the private sector – you cannot dismiss the value of modern management disciplines, financial accountability and consumer consciousness that we are seeking to build into the health service' (Hansard, 1989). As far as consultation with nurses and doctors was concerned, this was to be done after the publication of a variety of working papers, which were to provide more specific detail about the implementation at local levels.

Broadly, then, the process of consultation as described was very limited. Professional groups were not going to be allowed to influence the reforms in any major way, but they would be expected to deliver them. In turn, much of the detail in the legislation set out ground rules, expectations and rewards for delivery – trends and themes which we continue to see in today's health programme (DOH, 2010c).

Working for Patients (DOH, 1989c): Promises, opportunities and threats for professionals

The initial announcement of the proposed changes and the introduction of the market reforms suggested developments which held out promise and a positive future for some, but the opposite for others.

The pressure that existed to cut the costs of NHS spending, the continuing pressure to develop a managerial culture and commercialization, the search for cost-effective clinical effectiveness, a reassessment of skill mixes and possible labour substitutions and a determined effort to raise the calibre of untrained staff so that they could take on nursing roles all clearly contributed to a questioning of professional nursing expertise and status. The ever-increasing management control over the focus, content and degree of professional nurse care both purchased and provided within the internal healthcare market also had its own effects.

Efforts by nurses to professionalize further through practice and educational developments were often felt by them to be sidelined by the government, in spite of assertions to the contrary. The concern for meeting the aims and objectives of the NHS business appeared to many to supersede the internal professionalizing agendas of an increasingly challenged nurse workforce. Some nurses gave up the fight and left the NHS and nursing altogether, seeking a future in a more comfortable working environment or to retirement (Mills, 1998).

Having said that, this depressing picture did not apply to the whole of the nursing profession. Many also sought to strengthen their role, and to develop and change within the new environment. While

---

Box 11.2 *Working for Patients*: the proposed changes

- Greater satisfaction and rewards for those working in the NHS who responded successfully to local needs and preferences.
- The new organizations: the hospital trusts would harness the skills and dedication of their staff and would be setting their own conditions of service, pay rates and rewards for individual performances.
- Better use of professional staff and their skills.
- Provision of better training for non-professional support staff.
- An appraisal of the traditional practices of nurses would result in some roles previously carried out by doctors being passed to them and some clerical work removed.
- The nursing profession would become part of the resource-management initiatives to provide management with more information about nurse care activity and its cost.

acknowledging the difficulties of proving the value of professional nursing to manager and policy-makers alike, at the same time the changes provided the impetus to explore and explain the depth of the nature of nursing care, and in turn to develop innovative and high-quality services within the NHS. In a sense this was also an attempt to counter the anti-professional cries of some commentators who appeared to believe that anyone can be a nurse.

Efforts to 'professionalize'

During the periods we have visited so far, efforts were made to shift and to change the philosophy and process of professional nurse practice – in a sense, to explore and redefine its essence. According to Beardshaw et al. (1990), 'the changes involved moves to replace the task-based method of organising nursing work, with care more precisely tailored to individual patient needs'. The result of this would be 'to substitute a professional model of nurse organization for nursing's long established hierarchical, bureaucratic one', providing a means to move from 'old professionalism' to a 'new professionalism'.

Butterworth (1992) and Williams (1993) saw these developments as a challenge to the traditional biomedical ties of nursing to medicine. The domains of modern professional nursing were to encompass the wider emotional and social aspects of care, all issues which have an impact upon the health and well-being of the whole population.

In general terms these approaches are very much part of current professional nurse activity and understanding. These of course have had an impact not only upon all educational developments, including

---

Box 11.3 The attributes of a modern nursing profession

- the nurse and client are active partners in care decisions and delivery;
- the nurse as health educator has a goal of client empowerment;
- the client, not the task, is the central focus of care;
- care is individualized to meet the needs of the client;
- an understanding of the broad determinants of health and the holistic nature of client need necessitate an exploration of the physical, intellectual, emotional, social and spiritual needs of individuals, community and society;
- the client is seen as an individual in a broad social context (family, community and society), and this will influence and have an impact both positively and negatively on the health and well-being, response to illness, and recovery of that individual at any one time;
- the delivery of effective nursing care relies upon collaboration with other carers, both formal and informal, the client and other potential users of the health services.

(Maben and Griffiths, 2008)

the earlier Project 2000-style nurse training, but also on all the current developments around undergraduate and postgraduate nursing courses (Callanan, 2011; Corney, 2010). They also provided the impetus for a large number of nurse-led initiatives and allied activities to date. These have included nurse practitioner, specialist and consultant roles, non-medical prescribing and social enterprise initiatives, to note but a few. So, in spite of the often 'inhospitable terrain' of the NHS, nurses have, and are, pursuing professional status by many means, and, as before, are being supported by the government to push forward in this way and to make a difference, both for themselves and for the NHS (CNO, 2009; NHS Employers, 2009b; Milton, 2010c).

Activity: discuss with your fellow students or colleagues

- Can you relate these developments to your own experience?
- Can you defend the professional nature of your care with examples from your own practice?

The threat remains?

History has shown us that professional nurses have always, in the main, managed to rise to a challenge. It is clear from our past observations, however, that any future professional development will depend upon how much real support nurses are given by the government of the day and thus by management. Emphasis has regularly been placed on the value of the nursing profession to the future of the NHS and to the provision of high-quality health-promoting care (Wilson, 2004; DOH, 1997; Milton, 2010d). At the same time, support and interest has clearly developed (and is still developing) in skill mixing and also in the substitution of the financially costly nursing profession by a generic carer workforce as envisaged in 1996 (Manchester University, 1996). This idea, as we know, envisaged a healthcare workforce made up of an appropriately planned mix of differently skilled carers, remunerated according to skill level achieved, and employed because of their appropriateness to the needs of the care situation at any particular time. Such flexibility of employment, with the ability to skill mix and thus to contain costs, clearly holds appeal, not least to those who view nurse professionals as inappropriate and expensive rigidities within the healthcare employment market – no doubt a clear concern for today.

In many respects, the discussions around the need for skill mixing, flexibility of working and the fairness of pay linked to skills delivered very much mirrors the arguments made about the ambulance workers' pay in the early 1980s. It was said then that, as the skill levels involved varied from employee to employee – that is, broadly, from taxi driver to paramedic – there was no reason to pay everyone in the service at the same level. Those who delivered at a high level of skill and knowledge – for example, the highly skilled paramedics – deserved their titles and the financial rewards commensurate with their contribution to healthcare delivery. Those, however, who transported people to and from home and healthcare settings should be remunerated for their passenger transport role and be given a lower status than their more able colleagues.

Similarly, within the nursing profession there have been moves to differentiate between roles, tasks and financial rewards, not least through nurse regrading, banding and skill mixing within teams. In a sense, we can see how these moves over time have effectively divided up and emphasized different levels of skill and knowledge across the whole of the care workforce within the NHS (NAO, 2009). These sorts of moves have set apart and highlighted the well-skilled and higher-status elite minority of nurses, whether at practitioner, manager or academic levels. By contrast, their lesser-skilled and lower-status majority counterparts have been differently rewarded for their lower-level skill and knowledge-based contributions.

The status and role of professional nurses is currently still being examined. After all, qualified nursing care continues to remain a costly resource in the NHS budgeting equation. Times have long changed in terms of nurse employment policy. In place of reward for loyalty and expertise, all organizations are looking for innovation, flexibility, responsibility and accountability, and much more besides. Because of this, no matter how well the profession redefines itself, nursing, as in any other part of the labour market, will continue to be under close scrutiny and subject to vigorous questioning as to its value and special status within the healthcare setting – not least within one that has been described as 'facing a funding ice age' (Meehan, 2009) and the 'last stage before the [NHS] tanker slows down and finally retrenches' (Edwards, 2009).

The emergence of this scenario needs to be taken seriously. It has developed incrementally over the past two decades and without a doubt will continue to gain pace and strength. Three outcomes seem likely:

1 The professional nurse of the future will offer a defined set of high-level characteristics in education, practice skills and knowledge.
2 This nurse will be part of a small elite group, all of whom will be graduates and who will be classed as 'full professionals'.
3 The great majority of other carers will offer flexible and mixed packages of skills and knowledge, but will not be classed or paid as professionals. Their care work will be coordinated by professional nurses.

What is our strategy now?

The need for compassionate nursing is as strong as it has ever been. Nurses are a central resource in the NHS and are crucial to the delivery of 21st-century healthcare. They are in a powerful position to improve the experience of patients, the quality of care and health outcomes across the whole range of health services. Society is changing and so is the NHS and the need for expert nursing care has never been greater. (Maben and Griffiths, 2008: 5)

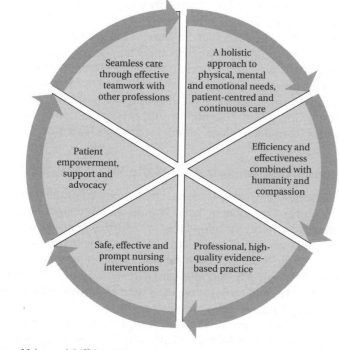

Source: Maben and Griffiths, 2008

Figure 11.4 Good-quality nursing care

The statement above is a good starting point for planning a way forward to harness the support of the public, other professionals and politicians in our aim to rejuvenate the professional nurse role and to ensure the delivery of good-quality nursing care within the NHS for the foreseeable future (see Figure 11.4).

The NHS: its needs and wants

The NHS is currently undergoing major change in both structure and organization, set against a tightening financial regime right across the whole of the public sector. This sharp reality has set in train important changes in NHS care services, which are focused on financial delivery and deficit reduction. The growing cost of meeting the major health challenges of rising obesity, for example, and consequent long-term needs, coupled with efforts to reduce health inequalities, are all combining to force the development of new services and approaches.

There is a growing encouragement of self-care for people with long-term conditions and greater demands for 'complementary approaches' to meeting health needs. Patient demand for choice is growing and is being encouraged, not least in relation to health advice, care packages, treatments, access for care arrangements and personal health budgets (Coyle, 2011).

Growing and increasingly diverse roles for the third and private sectors are being welcomed into the NHS, especially for secondary care. All services currently provided are gaining from the substantial benefits of improved information technology, with information for patients, and about patients, on effectiveness and healthcare performance. There is also a growing use of 'telecare' to support care at home, and new applications for biotechnology, bioengineering and robotics.

Management and organization of the NHS

The management and organizational changes are continuing to make for a turbulent environment in the NHS. Substantial changes in the pattern of hospital services are happening, with further concentrations on specialist services and reduced lengths of stay, and with provision at or near home for the more generalist services. There is now an increased incidence of day surgery and aftercare. Greater coordination of care between the NHS and social services is now an important means of caring for people outside the acute sector.

Government policy continues to focus on outcomes and the measurement of effectiveness, reducing variations in performance, improving safety, quality and productivity, and the design of more effective incentive systems, with the engagement of both the medical and nursing professions in delivering these across the services.

Nurses

For professional nurses, the Coalition programme of health reform within the NHS has, on the one hand, caused degrees of concern and dismay, while, on the other, it has opened up possibilities for new ventures. Nurses have been given the opportunity to direct and lead care both within and outside the NHS and have been encouraged and supported to take a more entrepreneurial stance and to use their undoubted skills and knowledge in new-style working. See the report of the Prime Minister's Commission on the future of nursing and midwifery in England published on 12 April 2011.

The need to consider the future for professional nursing within this new-style NHS remains, however, a major concern, particularly given the influx of a diversity of support workers and new sectors, both in their own way challenging the need to employ professional nursing care. Qualified nurses are, as a result, having to provide greater supervision of the care delivered by healthcare assistants. At the same time, they are expected to develop specialist and advanced professional nurse roles, with a blurring of professional and sector boundaries – an issue which is of concern to many because of the continuing failure to regulate advanced practice and the potential challenge to public safety.

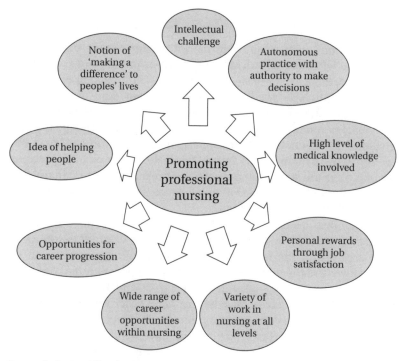

Source: Foskett and Hemsley-Brown, 1998

Figure 11.5 Messages to promote professional nursing as a career to young people

As Professor Dickon Weir-Hughes has said: 'If people go into a walk-in centre, they do not know whether the person treating them has done a weekend course or a Master's degree. They have no idea about the skills they can expect'. Maclaine agrees with this, noting that the general public assumes that if a person has a fancy title they have done something to achieve it (see Waters 2011a). Such required initiatives and emerging roles for all nurses, however, are in response to both government reform changes and healthcare demands, which dictate flexibility and innovatory high-level practice across the professional nursing workforce in the acute, primary and community care sectors.

There is a continuing need to give a high profile to recruitment and retention of the future professional nurse workforce. Students need to be well supported in practice – both to learn how to provide high-quality care and also to ensure an enthusiastic professional workforce for the future. The younger generation needs to be encouraged to see nursing as a top career choice, one which is perceived as a worthwhile career for talented people with aptitude and motivation. Importantly, the non-visible aspects of nursing (intellectual and decision-making) need to be made more clearly identifiable (see Figure 11.5).

So, what's the plan?

The Coalition's 2010 health reforms set in train major changes right across the NHS world, providing both opportunities and risks for all concerned, not least for professional nurses. The further opening up of the market into NHS care has provided the opportunity to reconfigure services, to enter new markets, to innovate and to create new ways of working. For nurses, there are opportunities to lead and shape the new systems for the benefit of the patients, to manage the inherent risks and to flourish with them within a new-style NHS. However, as in previous periods of health service change, those who look to a future in nursing within a flourishing profession will have to use their influence, skills and knowledge to make it happen.

The context has been set for the NHS and patients have expressed what they want from their nursing care. These can all be matched (and are) within the lexicon of professional nursing practice at its best. However, the negative issues around poor standards of care have, in recent times, often destroyed trust and belief in the profession's ability to claim primacy in care provision (Care Quality Commission, 2011; Parliamentary and Health Service Ombudsman, 2011). These incidents of failure to care have not only caused a great deal of harm to those affected, but have severely damaged the profession's image in the eyes of the public. As with politicians, reputation is all.

Similarly now in nursing, there is much work to be done in demonstrating the value of keeping the professional nurse at the centre of NHS care. There is a need to demonstrate a commitment to the new NHS environment, however difficult, by being part of it and creating innovative schemes which reflect all the essential and special qualities of professional nursing and which help the patients and the public to gain the services they require and the help they may need to take control of their own health and well-being. By these means, we can hope to demonstrate the value of high-quality nursing care and to win back the support of the public as we seek to ensure a healthy future for the nursing profession in the coming decades.

Conclusion

This chapter has considered a variety of issues around the nature of professionalism, with specific emphasis on nursing. The policy backcloth of NHS reforms appears to have produced dissonance between, on the one hand, the public statements of support for enhanced professional nurse practice and, on the other, the actual pressures upon that role. It is this dissonance that must continue to cause concern for the future of nursing as a profession. In light of the current policy moves towards a much more fragmented environment for care, can we maintain hope for the future even outside the NHS? Are we worried about the growth in non-professional carers or, indeed, the need for a degree qualification to be a nurse?

Initial responses to this may be upbeat. After all, the many perceived and real barriers to professional development have failed to halt the creation of innovative and relevant nurse responses to the ever-challenging policy agendas. Many new high-level skills have been developed in order to improve the standards of care offered and to deliver the types of nurse-led initiatives required by successive governments.

There appear to be opportunities opening up within the NHS for those nurses who have the professional skills and willingness to rise to the challenges. That said, while many will work to hold onto the status of being a professional nurse, there is no easy road ahead. The future is likely to be rough. What is known, however, is that nurses, in whatever field, can and do make a positive difference to the healthcare experiences of individuals whether at primary, secondary or tertiary levels. As Dr Jane Williams puts it: 'Work hard, look for opportunities. Make sure you step out of your comfort zone, and particularly from a nursing point of view, push the boundaries of what people think nurses can and should be doing. It is not always comfortable, but unless you try these things you don't challenge people's thinking' (in Munro, 2011a).

We need to look back at Asvall's statement cited at the beginning of this chapter. While in no doubt as to the importance and incredible potential of the professional nurse contribution to society, he reminds us that society and governments also have a duty to provide nurses with the recognition they deserve and the working conditions they need to carry out their unique role. The future for professional nursing rests not just within itself, but also in a reciprocal partnership with the whole community.

Learning outcomes

- an understanding of the concept of professionalism and what this means for nurses;
- an understanding of the implications of current policy developments for the nursing profession and its future;
- the importance of continually refreshing and developing professional skills and knowledge.

Further reading

Bishop, V. (ed.) (2009) *Leadership for Nursing and Allied Health Professionals*. Open University Press.

Bostridge, M. (2009) *Florence Nightingale: The Woman and her Legend*. Penguin Books.

Hall, C. and Ritchie, D. (2009) *What is Nursing? Exploring Theory and Practice*. Learning Matters Ltd.

McKimm, J. and Phillips, K. (eds) (2009) *Leadership and Management in Integrated Services.* Learning Matters Ltd.

Sellman, D. and Snelling, P. (2010) *Becoming a Nurse.* Pearson-Education Ltd.

Williamson, G. R., Jenkinson, T. and Proctor-Childs, T. (2008) *Nursing in Contemporary Healthcare Practice.* Learning Matters Ltd.

12 Learning from the Past, Looking to the Future

'The need for compassionate nursing is as strong as it has ever been. Nurses are a central resource in the National Health Service . . . and are crucial to the delivery of 21st-century healthcare. They are in a powerful position to improve the experience of patients, the quality of care and health outcomes across the whole range of health services. Society is changing and so is the NHS and the need for expert nursing care has never been greater.'

(Maben and Griffiths, 2008)

'To survive, the NHS will need to continually reinvent itself, as it has been doing since 1948, just like all the most durable British institutions – parliament, monarchy, BBC and Marks & Spencer. Personally, I hope and believe that it can do so, so that a decade from now it will be in rude health, alive and kicking and celebrating its three score years and ten.'

(Stevens, 2008: 110)

The discussions in this book have addressed two important issues:

1 The policy developments within the NHS from 1948 and their likely form and focus as we move into the second decade of the twenty-first century.
2 The past, present and potential future development of the nursing profession.

In earlier works I have encouraged nurses to be more actively involved in the debates about the future of the NHS in order to shape their own professional destiny (Fatchett, 1994, 1998, 2002). The discussions in this book have built upon that precedent. It is to be hoped that it will act as a further catalyst for an informed and practical response to what is currently happening both to the NHS and to the professional role of nursing. The backcloth to all the chapters has been that of profound policy changes within the NHS, instituted by successive governments since 1948. These have seen the creation of a quasi-market in health-care, with the separation of purchaser and provider roles, a mixed economy of care provision and the development of an underpinning ethos which is both commercialized and competitive in nature.

In tandem with this major and systematic overhaul of the health services, we have seen what appears to be a redefinition of professional nurse practice. The intellectual development of nurse education and training has moved apace over the past century. The move towards an all-graduate profession by 2013 is now a reality, backed up by a grow-ing army of cheaper support workers across all disciplines, employed to carry out 'non–nursing' work.

Opinions vary about this move, both for and against (Meehan, 2009). Interestingly, such a development would probably not have appealed to the highly intellectual Florence Nightingale (Bostridge, 2009). Although she was a great believer in the importance of a well- educated nurse workforce, she also understood the value of maintaining very high standards in basic nursing activities. Mary Spinks, Director of the Florence Nightingale Foundation, notes: 'She passionately believed that nurses should be well educated, but she would have been appalled to see "non-nursing" duties being contracted out to save money. She would have insisted that nurses are responsible for ensuring that hands-on care is carried out knowledgeably and with the utmost care and compassion' (in Whyte, 2010b) – a forerunner surely of the current privacy and dignity campaigns (DOH, 2006e, 2009e).

In any event, how worrying that this particular policy theme should continue to be necessary as an issue for professional nurses today. If the basic standards are perceived as apparently missing from the care lexicon of our potential professional nurse team leaders, what hope can we have for a promised future of high-quality care? Nightingale's belief may hold some truth when she said: 'While the intellectual foot has made a step in advance, the practical foot has remained behind' (Nightingale, 1860). That said, it is surely better to reflect, to accept, to learn and to respond if things are not working or are done badly. Most important is the need to continue our professional learning long after qualification and registration (Casey and Clark, 2009) As Nightingale (1860) put it: 'Nursing is a thing, which, unless we are making progress every year, every month, every week, (every day), take my word for it, we are going back.'

It is because of this that all nurses should have a clear interest in understanding the background to the situation in which they currently find themselves – not least if they aspire to any future role enrichment for the nursing profession and also for an NHS providing high-quality care for all. As a consequence, the discussions included have aimed to provide both an underpinning of relevant knowledge and an encour-agement to develop both political and influencing skills. Each chapter has highlighted different, but linked, policy issues of importance and their current relevance to the nursing profession of whatever country in the UK, discipline or circumstance. So what have we discussed?

The concepts of policy and policy-making and the role of the nurse

Chapter 2 explored the concepts of policy and policy-making and the potential for all nurses to be involved in both influencing and imple-menting the health agenda. With so many new and emerging policy imperatives, we all need to consider the implications of these and to introduce imaginative solutions to meet the economic, workforce and practice-related challenges ahead.

Why should we do this? Because our professional experience and knowledge equips us all to push, at many different levels, for a relevant and constructive balance in what is done, who requires our care and how things might be done better. Having changes imposed and instructions handed down can feel very disempowering. It often also inspires less support and ownership. Even really good ideas can seem hard to put into action.

So, as we continue to face a period of unprecedented change for both the NHS and to the future role of the professional nurse, now is surely the time to make a significant contribution to the policy-making agenda. As Carter (2010b) said: 'As health looks set to remain at the top of the political agenda, nurses are ideally placed to provide an invaluable link between patients and those who aspire to govern.'

Policy developments and reform in the NHS

'If politicians want to avoid repeating past NHS mistakes, they should make sure they listen to historians' (Timmins, 2008). Chapters 3 and 4 set out to provide a context and broad backcloth against which all subsequent discussions would be set. The early years of the NHS were outlined; these led into a long period of Conservative health reform, with the introduction of general management and an internal health care market. Four successive secretaries of state for health applauded and supported this new approach, seeing within it a modern success story replacing the failure of previous decades. They drew attention to the previous decades of inefficiencies, the long waiting lists, the seeming inability of health professionals to listen and to respond to the voices of the patients, the lack of knowledge about service costs, outcomes and levels of quality achieved. For those responsible for the reforms, the introduction of the quasi-market model to the NHS of the 1990s was lauded as both an improvement and as a massive achievement of which everyone involved could be justifiably proud.

The incoming Labour government of 1997 inevitably concentrated upon the negative aspects of the previous governments' health programmes and the introduction of this more commercialized focus into the NHS. It looked to the reductions in and removal of some NHS services; it condemned the perverse distortions in care provision, with two tiers of services between budget and non-budget-holding general practices; it observed the widening inequalities in healthcare provision and health standards; it criticized the greater concern which had been shown for financial cash flows rather than meeting patient need; it remarked on the increasing competitiveness and secrecy between professionals and organizations, and a consequent inability to work together well in multidisciplinary teams; it focused on the lack of democratic representation within the NHS and of real involvement and choice for patients and the public; and it reflected on the demoralization of staff across the NHS and the increased diminution and downplaying of professional contributions, not least from the nursing profession.

New Labour under Tony Blair and Gordon Brown claimed to offer a different agenda, one which, it was argued, would begin to address the negative and perverse outcomes of previous years, and sustain and develop a strong new NHS (DOH, 1997). It also offered a promising future for professional nursing, with the potential for ever greater growth and development. That said, after more than 13 years of Labour governments' health policies, we can all now look back and make a judgement on the delivery of their promises both for the NHS and for nursing.

The market mechanisms which had been introduced to the NHS by the successive Conservative governments of 1979–97 bloomed and grew under the Labour governments of 1997–2010. Their health programmes saw both investment and then cost containment. There was a massive expansion in nurse-led activities. At the same time, there was a growth in the employment of healthcare support workers across all professional disciplines, together with an increasing interest in services from the private and third sectors. These moves represented once again another threat to the long-term security of the traditional professional nurse role and also to the future and overarching responsibility for the health of the population by a *national* health service.

Activities were increasingly controlled and regulated by such bodies as the National Institute of Clinical Excellence (NICE), the Modernisation Agency, the Health Care Commission and the Care Quality Commission. The requirement to provide ever more specific evidence of meeting a seemingly growing number of quality indicators, targets and outcomes was linked to financial and other support. Failure to achieve these, or indeed appearance at the lower end of national or regional scales, resulted in being 'named and shamed', management takeover and closure. All were combined to define and to deliver the Labour government's policy agenda for health in the pursuit of high-quality care, innovative services and high productivity.

For all professionals, including nurses, there was a shift away from the traditional central control and job 'security for life' approach to one of individual responsibility for continuing professional development, regular reappraisal of fitness to practise and continuing employment. Professional responsibility for which evidence was sought was about demonstrating professional leadership of innovative work and proving the centrality of the quality agenda within all patient experiences (Burnham, 2009b; Darzi, 2009a, 2009b).

Sadly, a series of very unfortunate headlines around poor and dangerous practice within the NHS during this period provided stories to challenge the special nature of professional nurse care and to diminish trust and increase wariness in the eyes of the public and government.

High-profile stories had shown that some nurses failed to care and even killed (Parliamentary and Health Service Ombudsman, 2011). These incidents shocked us all and are certainly a major contradiction to the values on which the nursing profession is based.

Some have surmised that the changing complexity in the context of NHS care, with its increasingly technological environment, has somehow confounded or disorientated the professional nurse focus, providing a reason or an excuse for poor standards of care. Others like myself would disagree. A minority of nurses have shamed themselves and the profession, but the majority work hard to deliver high-quality and safe care in spite of many difficult and challenging situations. That said, there is every need, as Nightingale said, to learn and relearn so that we can rise to the ongoing challenges we currently face in whichever situation we find ourselves and our patients.

The Coalition's programme

Darzi's prophetic words, spoken as the Labour government under Gordon Brown approached election loss in 2010, remain an apt statement for us all as we currently deliver the Coalition's programme for the NHS:

> Now the NHS is entering the next phase. Arguably, this is the most difficult and also the most exciting period – transforming the NHS into a high-quality, high-performance system engaged in a continuous cycle of improvement, whose staff readily evaluate and raise their performance , so that the best is available for all. (Darzi, 2008)

The Coalition government's White Paper on health reform, *Equity and Excellence : Liberating the NHS*, published on 12 July 2010, set out the most significant reorganization of the NHS in its history. It focused on the government's wish to reduce bureaucracy by shifting power from the centre to GPs and the patients, moving £80 billion into the hands of groups of GPs (consortia) to commission health services. In announcing the proposed reforms, Andrew Lansley told Parliament of his plans for all hospital trusts to become or be part of a foundation trust. He reiterated three key principles:

1 Patients were to be at the heart of the NHS.
2 The measurement of services and quality standards were to change from targets and processes to defined outcomes.
3 Professionals were to be empowered, particularly GPs.

The White Paper set out an ambitious timetable for action. By April 2012:

* the establishment of an NHS Commissioning Board;
* the establishment of new local authority health and well-being boards;
* the development of Monitor as an economic regulator.

The new commissioning systems were expected to be in place by April 2013, by which time the primary care trusts and strategic health authorities would have been abolished.

While the new agenda was set out for the future, there was clearly no easy ride being offered to anyone, be it professional nurse, member of the public or indeed the NHS as a whole. We were warned that after a decade of growth in healthcare expenditure in the UK, we now faced 'a period of austerity'. The reforms, and the inevitable changes to follow, will in all likelihood start to determine the growth or demise of both the NHS as a *national* health service provider and the profession of nursing as we now know it. It is for these reasons that we all need to find the solutions and the energy to influence and become part of the policy-making process. By these means, we can redefine and consolidate professional nursing care within the newly evolving and, it is to be hoped, surviving NHS.

As Maben and Griffiths said in 2008 (and still relevant today):

> It is in the context of this wide-ranging [reform] programme that nursing faces the challenge of re-affirming its role, and describing 'an aspiring portrait of the modern nurse rooted in the values of nursing and the profession' re-defining nursing care and establishing nurses as advocates, champions and guardians of quality.

Working in partnership and delivering the policy agendas

As we saw in Chapter 5, the promotion of partnerships in healthcare delivery has assumed ever-greater importance in recent decades. That said, effective and successful collaborative ventures have proved at times to be very hard to achieve. During the period of the internal market reforms in the 1980s and 1990s, health and social carers faced some difficult challenges as they tried to implement policies, the aims of which often seemed implicitly to be in conflict. On the one hand, nurses and other healthcare workers were told to collaborate, but, on the other, the competitive internal healthcare market had created an environment not immediately conducive to multi-agency collaboration.

The contractual, financial imperatives of the internal market seemingly created a 'low-trust environment' – as theoretically explained by Flynn in 1996. In this situation of 'low trust', multidisciplinary or multi-sectoral working are not central to participants' immediate agendas, and, in practice, are antipathetic to the 'high-trust' environment which is believed to be essential to effective partnerships in care.

The incoming Labour government in 1997 appeared to offer an easier, less competitive future (DOH, 1997). Its programme of new NHS initiatives was strongly underpinned by the need for partnerships in care. Nevertheless, more than a decade on, the NHS world has changed into an even more competitive and financially led organization. The need to work in partnership with the diverse economy of care providers is now absolutely central to the delivery of effective and high quality healthcare (Darzi, 2009a; DOH, 2010c).

It is to be hoped that the developing commercialized healthcare environment of today does not, as in the recent past, lead to an ever more 'low-trust environment'. To counter this possibility, professionals and others need to be helped to learn how to work better together, especially in the potentially innovative, unusual and diverse scenarios of the NHS future as envisaged by the current government. Professionals and non-professionals importantly have to start by giving credit and value to each others' contributions, as the diverse and multi-sectoral health and social care teams and activities continue to grow and develop and become an inevitable fact of life (Stapleton, 2009).

Policy and information technology: the developing future

In Chapter 6 we explored the developing relationship between technology and the NHS, noting the many and varied applications for information, communication and care delivery. These continue to grow and develop apace as knowledge extends the realms of possibility and policy remit (MacLeod, 2010; Sample, 2010). Nurses are encouraged to navigate the complexity of this increasingly technological environment that is contemporary healthcare in the NHS, and to deliver the high-quality healthcare expected by the public, the profession and the government alike. Ham (2010) reminded us of the importance of not shying away from technological advances, but of using them to our advantage to maintain our professional roles, to refresh and modernize our knowledge, and to remain important players in an increasingly technologically literate society.

Policies and practice for the empowerment of the users

In spite of avowals to the contrary, the health reforms of the Conservative governments in the 1980s and 1990s, as we saw in Chapter 7, did not appear to empower the users of the services. Indeed, it has been argued that, far from being the powerful players in the NHS equation, they were mere pawns in the development of the competitive relationship within and between purchaser and provider bodies. In a similar vein, consumer power was reduced because democratic representation on planning and decision-making bodies were severely constrained. In turn, the patient charters were seen as nothing more than paper lists of stated intention, lacking financial and legislative backing, and were not, in any case, created by the users themselves. Inequalities in healthcare provision, the development of two-tier services, 'postcode lotteries', cancellation of operations, budgets running out and treatments removed from NHS activity were all seen in combination as creating a worse, rather than a better, deal for the consumers.

It is useful to reflect on how many of these aspects remain just as relevant today. That said, many successful new projects to empower the users have been introduced and developed during the past decade of Labour governments. But in practice greater progress is still needed to achieve a change in the power balance in the relationship between professional carer and members of the public – the users. The current Coalition government aspires to greater progress with the often-repeated mantra of 'no decision about me, without me' (DOH, 2010c).

Implementation of policy is not just about tick-box responses or mission statements stuck up on walls. It involves the promotion of shared values within teams with an agreed understanding of what user empowerment means for all the parties involved (Redding, 2009). It is about listening to the users, their 'expert' views, choices and concerns. It is about turning this feedback into a tool for quality improvement (Waters, 2009). Saddler (2009) reminds us all of the importance of listening, understanding and responding to the users – themes which permeate all current policy agendas.

At the same time, all practitioners need to feel similarly valued. According to research, there is a significant relationship between positive staff feedback and positive patient and user experience (Raleigh et al., 2009). Stockwell (2010) believes that 'nurses who feel undervalued become careless and unkind'. In her terms, supportive leadership is vital to delivering the high-quality care we wish to give and the care users wish to receive. Implementing this particular policy agenda in the challenging and changing NHS environment of today will require great determination, not least amongst the complexity of other important and competing policy imperatives all seemingly demanding our immediate attention.

Building a healthier nation and reducing health inequalities

As we saw in Chapter 8, health policy in the NHS over time has been imbued with two major themes:

- the improvement of the nation's health;
- the reduction of health inequalities.

Exploration of these themes has noted the high degree of policy challenge in attempting to make effective inroads into a complex mire of issues, not least of types which morph and change on an almost daily basis. The attempts made to date by the NHS have clearly only scratched the surface of need. Health inequalities continue to widen, while ever greater effort goes into health promotion activity (European Commission, 2009; NAO, 2010; Marmot, 2010; DOH, 2010d).

In recent decades the policy support for a stronger public health agenda and a reduction in health inequalities has been made clear. That said, although strides have been made and many successes achieved, the problems and challenges continue. Allied to this is a developing 'victim-blaming' culture within society, one which reverberates to the Victorian sounds of 'stand on your own two feet' (Burns et al., 2009). This may reflect the economic downturn of today, a 'period of austerity in the NHS' and concerns about using public expenditure wisely and effectively in the future. Community nurses and other public health professionals need to be alert. The perception that health promotion and preventative work within the NHS are more acceptable areas to cut or remove than acute services is still alive (NHS Confederation, 2010c). While politicians and currently stated policy may suggest the opposite (DOH, 2010c), it is worthwhile learning and remembering the lessons of fairly recent history (Fatchett, 1994, 1998).

The Coalition decision in 2010 to transfer public health teams to local authorities in an effort to improve population-wide health and reduce health inequalities held some promise. Potentially, it offered many benefits to nurses for widening their health promotion vision and activity, working in partnership with other colleagues more closely allied to all the broader health and well-being parts of people's lives – education, housing, social services, employment, transport, justice system and the police, to name but a few. That said, other changes within the NHS were potentially worrying. As valued health promoters (Milton, 2010d), many community nurses felt concern at the functional split of primary and acute care from local authority public health teams. New employers, for example, the acute foundation trusts or private sector bodies could sideline this aspect of their work in order to address other pressing health issues for their own organizations.

Currently, there are many moves to create a diverse community of care providers across all sectors. This may well ease the way to change or dissipate care delivery teams outside the acute NHS sector and to pass (as has happened before) responsibility for what might be perceived as more nebulous healthcare work to others. While the pursuit of good health for the whole population benefits the economy in the long run, cutting public health work and reducing the employment of community practitioners in this field has been seen, and is seen, as an easy option for financial retrenchment.

It is important to remember that the major policy challenge of promoting the health of the nation and, in turn, reducing health inequalities requires an all-embracing response – one that is led ideally by the NHS. A programme of such magnitude needs to be well managed and resourced. It is a risk to pass this agenda to the vagaries of a mixed economy of providers, who may or may not see the complex issues involved as an important or prime responsibility. Again, the onus is on all of us as professional nurses to influence the potentially negative agendas which face our users and patients, in particular to ensure public health as a discipline is kept safe and developed in overarching NHS hands.

Diversity and policy

Chapter 9 explored the need for a diversity-sensitive NHS, one which is clearly committed to equality, diversity and human rights throughout the system. It was seen that the achievement of such an important aim has to be recognized and understood from policy development, through service delivery and to patient care. It is about acknowledgement of and responsiveness to the different experiences, aspirations and needs of staff, patients and the public alike.

Sadly, in spite of laws, government policy and professional codes, the achievement of such a laudable aim appears to be lacking within the NHS. There are barriers to its success which need to be overcome, not least its perceived lack of importance in the pecking order for serious action. Although some parts of the NHS are making progress and see the promotion of a diversity-sensitive environment as core business, it is evident that the developing health reforms are focused on organizational change and cost containment. In light of this, it is clear that, as professional nurses, we need to take responsibility for ensuring that we work with others to ensure a viable, sensitive and responsive service for all our different patients and colleagues. In addition, we have a responsibility to challenge those who ignore, forget or do not understand this important duty of respect and equal treatment for patients, the public and work colleagues alike.

Supporting people with long-term conditions

In Chapter 10, we reflected on the major health challenge facing this country – that of the ever-rising number of people of all ages with a long-term condition (LTC). This is not a new agenda, as previous governments have tried in many different ways to address the issue and to stem the growing numbers – unfortunately, to little avail.

The current financial environment is set to provide a very difficult backcloth for sorting out new ways of caring and supporting this still-growing group in the population. The period of serious retrenchment in public spending, coupled with massive organizational changes and uncertainties right across primary and community care, must be of great concern to the many very vulnerable patients who until now have relied on substantial support from a wide range of public sector bodies – all currently under great pressure to cut services and reduce costs.

The Coalition government has promised to aspire to an NHS that can deliver high-quality care to all patients, in all areas, all the time (DOH, 2010c). It is to be hoped that the care of people with LTCs remains at the forefront of the government's health policy agenda. It is also to be hoped that the nursing profession is able to continue and to develop its effective contributions to date with the many patients with a LTC. While it still remains difficult to know exactly what the future NHS will look like, and who will be employed to care, professional nurses will surely be crucial to its success.

Policy and professionalism: developments explored

Chapter 11 discussed the precarious nature of nurse professionalism. It also acknowledged the clear strides made by many nurses against a difficult backcloth of organization and management change over a sustained period of time (Gray, 2009; Fernandez, 2009; Hazell, 2009; Snow, 2009a). The period broadly covered has witnessed significant efforts to reduce the power of the professional bodies in the health service, and not least that of nursing. In tandem, enthusiasm for the development and employment of non-professional carers has grown over time and is currently a very live issue for the increasingly financially challenged NHS (Dean, 2009b).

The demands on professional nurses are high and growing, with many proverbial hoops to jump through in the pursuit of financial reward or professional enrichment (Beasley, 2009; Carter, 2009). The requirement to improve the quality of care, increase flexibility and productivity, introduce innovative practice and services and be a health promoter is a very demanding agenda. It requires skills of effective leadership, accomplished teamworking, an ability to manage change, good technological dexterity and research proficiency (Butterworth, 2009). A graduate standard of education at Bachelor's or Master's level is also now an accepted expectation for professional nurses (Casey and Clark, 2010; Dean, 2009c; Meehan, 2009).

However, a word of warning is needed. Training and education have always been favoured targets for cost-containment in the NHS. Training budgets have been raided in the past to help balance the books (Buchan, 2009). Vying with the power of medical education for NHS funding is likely to remain a difficult process for nurses, when competing for scarce funds for continuing educational development opportunities. It is worthwhile remembering that while the focus of any health policy can look supportive and be aimed at improving the quality of care, the reality in financial terms may result in something that is unachievable or perverse (Dean, 2009c). In the case of continuing professional development and education – if one group wins, the other loses.

We have also looked at the currently growing population of support carers and assistants and considered the survival of the professional nurse role. Whereas research (NNRU, 2009b) has demonstrated the link between qualified nurses and better health outcomes, the development of a non-professional workforce of carers holds a continuing appeal to cost-conscious politicians and NHS managers. As such, the Chief Nursing Officer, Christine Beasley, regularly stressed the urgency

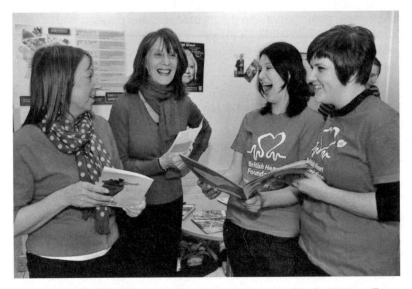

12.1 Anita (centre) with lecturer colleague and nursing students in 2011 – still enjoying nursing!

of explaining very clearly to the public the value of maintaining and supporting the high-level contributions of the nursing profession (Beasley, 2009)

Sadly, the portrayal of nursing in the media, the tabloids and popular journals still often seems to promote a very old-fashioned, limited and stereotypical image of nursing, which clearly perpetuates subliminal and unhelpful messages to the public and politician alike. This situation calls for nurses to use their influencing skills to ensure that the unique, higher-level contributions of the twenty-first-century nurse is made visible to both the public and politicians. As argued by Butterworth (2009), there is a need to foster and to combine both academic and practice skills; not only to develop work and services to a higher level and to improve quality, but also to explore and promote a greater understanding of the value and merit of professional nursing and the need to maintain that role and expertise.

We may all at times conclude that the complexity of health needs, the problems we face and the possibilities for care available (if not finance) defy solution and energy. However, do not give up! It is clearly incumbent on us all to seize these agendas, to be architects of our future, to ensure high-quality professional nursing care is there for our children and grandchildren in the future, ideally within a strong and healthy NHS.

Learning from the past, looking to the future

For many, the highlight of a day at a theme park is to enjoy the latest dare-devil ride: the greater the turbulence, the greater the enjoyment. For nurses, life in recent decades has been very much like the theme park rollercoaster ride. There is no evidence to suggest that there will be any change to this in the future. On the contrary, the best advice for all nurses would be to tighten their seatbelts.

The current climate of change offers opportunities, challenges and threats and may hold little appeal for those who find the quiet life of stability rather more seductive. Change, however, there will be: professional roles will be redefined and new contexts for practice introduced. It may well be possible to develop a true, new professionalism which better reflects and is more responsive to the healthcare needs of the twenty-first-century UK.

Such opportunities, of course, can only be seized through engagement. If there is one theme, indeed plea, contained in this book, it must be that it is in nurses' own interests to be engaged in the policy changes that are taking place, and which will shape their role and the way in which it interacts with others in society. Passive indifference or sullen opposition are not options; only through constructive engagement can the professional nurse's role be extended and enhanced, and nursing achieve greater esteem and value. After all, the rollercoaster always excites, challenges and reaches its promised destination. Enjoy the ride – I am!

References

Abel-Smith, B. (1976) *Value for Money in Health Services*. Heinemann.

Abel, G., Hampshaw, S., Stringer, M. D., Beck, J. M. and Puntis, J. W. L. (1995) Home gastrostomy feeding in children. *Clinical Nutrition* 14(2): 41.

Acheson Committee (1988) *Public Health in England*. DHSS.

Ackers, L. and Abbott, P. (1998) *Social Policy for Nurses and the Caring Professions*. Open University Press.

Adshead, F. and Behan, D. (2007) *The Role of Public Health in Supporting the Development of Integrated Services*. National Institute for Mental Health in England.

Agnew, T. (1995) League tables 'bad for staff morale'. *Nursing Times* 91(28): 9.

Alcock, C., Payne S. and Sullivan M. (2000) *Introducing Social Policy*. Prentice Hall.

Allen, J. (2011) Read the report, talk about it – then take action. *Nursing Standard* 25(26): 26–7.

Allsop, J. (1995) *Health, Policy and the NHS: Towards 2000*, 2nd edn. Longman.

Amadi, O. (2010) Empty promises. *Nursing Standard* 24(50): 26–7.

Andrews, J. (2009) The right incentive. *Nursing Standard* 24(4): 61.

Armstrong, G. (2005) Modern matron: Improving the patient experience. Presentation at Leeds Metropolitan University, April.

Ashton, J. and Seymour, H. (1988) *The New Public Health*. Open University Press.

Baggott, R. (1994) *Health and Health Care in Britain*. St Martin's Press.

Baggott, R. (2007) *Understanding Health Policy*. Policy Press.

Bailey, L. (2010) Any NHS overhaul needs to be tested. *Nursing Standard* 24(49): 26–7.

Ball, M. J. and Callen, M. F. (eds) (1984) *Aspects of the Computer-Based Patient Record*. Springer-Verlag.

Baly, M. (1995) *Nursing and Social Change*, 3rd edn. Routledge.

Barklem, H. (2010) Specialist jobs in jeopardy as efforts to save money intensify. *Nursing Standard* 25(10): 8.

Barnett, S. (2008) Foreword. In *The NHS Confederation, New Providers: New Solutions*. The independent sector partnering with the NHS (www.nhsconfed. org/Publications/Documents/IS_showcase_report_2009.pdf).

Barr, J. and Dowding, L. (2008) *Leadership in Health Care*. Sage.

Batty, D. (2009) The right person for the job. *Guardian*, 16 September, p. 2.

Beardshaw, V. and Robinson, R. (1990) *New For Old? Prospects for Nursing in the 1990s*. King's Fund.

Beasley, C. (2009) Public's old-fashioned image of nurses needs to be updated. *Nursing Standard* 24(7): 11.

Beasley, C. (2010) Helping patients make an informed choice is vital. *Nursing Standard* 24(44): 24.

Beecher-Stowe, H. (1852) *Uncle Tom's Cabin*. John Hewett & Co.

Behan, D. (2008) Foreword. In DOH, *Raising the Profile of Long-Term Conditions Care: A Compendium of Information* (http://www.dh.gov.uk/prod_consum_dh/ groups/dh_digitalassets/documents/digitalasset/dh_082067.pdf).

Belfast Health and Social Care Trust, University of Ulster, South Eastern Health and Social Care Trust (2011) Key performance indicators for nursing and midwifery care. In press.

Bennett, C., Perry, J. and Lawrence, Z. (2009) Promoting health in primary care. *Nursing Standard* 23(47): 48–55.

Bennett, S., Maton, K. and Kervin, L. (2008) The 'digital natives' debate: A critical review. *British Journal of Educational Technology* 39(5): 775–86.

Benzeval, M., Judge, K. and Whitehead, M. (eds) (1995) *Tackling Inequalities in Health: An Agenda for Action.* King's Fund.

Bernard, P. J., Hammand, M. V., Morton, J., Long, J. B. and Clark, I. A. (1981) Consistency and compatibility in human-computer disclosure. *International Journal of Man Machine Studies* 15: 87–134.

Best, G., Brazil, R. (1997) The personal touch. *Health Service Journal*, 16 October, p. 25.

Bevan, H. (2004) Realising the potential of the ten high impact changes (http://www.institute.nhs.uk/quality_and_value/introduction/article_7.html).

Beveridge, W. (1942) *Social Insurance and Allied Services.* HMSO.

Biggs, S. (1993) User participation and interprofessional collaboration in community care. *Journal of Interprofessional Care* 7(2): 151–9.

Billingham, K. (1989) 45 Cope Street – working in partnership with parents. *Health Visitor* 62(5): 156–7.

Bishop, V. (ed.) (2009) *Leadership for Nursing and Allied Health Professionals.* Open University Press.

Black, D. (1980) *Inequalities in Health: Report* of a *Research Working Group.* DHSS.

Blake, H. (2008a) Innovation in practice: mobile phone technology in patient care. *British Journal of Community Nursing* 13(4): 162–5.

Blake, H. (2008b) Mobile phone technology in chronic disease management. *Nursing Standard* 23(12): 43–6.

Blake, H. (2008c) Using technology in health promotion interventions. In M. R. Blakely and S. M. Timmons (eds), *Life Style and Health Research.* Nova Publishers.

BMJ (2010) Inequalities in mortality in Britain today greater than those during 1930s economic depression. BMJ Group, press release, 23 July.

Boarden, N. and Rillands, M. (1997) *Primary Care: Making Connections.* Open University Press.

Booth, R., Wachman, R. and Vasagar, J. (2010a) Austerity drive will hand billions to private sector. *Guardian*, 17 July, pp. 1–2.

Booth, R., Wachman, R. and Vasagar, J. (2010b) Outsourcing firms prepare for bonanza of contracts from public service providers. *Guardian*, 17 July, p. 1.

Boseley, S. (1998) Dobson pledges to cut illness gap. *Guardian*, 6 February, p. 10.

Bostridge, M. (2009) *Florence Nightingale: The Woman and her Legend.* Penguin Books.

Bow Group (2010) Equity and excellence: Opportunities and challenges. *NHS Confederation Health Policy Digest* 50, 24 August.

Bradford University (2011) Making diversity interventions count in organisational performance and service delivery (http://www.brad.ac.uk/health/CentreforInclusionandDiversity/Events/Conferences/).

Brindle, D. (1997) Fall in life expectancy among the worst off. *Guardian*, 9 September.

Brindle, D. (2010) Health services face a vertical challenge. *Society Guardian*, 24 March, p. 4.

Broome, A. (1998) *Managing Change.* Macmillan.

Brown, J. (1996) Robot nurses nonsense. *Nursing Standard* 10(47): 10.

Buchan, J. (2009) Safeguard learning. *Nursing Standard* 23(50): 26–7.

Buchan, J., Jobanputra, R., Gough, P. and Hutt, R. (2005) Internationally recruited nurses in London: Profile and implications for policy. King's Fund (http://www.kingsfund.org.uk/publications/internationally.html).

Burnham, A. (2009a) Burnham urges us to get dancing. NHS Confederation press summaries, 13 August.

Burnham, A. (2009b) Corner shops urged to sell more fruit and veg. *Daily Telegraph*, 28 July.

Burnham, A. (2009c) Embrace new era of redesign to take the NHS from good to great. *Health Service Journal*, 29 October, pp. 12–13.

Burnham, A. (2009d) Health headlines: Lord Darzi resignation. *Financial Times*, p. 1.

Burnham, A. (2009e) Institute of Healthcare Management, 30 September.

Burns, D., Costello, J., Haggart, M., Longshaw, K. and Thornton, R. (2009) The public health challenge of obesity: Is it the new smoking? *Journal of Community Nursing* 23(11): 4–9.

Butler, J. (1992) *Patients, Policies and Politics*. Open University Press.

Butler, P. (1997) Green shoots. *Health Service Journal*, 23 October, p. 13.

Butterworth, T. (1992) Clinical supervision as an emerging idea in nursing. In T. Butterworth and J. Faugier (eds), *Clinical Supervision and Mentorship in Nursing*. Chapman and Hall.

Butterworth, T. (2009) Championing research. *Nursing Standard* 23(40): 62–3.

Butterworth, T. and Bishop, V. (1995) Identifying the characteristics of optimum practice. *Journal of Advanced Nursing* 22: 24–32.

Caines, E. (1993) Goodbye nurses. *Nursing Standard* 10(39): 18.

Cairns-Berteau, M. (1991) LA flaw. *Nursing Times* 87(5): 36–8.

Callanan, C. (2011) Raising the standards. *Nursing Standard* 25(26): 62/63.

Cameron, D. and Clegg, N. (2010) *The Coalition: Our Programme for Government. Freedom, Fairness, Responsibility*. HM Government (http://www.direct.gov.uk/prod_consum_dg/groups/dg_digitalassets/@dg/@en/documents/digitalasset/dg_187876.pdf).

Campbell, D. (2009a) GPs in drive to prevent 10,000 cancer deaths. *Guardian*, 30 December, p. 1.

Campbell, D. (2009b) Head of NHS Watchdog resigns after criticism of patient care monitoring. *Guardian*, 5 December, p. 4.

Campbell, D. (2009c) No progress without prevention. *Health Service Journal*, 11 June, p. 17.

Campbell, D. (2010) Walking a tightrope. *Society Guardian*, 7 July, p. 5.

Care Quality Commission (2011) *The State of Health Care and Adult Social Care in England*. The Stationery Office.

Carlisle, D. (2008) Creating the perfect acute hospital. *Health Service Journal*, 17 January.

Carter, P. (2009) Nurses feel too busy to provide appropriate level of care. Manifesto: Royal College of Nursing, 19 October.

Carter, P. (2010a) An honest prognosis. *Society Guardian*, 29 September, p. 5.

Carter, P. (2010b) Nursing counts: Health, nursing and the next general election. Royal College of Nursing (http://generalelection.rcn.org.uk/).

Casey, D. and Clark, L. (2010) Professional development for registered nurses. *Nursing Standard* 24(15): 35–7.

Castells, M. (2000) *The Information Society: Issues and Illusions*. Polity.

Catton, H. (2010) Questions, questions, questions: The NHS White Paper paints an uncertain picture. *Nursing Standard* 24(50): 12–13.

Cavender, A. (2011) Sexually sidelined. *Nursing Standard* 25(22): 26–7.

Central Statistics Office (1993) *Social Trends 23*. HMSO.

Chadda, D. (1998) Survey confirms health inequalities. *Health Service Journal*, 15 January.

Chambers, E., Clarke, A. and Cooke, J. (2009) Patient and public involvement in community research. *Journal of Community Nursing* 23(7): 10–16.

Charman, K. (2009) Move to improve support workers' competencies as their role widens. *Nursing Standard* 24(10): 9.

Chifulya, S. (2010) Inspiring stories. *Nursing Standard* 25(5): 72.

Civil Service (1999) *Modernising Government*. Policy Hub (http://www.nationals-chool.gov.uk/policyhub/docs/modgov.pdf).

Civil Service (2002) *Reforming Our Public Services: Principles into Practice*. Policy Hub.

Civil Service (2008) *Better Policy-making*. Policy Hub (http://www.nationalschool.gov.uk/policyhub/better_policy_making/).

Clark, J. (2008) Embrace new technology or others will decide how we end up using it. *Nursing Standard* 22(17): 32.

Clarke, K. (1989) Statement: NHS Review. Hansard 146(39), 31 January.

CNO (Chief Nursing Officer) (2009) New thinking needed to bolster care. CNO bulletin, October.

CNO (Chief Nursing Officer) (2009) New thinking needed to bolster care. CNO Bulletin, October, p. 2.

CNO (Chief Nursing Officer) Directorate (2011) College criticises plan to end BME patient reports. *Nursing Standard* 25(27): 10.

Cole, E. (2010) Left out of the loop. *Nursing Standard* 24(46): p. 1.

Cole, E. (2011) Pensions under threat. *Nursing Standard* 25(26): 1.

Colebatch, H. K. (2002) Policy, 2nd edn. Open University Press.

Colin-Thome, D. (2008) Foreword. In DOH, *Raising the Profile of Long-Term Conditions Care: A Compendium of Information* (http://www.dh.gov.uk/prod_consum_dh/groups/dh_digitalassets/documents/digitalasset/dh_082067.pdf).

Command 1986 (1992) *The Health of the Nation: A Strategy for Health in England*. HMSO.

Command 7047 (1997) *Prevention and Health*. HMSO.

Community Outlook (1989) Hidden opportunities. *Nursing Times*, March.

Cooper, C. (2010) Remote control. *Nursing Standard* 25(9): 18–19.

Corney, B. (2010) An all graduate profession? *Journal of Community Nursing* 24(2).

Covey, S. (1989) *The Seven Habits of Highly Effective People*. Simon and Schuster.

Coyle, A. (2011) Personal health budgets and the role of nursing. *Nursing Standard* 25(26): 35–9.

Crinson, I. (2009) *Health Policy: A Critical Perspective*. Sage Publications.

Crisp, N. (2009) What would a new Griffiths bring? *Health Service Journal*, 4 June, p. 17.

Crowe, D. (2009) A more hands-on role. *Nursing Standard* 24(9): 22–3.

Cruickshank, J. (2010) There may be trouble ahead. *Health Service Journal*, suppl., 10 June, pp. 1–2.

Crumbie, A. (2010) The dismantling of structures is unnerving. *Nursing Standard* 24(49): 28.

Cullum, P. (2005) *Future Services: Taking the Voice of the Users to the Heart of the Public Service Reform Debate*. National Consumer Council (http://www.cfps.org.uk/userfiles/file/cfps2005-philipcullum%5B1%5D.pdf).

Cuthbert, S. and Quallington, J. (2008) *Values for Care Practice: Health and Social Care Theory and Practice*. Reflect Press.

Daily Telegraph (2010) GP consortia could hand over duties to private firms. 22 July.

Darzi, A. (2008) *High Quality Care for All: NHS Next Stage Review*, final report. DOH, 30 June.

Darzi, A. (2009a) *High Quality Care for All: Our Journey So Far*. DOH, June.

Darzi, A. (2009b) Savouring full-bodied reforms. *Health Service Journal*, 25 June, p. 17.

Darzi, A. (2009c) Why innovation matters today. *British Medical Journal*, 22 July.

Davies, C. (1995) *Gender and the Professional Predicament in Nursing*. Open University Press.

Davies, C. (1996) Cloaked in a tattered illusion. *Nursing Times* 92(45): 44–6.

Davies, C. (ed.) (2003) *The Future Health Workforce*. Palgrave Macmillan.

Davies, P. (2009) The power and the glory. *Health Service Journal*, 4 June, pp. 24–6.

Davis, C. (2008) Where age is no barrier. *Nursing Standard* 22(49): 18–19.

Davis, C. (2010) Joint approach to arthritis care. *Nursing Standard* 24(39): 22–3.

Dean, E. (2009a) The bedrock of children's services, so why are there not enough of them? *Nursing Standard* 23(9): 13–14.

Dean, E. (2009b) The future of nursing: Conservative style. *Nursing Standard* 23(40): 12–13.

Dean, E. (2009c) What will all-graduate entry to nursing mean to the profession? *Nursing Standard* 23(42): 12–13.

Dean, E. (2010a) Health charities launch fight to keep specialist nurses threatened by cuts. *Nursing Standard* 24(19): 12–13.

Dean, E. (2010b) Nurses feel left out of plan to give GPs control of £80bn spending. *Nursing Standard* 24(46): 6.

Dean, E. (2010c) Thousands of posts to disappear as the NHS austerity drive begins. *Nursing Standard* 24(41): 12–13.

Dean, E. (2010d) Training is a 'lottery' for HCAs. *Nursing Standard* 24(18): 12–13.

Dean, E. (2010e) Unions warn that wards, services and jobs are already under threat. *Nursing Standard* 24(49): 6.

Dean, E. (2011a) Cuts to health services leaves region's staff at breaking point. *Nursing Standard* 25(20): 12–13.

Dean, E. (2011b) NHS director assures BME staff they will not bear brunt of cuts. *Nursing Standard* 25(21): 10.

Dean, E. (2011c) Posts remain unfilled despite assurances about cuts. *Nursing Standard* 25(26): 12–13.

Dean, E. (2011d) Unions slam recommendation to reduce nurse–patient ratio. *Nursing Standard* 25(18): 11.

Dean, E. (2011e) Workforce planning shake-up prompts fear of staff shortfall. *Nursing Standard* 25(19): 12–13.

Dean, E. and Kendall-Raynor, P. (2010) Community nurses face a future where change is the only certainty. *Nursing Standard* 24(46): 12–13.

Dean, E. and Kendall-Raynor, P. (2011) RCN launches pre-budget letter campaign against frontline cuts. *Nursing Standard* 25(26): 5.

Denny, E. and Earle, S. (2008) *Sociology for Nurses*. Polity.

DHSS, Department of Health and Social Security (1976) *Prevention and Health: Everybody's Business. A Reassessment of Public and Personal Health*. HMSO.

Dinsdale, P. (1998) Pilot lights new way forward. *Guardian*, 4 February, p. 7.

DOH (Department of Health) (1987) *Promoting Better Health*. Command 249, HMSO.

DOH (Department of Health) (1989a) *Caring for People: Community Care in the Next Decade and Beyond*. Command 849, HMSO.

DOH (Department of Health) (1989b) *National Health Service Review Working Papers*. HMSO.

DOH (Department of Health) (1989c) *Working for Patients*. Command 555, HMSO.

DOH (Department of Health) (1992) *The Patient's Charter*. HMSO.

DOH (Department of Health) (1995) *Written Complaints by or on Behalf of Patients, 1993–1994*. DOH.

DOH (Department of Health) (1996) *The National Health Service: A Service With Ambitions*. Command 3425, HMSO.

DOH (Department of Health) (1997) *The New NHS: Modern, Dependable.* Command 3807, HMSO.

DOH (Department of Health) (1998a) *A First Class Service: Quality in the New NHS.* DOH.

DOH (Department of Health) (1998b) *Our Healthier Nation: A Contract for Health. A Consultation Paper.* The Stationery Office.

DOH (Department of Health) (1998c) *Partnership in Action: New Opportunities for Joint Working Between Health and Social Services. A Discussion Document.* DOH.

DOH (Department of Health) (1998d) *The Health of the Nation: A Policy Assessed.* The Stationery Office.

DOH (Department of Health) (1999a) *Making a Difference: Strengthening the Nursing, Midwifery and Health Visiting Contribution to Health and Healthcare.* DOH (http://www.publications.doh.gov.uk/pub/docs/doh/nursum.pdf).

DOH (Department of Health) (1999b) *Patient and Public Involvement in the New NHS.* DOH.

DOH (Department of Health) (1999c) *Reducing Health Inequalities: An Action Report.* DOH.

DOH (Department of Health) (1999d) *Saving Lives: Our Healthier Nation.* The Stationery Office.

DOH (Department of Health) (2000a) *Improving Working Lives Standard.* DOH.

DOH (Department of Health) (2000b) *The NHS Plan: A Plan for Investment, a Plan for Reform.* DOH.

DOH (Department of Health) (2000c) *Research and Development for a First Class Service.* DOH.

DOH (Department of Health) (2001a) *The Essence of Care: Patient-Focused Benchmarking for Healthcare Professionals.* DOH.

DOH (Department of Health) (2001b) *The Expert Patient: A New Approach to Chronic Disease Management for the 21st century.* The Stationery Office.

DOH (Department of Health) (2001c) *Governance Arrangements for NHS Research Ethics Committees.* DOH.

DOH (Department of Health) (2001d) *A Research and Development Strategy for Public Health.* DOH.

DOH (Department of Health) (2002a) *Delivering the NHS Plan.* HMSO.

DOH (Department of Health) (2002b) *Liberating the Talents: Helping Primary Care Trusts and Nurses to Deliver the NHS Plan.* DOH.

DOH (Department of Health) (2002c) *Learning From Bristol: The Department of Health's Response to the Report of the Public Inquiry into Children's Heart Surgery at the Bristol Royal Infirmary 1984–1995.* Command 5363, HMSO.

DOH (Department of Health) (2003a) *Modern Matrons: Improving the Patient's Experience.* DOH.

DOH (Department of Health) (2003b) *Tackling Health Inequalities: A Programme for Action.* DOH.

DOH (Department of Health) (2004a) *Choosing Health: Making Healthy Choices Easier.* DOH.

DOH (Department of Health) (2004b) *Improving Chronic Disease Management.* DOH.

DOH (Department of Health) (2004c) *Commissioning a Patient-led NHS.* DOH.

DOH (Department of Health) (2004d) *Managing Change in the NHS.* DOH.

DOH (Department of Health) (2004e) *National Standards, Local Action.* DOH.

DOH (Department of Health) (2004f) *The NHS Improvement Plan: Putting People at the Heart of Public Services.* Command 6268, The Stationery Office.

DOH (Department of Health) (2004g) *Chronic Disease Management: A Compendium of Information.* DOH.

DOH (Department of Health) (2005a) *Public Attitudes to Self Care: Baseline Survey* (MORI). DOH.

DOH (Department of Health) (2005b) *National Service Framework for Long-Term Conditions.* HMSO.

DOH (Department of Health) (2005c) *Now I Feel Tall: What a Patient-Led NHS Feels Like.* DOH.

DOH (Department of Health) (2005d) *Supporting People with Long-Term Conditions: An NHS and Social Care Model to Support Local Innovation and Integration.* DOH.

DOH (Department of Health) (2006a) *A Stronger Local Voice.* DOH.

DOH (Department of Health) (2006b) *Best Research for Best Health: A New National Health Research Strategy.* DOH.

DOH (Department of Health) (2006c) *Our Health, Our Care, Our Say: Making It Happen.* DOH.

DOH (Department of Health) (2006d) *Our Health, Our Care, Our Say: A New Direction for Community Services.* Command 6737, HMSO.

DOH (Department of Health) (2006e) *Dignity in Care.* DOH.

DOH (Department of Health) (2006f) *Your Health, Your Care, Your Say: Research Report.* DOH.

DOH (Department of Health) (2007a) *Local Involvement Networks (LINks) Explained.* DOH.

DOH (Department of Health) (2007b) *Our NHS Our Future: NHS Next Stage Review. Interim Report.* DOH.

DOH (Department of Health) (2007c) *Patient and Public Involvement in the NHS.* DOH.

DOH (Department of Health) (2007d) *NHS Foundation Trusts: A Guide to Developing HR Systems and Practices.* DOH (http://www.dh.gov.uk/en/Publications andstatistics/Publications/PublicationsPolicyAndGuidance/DH_077171).

DOH (Department of Health) (2008a) *High Quality Care for All: NHS Next Stage Review. Final Report.* DOH.

DOH (Department of Health) (2008b) *The NHS Constitution: Securing the NHS for Generations to Come.* DOH.

DOH (Department of Health) (2008c) *Raising the Profile of Long Term Conditions Care: A Compendium of Information* (http://www.dh.gov.uk/prod_consum_dh/ groups/dh_digitalassets/documents/digitalasset/dh_082067.pdf).

DOH (Department of Health) (2009a) High Impact Changes. Care Services Improvement Partnership, DOH.

DOH (Department of Health) (2009b) *High Quality Care for All: Our Journey So Far.* DOH.

DOH (Department of Health) (2009c) *Listening, Responding, Improving: A Guide to Better Customer Care.* DOH.

DOH (Department of Health) (2009d) *NHS 2010–2015: From Good to Great. Preventative, People-Centred, Productive.* DOH.

DOH (Department of Health) (2009e) *The Dignity in Care Campaign.* DOH (www. dignityincare.org.uk/DignityCareCampaign/).

DOH (Department of Health) (2009f) *The Report on the National Patient Choice Survey.* DOH.

DOH (Department of Health) (2009g) *Transforming Community Services: Enabling New Patterns of Provision.* DOH.

DOH (Department of Health) (2009h) *World Class Commissioning: An Introduction.* DOH.

DOH (Department of Health) (2010a) *The NHS Constitution for England.* DOH.

DOH (Department of Health) (2010b) Speech by the Rt Hon Andrew Lansley, CBE, MP, Secretary of State for Health, 8 June 2010.

DOH (Department of Health) (2010c) *Equity and Excellence: Liberating the NHS*. DOH.

DOH (Department of Health) (2010d) *Healthy Lives, Healthy People: Our Strategy for Public Health in England*. Command 7985, HMSO.

DOH (Department of Health) (2010e) *The NHS: Quality, Innovation, Productivity and Prevention Challenge. An Introduction for Clinicians*. DOH.

Donaldson, L. (2010) Foreword: Richer than ever in data. *Health Service Journal* – Health Intelligence supplement, 27 May.

Dorling, D. (2010) *Injustice: Why Social Inequality Persists*. Policy Press.

Downey, R. (1993) Call for freeze on student intakes. *Nursing Times* 89(14): 6.

Drake, L. (2010a) Braced for another round of musical chairs. *Nursing Standard* 24(49): 28.

Drake, L. (2010b) A chance to shape community services. *Nursing Standard* 25(14): 26–7.

Duffin, C. (2010) A local crisis. *Nursing Standard* 24(49): 23.

Durkheim, E. (1951) *Suicide: A Study in Sociology*. Free Press.

Economist, The (1997) Dobson's Choice. The internal market is dead. Long live the market. 11 December.

Editorial (1989) *Nursing Times* 85(12): 3.

Editorial (1991) Stealthy is not very healthy. *Guardian*, 20 May.

Editorial (1997) Blair's affordable vision. *Guardian*, 1 October.

Edwards, N. (2009) Rise in number of NHS staff. *Financial Times*. 16 December.

Elliott, L. and Wintour, P. (2011) Budget 2011: Forget the cuts, just fill up your petrol tanks. *Guardian*, 23 March.

EPP (Expert Patients Programme) (2011) *Healthy Lives Equal Healthy Communities: The Social Impact of Self-Management* (http://www.expertpatients.co.uk/sites/default/files/publications/healthy-lives-equal-health-communities-social-impact-self-management.pdf).

Equality and Human Rights Commission (2009) *The Public Sector Equality Duties and Financial Decisions* (http://www.equalityhumanrights.com/uploaded_files/PSD/31_psdandfinancialdecisions.pdf).

Etzioni, A. (1969) *The Semi-Professions and their Organization: Teachers, Nurses, Social Workers*. Free Press.

European Commission (2009) *Health Inequalities*. NHS European Office.

Farrar, M. (2009) QUIPP needs to become woven into the NHS's DNA. *Health Service Journal*, 10 September.

Fatchett, A. (1994) *Politics, Policy and Nursing*. Baillière Tindall.

Fatchett, A. (1996) A chance for community nurses to shape the agenda. *Nursing Times* 92(45): 40–2.

Fatchett, A. (1998) *Nursing in the new NHS: Modern, Dependable?* Baillière Tindall.

Fatchett, A. (2000) DAZLing success. *Nursing Times* 14(51): 14.

Fatchett, A. (2002) Advancing nursing practice in cancer and palliative care. In D. Clark, J. Flanagan and K. Kendrick (eds), *Cancer and Palliative Care Nursing: The Influence of Policy*. Palgrave Macmillan.

Fernandez, J. (2009) Nurse-led detox in primary care. *Journal of Community Nursing* 23(8): 18–22.

Financial Times (2010) Cameron's speech strongest on Big Society. 6 October.

Flatman, B. (2010) There may be trouble ahead. *Health Service Journal Supplement*, 10 June, pp. 1–2.

Flynn, P. (1997) Public health in Europe (employment and social affairs). European Commission, Luxembourg Office.

Flynn, R., Williams, G. and Pickard, S. (1996) *Markets and Networks. Contracting in Community Health Services*. Open University Press.

Foot, M. (1973) *Aneurin Bevan*, vol. 2. Davis Poynter.

Ford, S. (2010) Marmot might be fair, but will it be feasible? *Health Service Journal*, 4 March, pp. 12–13.

Foskett, N. H. and Hemsley-Brown, J. V. (1998) *Perceptions of Nursing as a Career*. University of Southampton.

Fowler, N. (1984) *Hansard* (1286): 168.

Fox, A. (1974) *Beyond Contract*. Faber & Faber.

Fradd, L. (2011) A united front. *Nursing Standard* 25(26): 26–7.

Francis, C. (2010) *The Mid-Staffordshire NHS Foundation Trust Inquiry. Independent Inquiry Into Care Provided by the Mid-Staffordshire Hospital Between January 2005–March 2009*. The Stationery Office.

Francis, G. (2011) Gillian fights prejudice against gypsies. *Nursing Standard* 25(25): 10.

Fraser, D. (1973) *The Evolution of the British Welfare State*. The Open University.

Friedson, E. (1970) *The Profession of Medicine*. Dodd Mead.

Fyffe, T. (2010) Care will suffer if you slash and burn, RCN warns politicians. *Nursing Standard* 25(7): 11.

Gaffney, K. (2008) Becoming a community matron. *Journal of Community Nursing* 23(1): 4–8.

Gaze, H. (1990) Sweeping change? *Nursing Times* 86(24): 27–8.

Gentleman, A. (2011) The human cost of the cuts. *Guardian*, 25 March, pp. 1, 14–19.

Giddens, A. (1998) *The Third Way*. Polity.

Glasby, J. and Dickinson, H. (2008) *Partnership Working in Health and Social Care*. Policy Press.

Glenn, L. (2010) Implementing change. *Journal of Community Nursing* 24(5): 10–14.

Godson, R. (2010) Too little time spent with patients in the community. *Nursing Standard* 24(44): 10.

Goldacre, B. (2009) *Bad Science*. Fourth Estate.

Goodchild, G. (1995) The Jack of all trades is master of none. *Nursing Times* 92(24): 24.

Gooding, L. (2009) Positively out of touch. *Nursing Standard* 23(22): 16–17.

Goodman, B. (2008) Language matters. *Nursing Standard* 23(15–17): 61.

Goodman, B. and Clemow, R. (2008) *Nursing and Working With Other People*. Learning Matters Ltd.

Goodman, B. and Clemow, R. (2010) *Nursing and Collaborative Practice*. Learning Matters Ltd.

Goodwin, S. (1989) Looking between the lines of the White Paper. *Health Visitor* 62(4): 103.

Gough, P. (1997) Time to grasp the nettle. *Nursing Times* 93(12): 26–7.

Gough, P., Maslin-Prothero, S. and Masterton, A. (1994) *Nursing and Social Policy*. Butterworth Heinemann.

Gould, M. (2010) More power to the patients. *Guardian Roundtable*, 12 May, p. 7.

Graham, H. (2007) *Unequal Lives: Health and Socioeconomic Inequalities*. Open University Press.

Gray, J. (2009) Commitment at its best. *Nursing Standard* 24(9): 1.

Green, S. (2007) *Involving People in Healthcare Policy and Practice*. Radcliffe Publishing.

Greener, I. (2009) *Healthcare in the UK: Understanding Continuity and Change*. Policy Press.

Greenwood, E. (1957) Attributes of a profession. *Social Work* 2(3): 44–5.

Greenwood, L. (2009) Conscript the public in war on bad health. *Health Service Journal*, 2 July, pp. 22–3.

Gregson, B., Cartlidge, A. and Bond, J. (1991) Interprofessional collaboration in primary care organisations. Occasional paper 52. The Royal College of Practitioners.

Griffith, R. and Tengnah, C. (2010) *Law and Professional Issues in Nursing*. Learning Matters Ltd.

Griffiths, J. (2010) Patient explanation. *Health Service Journal*, 10 June, pp. 17.

Griffiths, R. (1983) The NHS Management Inquiry Report. Letter to Norman Fowler, Department of Health, London.

Hadley, R. and Clough, R. (1996) *Care in Chaos*. Cassell.

Hafford-Letchfield, T., Leonard, K., Begum, N. and Chick, N. F. (2008) *Leadership and Management in Social Care*. Sage.

Hall, C. and Ritchie, D. (2009) *What is Nursing? Exploring Theory and Practice*. Learning Matters Ltd.

Halstead, J. (2010) GPs may not want to hold the purse strings. *Nursing Standard* 24(47): 28.

Ham, C. (2009) Lessons from the past decade for future health reforms. *British Medical Journal* 28.

Ham, C. (2010) *A High-Performing NHS? A Review of Progress 1997–2010*. King's Fund.

Ham, C. (2011) The era of patients on trolleys could be back. *The Times*, 19 January, p. 22.

Ham, C. and Hill, M. (1993) *The Policy Process in the Modern Capitalist State*, 2nd edn. Harvester Wheatsheaf.

Hamer, S. (2010) Making more of IT. *Nursing Standard* 25(7): 20–1.

Handley, A. (2009) How was your care? *Nursing Standard* 23(42): 24–5.

Handley, A. (2011) Fast track to efficiency. *Nursing Standard* 25(20): 18–19.

Hannah, K. J., Ball, M. J. and Edwards, M. J. A. (2006) *Introduction to Nursing Informatics*, 3rd edn. Springer.

Hansard (1989) HC Deb, 31 January, vol. 146, cc.165–90.

Harrison, S. and Snow, T. (2010) England defines advanced level role. *Nursing Standard* 25(12): 11.

Harrison, S., Hunter, D., Johnston, I. and Wistow, G. (1989) *Competing for Health. A Commentary on the NHS Review*. Nuffield Institute Reports, University of Leeds.

Hart, C. (1994) *Behind the Mask: Nurses, Their Unions and Nursing Policy*. Baillière Tindall.

Harteveldt, R. (2005) It is time to put a stop to health inequalities. *Nursing Times* 101(43): 14,

Hayes, N. (2010) Qualified to advise. *Nursing Standard* 24(19), January, pp. 62–3.

Hazell, T. (2009) Tony Hazell says the four countries can learn from each other. *Nursing Standard* 24(6): 24.

Health Policy Digest (2010) Commentary: Educating health professionals collaboratively for team-based primary care. 7 September.

Healy, P. (1996) President of BMA condemns idea of generic workforce as 'nonsense'. *Nursing Standard* 10(39): 7.

Healy, P. (1997) Uneasy bedfellows. *Health Service Journal*, 6 November, pp. 10–11.

Heaney, C. (2010) Focus on working with the third sector. *Practical Commissioning PULSE*, March, p. 27.

Hearnden, M. (2008) Coping with differences in culture and communication in health care. *Nursing Standard* 23(11): 49–57.

Heath, H. and Sturdy, S. (2007) Vulnerable adults: The prevention, recognition and management of abuse. *Nursing Standard* 21(40).

Heller, T. (1978) Restructuring the health service. Croom Helm.

Hetherington, P. (2010) The power broker. *Society Guardian*, 15 September, p. 5.

Hewitt-Taylor, J. (2010) Supporting children with complex health needs. *Nursing Standard* 24(19): 50–6.

Hill, M. (1990) *Understanding Social Policy*, 3rd edn. Blackwell.

Hills, J. (2010) *Inequality in the UK: The Data Behind the National Equality Panel.* London School of Economics.

Hills, S. (2009) Twelve steps to perfect competence. *Health Service Journal Supplement*, 25 June, pp. 6–7.

HM Government (2004) *Choice for Parents, the Best start for Children: A Ten Year Strategy for Childcare*. DWP.

HM Government (2010) *Freedom, Fairness, Responsibility. The Coalition: Our Programme for Government*. Cabinet Office.

Hoffenberg, R., Todd, I. P. and Pinker, G. (1987) Crisis in the National Health Service. *British Medical Journal* 295, p. 1505.

Holland, K. and Hogg, C. (2010) *Cultural Awareness in Nursing and Health Care*, 2nd edn. Hodder-Arnold.

Holliday, I. (1995) *The NHS Transformed*, 2nd edn. Baseline Books.

Hudson, B. (1997) Local differences. *Health Service Journal*, 18 September, pp. 31–3.

Hudson, J., Kuhner, S. and Lowe, S (2008) *The Short Guide to Social Policy*. Policy Press.

Hughes, K. (2005) *The Short Life and Long Times of Mrs Beeton*. Fourth Estate.

Hugman, R. (1991) *Power in Caring Professions*. Macmillan.

Hugman, R. (1995) Contested territory and community services. In K. Soothill, L. Mackay and C. Webb (eds), *Interprofessional Relations in Health Care*. Edward Arnold.

Hunter, D. (1993) To market! To market! A new dawn for community care. *Health and Social Care in the Community* 1(1): 3–10.

Hunter, D. (1997) The challenges of health care restructuring. *Nursing Times* 93(39): 67–70.

Hunter, D. J. (2008) *The Health Debate*. Policy Press.

Hurst, K. (2011a) Has nursing quality improved in the past quarter of a century? *Nursing Standard* 25(28): 15–16.

Hurst, K. (2011b) Where in England do older people feel most vulnerable? *Nursing Standard* 25(20): 15.

III (Institute for Innovation and Improvement) (2007) *Technology to Improve Service*. Developed in partnership with NHS Connecting for Health.

Integrated Care Network (2004) *Integrated Working: A Guide*. Short Run Press.

Ivory, M. (2010) Power to the people. *Society Guardian*, 17 March, p. 3.

Jay, M. (1997) The White Paper recognises that nurses have a critical contribution to make. *Nursing Times* 93(51): 3.

Jebb, P. (2010) Reforms are needed but timescale is unworkable. *Nursing Standard* 24(49).

Jelphs, K. and Dickinson, H. (2008) *Working in Teams*. Policy Press.

Jennings, M. (2010) A powerful appeal. *Nursing Standard* 25(5).

Johnson, C. (1994) Healthcare and social care boundaries. *Nursing Times* 90(26): 40–2.

Johnson, T. J. ((1972) *Professions and Power*. Macmillan.

Jones, S. (2010) Snowbound mum born after mum's online SOS. *Guardian*, 13 January, p. 5.

Jupp, B. (2000) *Working Together: Creating a Better Environment for Cross-Sector Partnerships*. Demos.

Kargar, I. (1993) Charter of charters. *Nursing Times* 89(2).

Karim, K. (2010) This proposed NHS restructuring is the biggest botched job to date. *Nursing Standard* 24(46): 33.

Keenan, B. and Atkins, C. (2011) Promoting mental health in older people admitted to hospitals. *Nursing Standard* 25(20): 46–56.

Kendall-Raynor, P. (2007) Two days a week to bring the NHS into line. *Nursing Standard* 21(32): 12–13.

Kendall-Raynor, P. (2009a) Caring in troubled times. *Nursing Standard* 23(38): 20–2.

Kendall-Raynor, P. (2009b) Lack of funding could undermine government's mental health vision. *Nursing Standard* 24(15–17): 11.

Kendall-Raynor, P. (2009c) Will measuring the quality of nursing improve patients' experiences? *Nursing Standard* 23(39): 12.

Kendall-Raynor, P. (2010a) School nurses and health visitors handed key role in delivering public health proposals. *Nursing Standard* 25(14): 6.

Kendall-Raynor, P. (2010b) Specialists being lost to general duties as employers cut costs. *Nursing Standard* 24(50): 7.

Kendall-Raynor, P. and Doult, B. (2010) Action to avert crisis needed as 27,000 posts earmarked for cuts. *Nursing Standard* 25(11): 5.

Kennedy, I. (2001) The Inquiry into the management of care of children receiving complex heart surgery at the Bristol Royal Infirmary (http://www.bristol-inquiry.org.uk/index.htm).

Kenny, C. (1997a) Leaflets to replace nurses. *Nursing Times* 93(25): 8.

Kenny, C. (1997b) Nurses the key to health savings. *Nursing Times* 93(34): 7.

King, O. (2010) Recession no excuse to move workplace diversity to back burner. *The Times*, 20 January.

King's Fund (2010a) *A High Performing NHS? A Review of Progress 1997–2010* (http://www.kingsfund.org.uk/publications/a_highperforming_nh.html).

King's Fund (2010b) Patient choice: How patients choose and how providers respond (http://www.kingsfund.org.uk/current_projects/patient_choice/).

Klein, R. (1980) Models of man and models of policy. Milbank Memorial Fund Quarterly/ *Health and Society* 58(3).

Klein, R. (1989) The Politics of the NHS. 2nd edn. Longman.

Knight, J. (2010a) Click for baby clinic. *Nursing Standard* 24(20): 18–19.

Knight, J. (2010b) Model for success. *Nursing Standard* 25(12): 62–3.

Körner (1982a) *First Report of the Steering Group on Health Services Information*. HMSO.

Korner (1982b) Korner Group urges changes in NHS statistics. *British Medical Journal* 285, 27 November, p. 1591.

Krotoski, A. (2011) Untangling the web. *Observer: The New Review*, 9 January, p. 24.

Kumar, K. (2005) *From Post-Industrial to Post-Modern Society*, 2nd edn. Blackwell.

Kurtz, J. and Nichol, R. (1992) A case for treatment. *Health Service Journal* 16(102): 25.

Lane Fox, M. (2010) UK Digital Inclusion Champion (www.marthalanefox.com).

Langlands, A. (2008) *Rejuvenate or Retire? Views of the NHS at 60*. The Nuffield Trust.

Lansley, A. (2009) A Conservative recipe for reform. *Health Service Journal*, 8 October, p. 16.

Lansley, A. (2010) Letter to executive and non executive directors in the NHS announcing the Health White Paper, 12 July.

Laurent, C. (1990) Taken to the cleaners? *Nursing Times* 86(19): 20.

Le Grand, J. (1982) *The Strategy of Equality: Redistribution and the Social Services*. George Allen and Unwin.

Leathard, A. (2004) *Going Inter-Professional: Working Together for Health and Welfare*. Routledge.

Leifer, D. (1996) Designing new workers for tomorrow's world. *Nursing Standard* 10(36): 14.

Levin, P. (1997) *Making Social Policy: The Mechanisms of Government and Politics, and How to Investigate Them*. Open University Press.

Lewis, I. (1997) Healthy, wealthy and wise. *Tribune*, 7 November.

Lewis, P. (2009) Nurse leaders say BME bias is still prevalent. *Nursing Standard* 24(5): 5.

Lewis, P. G., Potter, D. C. and Castles, F. G. (eds) (1978) *The Practice of Comparative Politics*. Longman.

Liddle, A., Adshead, S. and Burgess, E. (2008) *Technology in the NHS: Transforming the Patient's Experience of Care*. King's Fund, London.

Lindberg, J., Hunter, M. and Kruszewski, A. (1990) *Introduction to Nursing: Concepts, Issues, and Opportunities*. Lippincott, PA.

Lipsky, M. (1980) *Street-level Bureaucracy: Dilemmas of the Individual in Public Services*. Russell Sage Foundation, NY.

Lister, J. (2008) *The NHS After 60: For Patients or Profits?* Middlesex University Press.

Llewellyn, A. and Hayes, S. (2008) *Fundamentals of Nursing Care*. Reflect Press.

Llewellyn, A., Agu, L. and Mercer, D. (2008) *Sociology for Social Workers*. Polity.

Luker, K. and Orr, J. (eds) (1992) *Health Visiting: Towards Community Health Nursing*. Blackwell Scientific Publications.

Maben, J. and Griffiths, P. (2008) *Nurses in Society: Starting the Debate*. National Nursing Research Unit (NNRU), King's College London.

Machiavelli, N. (1532) *The Prince and The Discourses,* Introduction by Max Lerner. New York Modern Library, pp. 103–5.

MacLeod, K. (2010) Humanity will thank heaven that this creator of synthetic life is playing God. *Guardian*, 22 May, p. 38.

Mahon, A., (1992) Feature. Manchester University patient survey. *Health Service Journal*, 3 December.

Main, M. (2010) Right on the button. *Nursing Standard* 24(44): 61.

Manchester University (1996) *The Future Healthcare Workforce*. Health Service Management Unit (HSMU).

Mangan, P. (1993) Survival of the fittest. *Nursing Times* 89(6): 26.

Marmot, M. (2010) *Fair Society, Healthy Lives: The Marmot Review* (http://www.marmotreview.org/AssetLibrary/pdfs/Reports/FairSocietyHealthyLives.pdf).

Maslin-Prothero, S. and Masterson, A. (1998) Continuing care: Developing a policy analysis for nursing. *Journal of Advanced Nursing* 28(3): 548–53.

Maslin-Prothero, S. and Masterson, A. (2002) Power, politics and nursing in the United Kingdom. *Policy, Politics and Nursing Practice* 3(2): 108–17.

Mason-Whitehead, E., McIntosh, A., Bryan, A. and Mason, T. (2008) *Key Concepts in Nursing*. Sage.

Mason, P. (1993) Healthy living. *Nursing Times* 89(11): 16–17.

Mathieson, S. A. (2010) A bug in the system. *Society Guardian*, 13 January, p. 6.

McCallin (2001) Interdisciplinary practice: A matter of teamwork. An integrated literature review. *Journal of Clinical Nursing* 10(4): 419–28.

McCargow, R. (2010) Human resources. Value the 'collective difference'. *Health Service Journal*, 10 June, p. 19.

McCarthy, J. and Holt, M. (2007) Complexities of policy-driven pre-registration nursing curricula. *Nursing Standard* 22(10): 35–8.

McCormack, B. and Slater, P. (2009) Happy in their work. *Nursing Standard* 24(7): 80.

McCray, J. (ed.) (2009) *Nursing and Multi-professional Practice*. Sage.

McGowan, J. (2010) Do we need to be hearing this? *Health Service Journal*, 27 May, pp. 14–15.

McKimm, J. and Phillips, K. (eds) (2009) *Leadership and Management in Integrated Services*. Learning Matters Ltd.

Meehan, F. (1996) A lesson learned. *Journal of Community Nursing* 10(9): 1.

Meehan, F. (2009) The art and science of nursing practice. *Journal of Community Nursing*, December, p. 3.

Mencap (2004) *Treat Me Right: Better Care for People With Learning Disability* (http://www.mencap.org.uk/node/5880).

Merron, G. (2010) NHS better equipped to tackle local health inequalities. *Health Policy Digest* 23 March.

Mihill, C. (1992) Strategy for improvement or window dressing. *Guardian*, 9 July.

Mihill, C. (1993) Black returns to the fray in defence of the NHS. *Guardian*, 17 December, p. 9.

Milburn, A. (2000) *Summary Version of The NHS Plan: A Plan for Investment, a Plan for Reform*. DOH.

Millerson, G. (1964) *The Qualifying Associations: A Study in Professionalism*. Routledge and Kegan Paul.

Milliband, E. (2010) Only New Labour offers you a genuine big society. *Observer*, 25 April, p. 40.

Milligan, J. (2009) Read all about it. *Nursing Standard* 23(33): 28.

Mills, B. (1998) Degree of sacrifice. *Society Guardian*, 21 January, pp. 2–3.

Milton, A. (2010a) Health visitor employers to be determined locally. *Nursing Standard* 24(48): 7.

Milton, A. (2010b) Milton sure of nurse role in commissioning. *Nursing Standard* 24(48): 7.

Milton, A. (2010c) Nurses can adapt to new models of care. *Nursing Standard* 24(51): 12–14.

Milton, A. (2010d) Opportunity knocks, says Minister. *Nursing Standard* 24(46): 7.

Mitchell, M. (2010) A patient-centred approach to day surgery nursing. *Nursing Standard* 24(44): 40–5.

Modernisation Agency (2004) Ten High Impact Changes for Service Improvement and Delivery: A Guide for NHS leaders (http://www.ogc.gov.uk/documents/Health_High_Impact_Changes.pdf).

Moon, G. and Lupton, C. (1995) Within acceptable limits: Healthcare provider perspectives on Community Health Councils in the reformed National Health Service. *Policy and Politics* 23: 335–46.

Moore, A. (2011) Shaping the service to fit the person. *Nursing Standard* 25(22): 20–3.

Mullally, S (2005) *Review of the Nursing, Midwifery and Health Visiting Contribution to Vulnerable Children and Young Children*. DOH.

Munro, E. (2010) *Review of Child Protection: A Systems Analysis*. DfE .

Munro, R. (2011a) Scaling the peaks. *Nursing Standard* 25(28): 20–1.

Munro, R. (2011b) Smarter Solutions. *Nursing Standard* 25(26): 24–5.

Muscular Dystrophy Campaign (2010) in NHS Confederation Summaries, 25 August.

Myers, J. (2009) More work to be done. *Nursing Standard* 24(5): 1.

Naidoo, J. and Wills, J. (2005) *Health Promotion: Foundations for Practice*, 2nd edn. Baillière Tindall.

Naish, J. (2010) 21st century nurse. *Nursing Standard* 24(8): 22–3.

NAO (National Audit Office) (1989) *Report of the Controller and Auditor General: NHS Coronary Health*. HMSO.

NAO (National Audit Office) (2009) *NHS Pay Modernisation in England: Agenda for Change*. HMSO.

NAO (National Audit Office) (2010) in *NHS Confederation Health Policy Digest* 49(10).

National Consumer Council (2005) *Future Services: Taking the Voice of Users to the Heart of the Public Service Reform Debate*. NCC.

National Council for Palliative Care (2006) Introductory guide to end of life care in care homes. NHS End of Life Care Programme.

Nazroo, J. (2009) Ethnicity and health. *Health Matters* 76: 16–18.

News (2010) Privatisation of NHS Staff Agency 'makes no sense'. *Nursing Standard* 24(49): 6.

News (2011) Older people's care will top agenda at senior nurse meeting. *Nursing Standard* 25(26): 9.

NHS Confederation (2010a) Press summaries: Doctors and nurses axed at Department of Health, 21 September.

NHS Confederation (2010b) Press summaries: NHS IT programme to be scaled back, 10 September.

NHS Confederation (2010c) Press summaries: People with learning disabilities and mental health problems often do not get the services they should from the NHS, 21 September.

NHS Employers (2009a) *Managing Diversity, Making it Core Business* (http://www.nhsemployers.org/Aboutus/Publications/Documents/Briefing_60_Managing_diversity_making_it_core_business.pdf).

NHS Employers (2009b) *The Role of the Nurse* (http://www.nhsemployers.org/Aboutus/Publications/Pages/TheRoleOfTheNurse.aspx).

NHSME (National Health Service Management Executive) (1992) *NHS Reforms: The First Six Months.* HMSO.

NHSME (National Health Service Management Executive) (1993) *A Vision for the Future.* HMSO.

NHSME (National Health Service Management Executive) (1994) *The Operation of the NHS Internal Market.* HMSO.

Nightingale, F. (1860) *Notes on Nursing: What It Is and What It Is Not.* Appleton, NY.

NMC (Nursing and Midwifery Council) (2008) *The Code: Standards of Conduct, Performance and Ethics for Nurses and Midwives* (http://www.nmc-uk.org/Nurses-and-midwives/The-code/The-code-in-full/).

NNRU (National Nursing Research Unit) (2009a) *From Bench to Bedside. What Role for Nurses in Helping the NHS Make Better and Quicker Use of Technological Innovations?* King's College London.

NNRU (National Nursing Research Unit) (2009b) *Is There a Case for the UK Nursing Workforce to Include Grades of Qualified Nurses Other Than the Registered Nurse?* King's College London.

Nocon, A. (1994) Collaboration in community care in the 1990s Business Education Publishers, Sunderland, Tyne and Wear.

Normand, C. (1991) Economics, health and the economics of health. *British Medical Journal* 303: 1572–7.

North, N. and Bradshaw, Y. (eds) (1997) *Perspectives in Health Care.* Macmillan.

Nursing Standard (2004) Racism and the NHS, 19(6): 12–14.

Nursing Standard (2010a) In brief, 24(44): 9.

Nursing Standard (2010b) Notice board, 24(44): 63.

Nursing Standard (2010c) Tributes paid to equality campaigner, 24(41): 10.

Nursing Times (1992) Power to the people, 89(14): 32–3.

Nursing Times (1995) NHS league tables out this week, 90(26): 6.

Nursing Times (1996) Pandora's box of tricks. 92(15): 3.

Nursing Times (1999) HAZ it worked? 14(51): 13–15.

O'Connor, D. and Purves, B. (2009) *Decision Making. Personhood and Dementia: Exploring the Interface.* Jessica Kingsley Publishers.

Oliver, A. (2009) What to do about health inequalities policy in the United Kingdom. *Health Matters* 75: 12–15.

Ovretveit, J. (1997a) 'How to describe interprofessional working,' in J. Ovretveit, P. Mathias and T. Thompson (eds), *Interprofessional Working for Health and Social Care.* Palgrave Macmillan.

Ovretveit, J. (1997b) 'How patient power and client participation affects relations between professions', in J. Ovretveit, P. Mathias and T. Thompson (eds), *Interprofessional Working for Health and Social Care*. Palgrave Macmillan.

Parkin, P. (2009) *Managing Change in Healthcare: Using Action Research*. Sage.

Parliamentary and Health Service Ombudsman (2011) *Care and Compassion?* Report of the Health Service Ombudsman on ten investigations into NHS care of older people (www.ombudsman.org.uk/care-and-compassion).

Parsons, T. (1939) The professions and the social structure. *Social Forces* 17: 457–67.

Parsons, T. (1951) *The Social System*. Routledge & Kegan Paul.

Patients Association (2009) Patients not numbers. People not statistics (http://www.patients-association.com/Research-Publications/297).

Payne, M. (2000) *Teamwork in Multiprofessional Care*. Macmillan.

Pearce, L. (2011) Inspirational nurses vie for public's vote. *Nursing Standard* 25(29): 20–1.

Peckham, S. and Meerabeau, L. (2007) *Social Policy for Nurses and the Helping Professions*, 2nd edn. Open University Press.

Perry, J., Bennett, C. and Lapworth, T. (2010) Management of long-term conditions in a prison setting. *Nursing Standard* 24(42): 35–40.

Phillips, A. (2009) Dance tsar. NHS Confederation press summaries, 14 August.

Pike, S. and Forster, D. (1995) *Health Promotion for All*. Churchill Livingstone.

Plamping, D. and Delamothe, T. (1991) The Citizen's Charter and the NHS. *British Medical Journal* 303: 203–4.

Player, S. and Leys, C. (2008) *Confuse and Conceal. The NHS and Independent Sector Treatment Centres*. Merlin Press.

Pollitt, C. (1989) Consuming passions. *Health Service Journal* 99(5178): 1436–7.

Pollock, A. (2011) A Return to pre-NHS fear. *Guardian*, 17 June, p. 36.

Potter, J. (1988) Consumerism and the public sector: How well does the coat fit? *Public Administration* 66: 149–64.

Powell, M. (2000) New Labour and the Third Way in the British welfare state: A new and distinctive approach? *Critical Social Policy* 20(1): 39.

Prandy, K. (1965) *Professional Employees*. Faber and Faber.

Prensky, M. (2005) *Don't Bother Me Mom – I'm Learning!* Paragon House.

Price, B. (2010) Practical evidence in improving local healthcare policies and practices *Nursing Standard* 25(7): 39–46.

Puntis, J. W. L. (1995) Home parenteral nutrition. Archives of *Disease in Childhood* 72: 186–90.

Rafferty, A. M. (1992) Nursing policy and the nationalisation of nursing: The representation of crisis and the crisis of representation. In J. Robinson, A. Gray and R. Elkan (eds) *Policy Issues in Nursing*. Open University Press.

Rafferty, A. M. (1996) *The Politics of Nursing Knowledge*. London: Routledge.

Rafferty, A. M. (2009) The big issue: Nursing degrees. Today's nurses need to be caring and clever too. *Observer*, 22 November.

Raleigh, V. S., Hussey, D., Seccombe, I., et al. Do associations between staff and inpatient feedback have the potential for improving patient experience? An analysis of surveys in NHS acute trusts in England. *Quality & Safety Health Care* 18: 347–54.

Ramesh, R. (2010) How to bridge the divide. Healthcare: The future. *Guardian*, 23 June, p. 3.

Ramesh, R. (2011) Lansley's NHS will be unrecognisable. *Society Guardian*, 5 January, p. 4.

Ranade, W. (1997) *A Future for the NHS? Health Care for the Millennium*, 2nd edn. Longman Ltd.

Raynor, C. (2010) *How Did I Get Here From There?* Virago Press.

RCN (Royal College of Nursing) (2005) *Success with Internationally Recruited*

Nurses: RCN Good Practice Guidance for Employers in Recruiting and Retaining. Working Well Initiative (http://www.rcn.org.uk/__data/assets/pdf_file/0010/78625/002445.pdf).

RCN (Royal College of Nursing) (2010a) Pillars of the community: The RCN's UK position on the development of the registered nursing workforce in the community (http://www.rcn.org.uk/__data/assets/pdf_file/0007/335473/003843.pdf).

RCN (Royal College of Nursing) (2010b) Thousands of jobs at risk: Frontline first. *Nursing Standard* 24(49): 13.

RCN (Royal College of Nursing) (2011) College criticises plan to end BME patient reports. *Nursing Standard* 25(27): 10.

Redding, D. (2009) The standards glass is half empty. *Health Service Journal*, 20 August, p. 13.

Rillands, M. (1997) Book review. 'Primary Care: Making Connections'. *Health Service Journal*, October, p. 39.

Roberts, D. (2010) NHS chaos will be Cameron's poll tax. *Guardian*, 15 December, p. 35.

Robinson, J., Gray, A. and Elkan, R. (eds) (1992) *Policy Issues in Nursing.* Open University Press.

Robinson, R. (1989) New health care market. *British Medical Journal* 298: 437–9.

Rodgers, J. (1994) Collaboration among health professionals. *Nursing Standard* 9(6): 25–6.

Rogers, Everett M. (1962) *Diffusion of Innovation.* New York Free Press.

Ross, F. and Mackenzie, A. (1996) *Nursing in Primary Health Care: Policy into Practice.* Routledge.

Rowntree (2010) *Minimum Income Standard Report*, 6 July. Joseph Rowntree Foundation.

Saddler, J. (2009) The building blocks of quality. *Health Service Journal*, 23 July, p. 15.

Sadler, C. (2010) Shopping bad service. *Nursing Standard* 24(50): 20–2.

Salvage, J. and Heijnen, S. (eds) (1997) *Nursing in Europe. A Better Resource for Health.* WHO Regional Publications. European Series no. 74.

Sample, I. (2010) Synthetic life breakthrough could be worth over a million dollars. *Guardian* 21 May, p. 9.

Satchell, G. (2008) Matron gives modern NHS a check-up. *BBC Breakfast News* (http://news.bbc.co.uk/2/hi/health/7477420.stm).

Saunders, C. (1999) When you're 81, you don't care about diets. *The Times*, 8 June.

Schaffer, B. (1977) On the politics of policy. *Australian Journal of Politics and History*, 23: 146–55 .

SCIE (Social Care Institute for Excellence) (2006) *Dignity in Care.* Practice Guide 9, November (http://www.dorsetforyou.com/media.jsp?mediaid=157813&filetype=pdf).

Scott, G. (2001) Nursing Informatics. *Journal of Community Nursing* 15(3): 4–13 March.

Scott, G. (2009) Darling draws the line. *Nursing Standard* 24(15–17): 1.

Scott, G. (2009) New grounds for optimism. *Nursing Standard* 23(40): 1.

Scott, G. (2009) The cruellest cuts of all. *Nursing Standard* 23(4): 1.

Scott, G. (2010a) A time for regulation. *Nursing Standard* 24(39): 1.

Scott, G. (2010b) Cuts that will cost lives. *Nursing Standard* 24(44): 1.

Scott, G. (2010c) Defending the front line. *Nursing Standard* 25(10): 1.

Scott, G. (2011a) Fight for equality still on. *Nursing Standard* 25(22): 1.

Scott, G. (2011b) Four of the very best. *Nursing Standard* 25(29): 1.

Scottish Executive (2007) Adult Support and Protection (Scotland) Bill.

Scottish Government (2010) *NHS Scotland Quality Strategy* (http://www.scotland.gov.uk/Topics/Health/NHS-Scotland/NHSQuality/About).

Scriven, A. (2010) *Promoting Health: A Practical Guide*. Baillière Tindall.

Seedhouse, D. (1986) *Health: The Foundations for Achievement*. John Wiley.

Sefton, T. (2002) Recent changes in the distribution of the social wage, Case paper 62. Centre for Analysis of Social Exclusion.

Selincourt, de K. (1992) Power to the patients. *Nursing Times* 88(33): 18.

Sellman, D. and Snelling, P. (2010) *Becoming a Nurse*. Pearson Education Ltd.

Serrant-Green, L. (2010) A celebration of diversity. *Nursing Standard* 25(5): 1.

Sheldon, A. (ed.) (1980) *The Litmus Papers*. Centre for Policy Studies, London.

Shepherd, S. (2009) Know the figures behind the facts. *Health Service Journal*, 9 July, pp. 18–19.

Shipman Inquiry (2005) Systems failures and tasks for phase two, Section 14.16 (www.the-shipman-inquiry.org.uk/home.asp).

Shirkey, C. (2008) *Here Comes Everybody: How Change Happens When People Come Together*. Allen Lane.

Shirkey, C. (2010) *Cognitive Surplus: Creativity and Generosity in a Connected Age*. Allen Lane.

Shultz, R. and Harrison, S. (1983) Teams and top managers in the NHS: A survey and a strategy. Project paper no. 4. King's Fund.

Sin, C. H. (2008) Setting the standards for entry. *Nursing Standard* 23(10): 62.

Smith, C. (1996) A health service for a new century: Labour's proposals to replace the internal market in the NHS. *Health Service Journal*, 3 December.

Smith, J. (2010) Unfair treatment. *Nursing Standard* 24(20).

Smith, R., Gaster, L., Harrison, L., Martin, L., Means, R. and Thistlewaite, P. (1993) *Working Together For Better Community Care*. University of Bristol.

Snow, T. (2009a) Nurses help lead the transformation in delivery of community care services. *Nursing Standard* 23(43): 12–13.

Snow, T. (2009b) Workforce planning tops agenda to prevent shortfall of nurses. *Nursing Standard* 24(3): 12–13.

Snow, T. (2010a) All change on the training front. *Nursing Standard* 24(37): 12–13.

Snow, T. (2010b) Chief Nurse to push for profession's place on key NHS board. *Nursing Standard* 24(49): 12–13.

Snow, T. (2010c) Coalition government faces tough choices over nurses' pay and pensions. *Nursing Standard* 24(37): 12–13.

Snow, T. (2010d) Community nurses warn shift to HCAs is threatening patient care. *Nursing Standard* 25(13): 8.

Snow, T. (2010e) Project grants for award winners set to benefit BME communities. *Nursing Standard* 25(9).

Snow, T. (2011a) Government presses on with NHS overhaul despite serious concerns. *Nursing Standard* 25(19): 10.

Snow, T. (2011b) GPs and managers agree nurses must have a say in commissioning. *Nursing Standard* 25(20): 8.

Social Services Committee (1984) *Griffiths NHS Management Inquiry Report, 1983–4*. HMSO.

Soothill, K., Henry, C. and Kendrick, K. (1992) *Themes and Perspectives in Nursing*. Chapman and Hall.

Sprinks, J. (2010a) As complaints of poor care rise, patients' group offers solutions. *Nursing Standard* 25(9): 12–13.

Sprinks, J. (2010b) Drive to abolish 'politically motivated' NHS targets raises serious clinical issues. *Nursing Standard* 24(49): 14.

Stapleton, V. (2009) I was amazed by the skill and professionalism of paramedics. *Nursing Standard* 24(6): 27.

Stevens, S. (2008) *Rejuvenate or Retire? Views of the NHS at 60*, ed. Nicholas Timmins.

The Nuffield Trust (http://www.nuffieldtrust.org.uk/sites/files/nuffield/publication/rejuvenate-or-retire-nhs-at-60-jul08-final-web.pdf), pp. 107–10.

Stockwell, F. (2010) Nurses who feel undervalued become careless and unkind. *Nursing Standard* 24(19): 15.

Strachan-Bennett, S. (2004) Mental health nursing set for overhaul. *Nursing Times* 100(7): 2.

Straughan, T. (2008) Towards world-class quality of information for healthcare: Magic Touch: the revolution in information management. *Health Service Journal* 118 (October supplement): 6126.

Sturdy, D. and Heath, H. (2007) Keeping older people safe. *Nursing Standard* 21(40): 20 .

Stuttle, B. (2006) Technology acts as 'enabler' for safer, better healthcare. CNO.

Stuttle, B. (2007) Nurses back EPR: says new RCN IT survey. CNO Bulletin, p. 6.

Sutherland, K. and Coyle, N. (2009) Quality of healthcare in England, Wales, Scotland, Northern Ireland: An intra-UK chartbook. Health Foundation, March (http://www.health.org.uk/publications/quality-of-healthcare-in-england-scotland-wales-and-northern-ireland-an-intra-uk-chartbook/).

Sweeney, C. (2010) There may be trouble ahead. *Health Service Journal Supplement*, 10 June, pp. 1–2.

Thomas, B. and Warm, D. (2009) Providing support for the Informing Healthcare programme in Wales. *Nursing Standard* 23(26): 35–41.

Thomson, S. (1998) After Project 2000: What does the future hold for nursing education? *Nursing Times* 94(3): 60–1.

Timmins, N. (2002) A time for change in the British NHS: An interview with Alan Milburn. *Health Affairs* 21(3): 129–35.

Timmins, N. (2008) History matters. *Nursing Standard* 22(17): 22–4.

Toofany, S. (2005) Nurses and health policy. *Nursing Management* 12(3).

Toynbee, P. (2010) It is no careful plan. The NHS is being demolished at speed. *Guardian*, 17 July, p. 29.

Trevillion, S. (1995) Competent to Collaborate? Keynote speech, *Social Work and General Practice*, Centre for Advanced Interprofessional Education, April.

Tudor-Hart, J. (2010) NHS Confederation press summaries, 1 September.

Turnbull, J. and Chapman, S. (2010) Supporting choice in health care for people with learning disabilities. *Nursing Standard* 24(22): 50–6.

Turner, J. C. (1991) *Social Influence*. Open University Press.

Turner, T. (1998) The last nail. *Nursing Times* 84(16): 28–30.

Upton, T. and Brooks, B. (2000) *Managing Change in the NHS*. Open University Press.

Vize, R. (2009) One year down Darzi's road the way ahead looks a lot tougher. *Health Service Journal*, 25 June, p. 3.

Voluntary Organisation (1989) *Health Service Users and the NHS Review.* A statement from voluntary organisations. London.

WAG (Welsh Assembly Government) (2003a) *Informing Healthcare: Transforming Healthcare Using Information and IT.* NHS Wales.

WAG (Welsh Assembly Government) (2003b) *The Review of Health and Social Care in Wales.* NHS Wales.

WAG (Welsh Assembly Government) (2004) *Making the Connections: Delivering Better Services for Wales.* NHS Wales.

WAG (Welsh Assembly Government) (2005) *Designed for Living: Creating World Class Health and Social Care for Wales in the 21st Century.* NHS Wales.

WAG (Welsh Assembly Government) (2007) *Making the Connections: Building Better Customer Service: A Framework for Improvement.* NHS Wales.

WAG (Welsh Assembly Government) (2010) *Doing Well, doing Better: Standards for Health Services in Wales.* NHS Wales.

Wallace, C. and Davies, M. (2009) *Sharing Assessment in Health and Social Care – A Practical Handbook for Interprofessional Working.* Sage.

Walshe, K. (2009) Getting wrapped up in research. *Health Service Journal,* 23 April, p. 15.

Wanless, D. (2002) *Securing Our Future Health: Taking a Long-Term View.* DOH.

Wanless, D. (2006) Securing good care for older people: Taking a long-term view. *Social Care Review,* Kings Fund, pp. 4–5.

Waters, A. (2009) How are we doing ? *Nursing Standard* 23(43): 24–5.

Waters, A. (2011a) A role under scrutiny. *Nursing Standard* 25(26): 18/19.

Waters, A. (2011b) Meet my new sister. *Nursing Standard* 25(22): 18/19.

Watt, S. (1987) Applications of computers in nurse management. In B. Koch and J. Rankin (eds), *Computers and their Applications in Nursing.* Harper and Row.

Weber, M. (1966) *The Sociology of Religion.* Methuen.

Webster, C. (2002) *The National Health Service: A Political History.* 2nd edn. Oxford University Press.

Weekes, D. (2009) The business of diversity. *Nursing Standard* 24(5): 62–3.

Weekes, D. and Blakemore, S. (2009) Lung cancer specialists audit points to value of specialist practitioners. *Nursing Standard* 24(14): 7.

Weiner, M. E. and Petronella, P. (2007) The impact of new technology: Implications for social work and social care managers. In J. Aldgate, P. Healy, B. Pine, W. Rose and J. Seden (eds), *Enhancing Social Work Management.* Jessica Kingsley Publishers.

Welch, C. (1993) Now the bourgeoisie bang their spoons. *Independent,* 31 May.

West, R. (2009) NHS Golf tees off. *The Times,* 26 June.

White, C. (2009) Commission for all your patients. *Health Service Journal,* 27 August, pp. 18–19.

Whitehead, M. (1987) *The Health Care Divide: Inequalities in Health in the 1980s.* Health Education Council, London.

WHO (World Health Organization) (1946) Constitution. WHO, Geneva.

WHO (World Health Organization) (1978) *Declaration of Alma-Ata.* International Conference on Primary Health Care, 6–12 September (http://www.who.int/hpr/NPH/docs/declaration_almaata.pdf).

Whyte, A. (2010b) Relighting the Lamp *Nursing Standard* 24(18): 18–20.

Whyte, A. (2010a) Ardent Campaigners *Nursing Standard* 25(15): 16–18.

Wicks, D. (1998) *Nurses and Doctors at Work: Rethinking Professional Boundaries.* Open University Press.

Wildavsky, A. (1979) *Speaking Truth to Power: The Art and Craft of Policy Analysis.* Little, Brown.

Williams, J. (1993) What is a profession? Experience versus expertise In A. Beattie, M. Gott, L. Jones and M. Sidell (eds), *Health and Well-being : A Reader.* Open University Press.

Williams, J. (2007) *Rethinking the Future of Work.* Palgrave Macmillan.

Williamson, G. R., Jenkinson, T. and Proctor-Childs, T. (2008) *Nursing in Contemporary Healthcare Practice.* Learning Matters Ltd.

Williamson, G. R., Jenkinson, T. and Proctor-Childs, T. (2010) *Contexts of Contemporary Nursing,* 2nd edn. Learning Matters Ltd.

Willis, J. (1992) The price of health. *Nursing Times* 88(30): 24–6.

Willis, R. (2009) 90 years strong. *Nursing Standard* 24(14): 18–19.

Wilson, A. (1994) *Being Heard.* DOH.

Winkler, F. (1987) Consumerism in health care: beyond the supermarket model. *Policy and Politics* 15(1): 1–8.

Wintour, P. (2009) Britain's closed shop: Damning report on social mobility failings. *Guardian* 22 July, p. 4.

Wistow, G. (1992) Working together in a new policy concept. *Health Services Management* 88(1) 25–8.

Wright, S. (2008) Age of experience. *Nursing Standard* 23(15–17): 24–5.

Wright, S. (2010) One falls, we all fall. *Nursing Standard* 24(47): 26–7.

Wright, S. G. (1998) *Changing Nursing Practice*. Arnold.

Younger, P. (2010) Using Google Scholar to conduct a literature search. *Nursing Standard* 24(45): 40–8.

Websites

Appointments Commission: www.appointments.org.uk

Care Quality Commission: www.cqc.org.uk

Choose and Book: www.chooseandbook.nhs.uk

CNO bulletins: www.dh.gov.uk/cnobulletin

Department for Education: www.education.gov.uk

Department of Health: www.dh.gov.uk

Expert Patients Programme: www.dh.gov.uk

Long-Term Care Resources: www.ltca.org.uk

The National Archives: www.nationalarchives.gov.uk

Nursing and Midwifery Council: www.nmc-uk.org

Opportunity Now: www.bitcdiversity.org.uk

The Patients Association: www.patients-association.org.uk

UK Central Government and Local Authority Public Spending: www.ukpublicspending.co.uk

UK Legislation: www.legislation.gov.uk

Index

Boxes (b), figures (f) and tables (t) are indexed in **bold**.